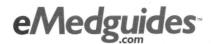

online and in-print Internet directories in medicine

Internal Medicine

AN INTERNET RESOURCE GUIDE

November 2001 — October 2002

Consulting Editor

John A. Flynn, M.D., M.B.A., F.A.C.P.

Associate Professor, Department of Medicine
Clinical Director, Division of General Internal Medicine
Johns Hopkins University School of Medicine

Visit **Internal Medicine**
at www.eMedguides.com

Access code: **1515**

eMedguides.com, Inc., a Thomson Healthcare company, Princeton, New Jersey

About the Editor
John A. Flynn, M.D., M.B.A., F.A.C.P.

Dr. Flynn holds the D. William Schlott Professorship in Clinical Medicine, and serves as the Clinical Director of the Division of General Internal Medicine, both at The Johns Hopkins University School of Medicine. A graduate of the University of Missouri-Columbia School of Medicine, Dr. Flynn joined a newly established Faculty Practice Group at Johns Hopkins in 1992, and now divides his time between teaching and clinical medicine. Between 1994 and 1999 he served as Director of Curriculum for Ambulatory Subspecialty Electives, and was recognized for his educational contributions by the American College of Rheumatology as recipient of its Clinican-Educator Award.

In addition to his Johns Hopkins responsibilities, Dr. Flynn has served as editor for *Clinical Evidence* and *Cutaneous Medicine: Cutaneous Manifestations of Systemic Disease*, and has published articles in *The New England Journal of Medicine, Arthritis Care and Research*, and *Chest*. Along with his membership in the ACP/ASIM, Dr. Flynn is a Fellow of the American College of Rheumatology, where he serves on the Education Committee.

Sales Department
eMedguides.com, Inc.
15 Roszel Road
Princeton, NJ 08540
tel   800-230-1481 x16
fax   609-520-2023
e-mail sales@eMedguides.com
web   http://www.eMedguides.com/books

This book is set in Avenir, BaseNine, Gill Sans, and Sabon typefaces and was printed and bound in the United States of America.

10 9 8 7 6 5 4 3 2 1

ISBN 0-9676811-7-0

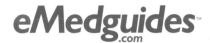

Internal Medicine
AN INTERNET RESOURCE GUIDE

John A. Flynn, M.D., M.B.A, *Consulting Editor*
Associate Professor, Department of Medicine
Clinical Director, Division of General Internal Medicine
Johns Hopkins University School of Medicine

Karen M. Albert, MLS,
Consulting Medical Librarian
Director of Library Services, Fox Chase Cancer Center

Daniel R. Goldenson, *Publisher*

Alysa M. Wilson, *Editor-in-Chief*

Karen B. Schwartz, *Managing Editor*

Ravpreet Syalee, *Production Editor*

Barbara Morrison, *Manuscript Editor*

Joyce Milione, Kim Seok, *Production Assistants*

Sue Bannon, *Designer*

eMedguides.com, Inc.,
a Thomson Healthcare company
15 Roszel Road, Princeton, NJ 08540

Daniel R. Goldenson, *General Manager*

Amy Ma, Ph. D., *Coordinator,*
Publication Development

Raymond Egan, Jr., *Coordinator,*
Marketing Administration

Book Orders & Feedback

Book orders • http://www.eMedguides.com/books
Phone orders • 800.230.1481 x16
Facsimile • 609.520.2023
E-mail • internal@eMedguides.com
Web • http://www.eMedguides.com/internal

2001–2002
Annual Editions

Allergy & Immunology
Anesthesiology & Pain Management
Arthritis & Rheumatology
Cardiology
Dental Medicine
Dermatology
Diet & Nutrition
Emergency Medicine
Endocrinology & Metabolism
Family Medicine
Gastroenterology
General Surgery
Infectious Diseases & Immunology

Internal Medicine

Neurology & Neuroscience
Nurse Practitioners
Obstetrics & Gynecology
Oncology & Hematology
Ophthalmology
Orthopedics & Sports Medicine
Osteopathic Medicine
Otolaryngology
Pathology & Laboratory Medicine
Pediatrics & Neonatology
Physical Medicine & Rehabilitation
Psychiatry
Radiology
Respiratory & Pulmonary Medicine
Urology & Nephrology
Veterinary Medicine

Disclaimer

eMedguides.com, Inc., hereafter referred to as the "publisher," has developed this book for informational purposes only, and not as a source of medical advice. The publisher does not guarantee the accuracy, adequacy, timeliness, or completeness of any information in this book and is not responsible for any errors or omissions or any consequences arising from the use of the information contained in this book. The material provided is general in nature and is in summary form. The content of this book is not intended in any way to be a substitute for professional medical advice. One should always seek the advice of a physician or other qualified healthcare provider. Further, one should never disregard medical advice or delay in seeking it because of information found through an Internet Web site included in this book. The use of the eMedguides.com, Inc. book is at the reader's own risk.

All information contained in this book is subject to change. Mention of a specific product, company, organization, Web site URL address, treatment, therapy, or any other topic does not imply a recommendation or endorsement by the publisher.

Non-liability

The publisher does not assume any liability for the contents of this book or the contents of any material provided at the Internet sites, companies, and organizations reviewed in this book. Moreover, the publisher assumes no liability or responsibility for damage or injury to persons or property arising from the publication and use of this book; the use of those products, services, information, ideas, or instructions contained in the material provided at the third-party Internet Web sites, companies, and organizations listed in this book; or any loss of profit or commercial damage including but not limited to special, incidental, consequential, or any other damages in connection with or arising out of the publication and use of this book. Use of third-party Web sites is subject to the Terms and Conditions of use for such sites.

Copyright Protection

Information available over the Internet and other online locations may be subject to copyright and other rights owned by third parties. Online availability of text and images does not imply that they may be reused without the permission of rights holders. Care should be taken to ensure that all necessary rights are cleared prior to reusing material distributed over the Internet and other online locations.

Trademark Protection

The words in this book for which we have reason to believe trademark, service mark, or other proprietary rights may exist have been designated as such by use of initial capitalization. However, no attempt has been made to designate as trademarks or service marks all personal computer words or terms in which proprietary rights might exist. The inclusion, exclusion, or definition of a word or term is not intended to affect, or to express any judgment on, the validity or legal status of any proprietary right that may be claimed in that word or term.

eMedguides.com Online

Instant access to every Web site in this book at www.eMedguides.com!

This volume, *in its entirety*, can be browsed online at eMedguides.com. Simply point and click to surf to the latest Web sites in your specialty! eMedguides.com is continually updated with URL and content changes, as well as new sites in each specialty. Start your search for medical information, in any specialty, with the trusted assistance of eMedguides.com.

THREE WAYS TO SURF WITH AN EMEDGUIDE:

FAST Drill down at eMedguides.com to the Web information you seek.

FASTER Find a site in the print edition and type the URL into your browser.

FASTEST Find a site in the print edition and type in the e-Link code instead of the URL (for example, go to site G-1234 by typing: www.eMedguides.com/G-1234).

GENERAL MEDICINE REFERENCE
Part Two of every book (General Medical Web Resources) is always available in the sidebar.

E-LINK WITH THE URL
Type in the e-Link code (found next to each entry in this book) after www.eMedguides.com/. You will go directly to the site you seek, even if the URL has changed.

TELL US ABOUT A SITE
When you find a terrific site, tell us about it. Fill out a simple form and we may add your site immediately to eMedguides.com, and we may include it in our next print edition too.

BUY MORE BOOKS
Quickly order books in any of our available specialties, including patient guides, from our online store.

FREE JOURNALS & ASSOCIATIONS
Hundreds of links to journals and associations in each of over 20 specialties are provided.

BROWSE THE TABLE OF CONTENTS
You can quickly find every topic using the full table of contents.

FULL PRINT EDITION, ONLINE
Click to view the sites in a topic. An access code is required; you can find it on the title page of this book.

E-LINK OR SEARCH
Enter an e-Link code (found next to each site in this book) or enter a text string to search the entire specialty.

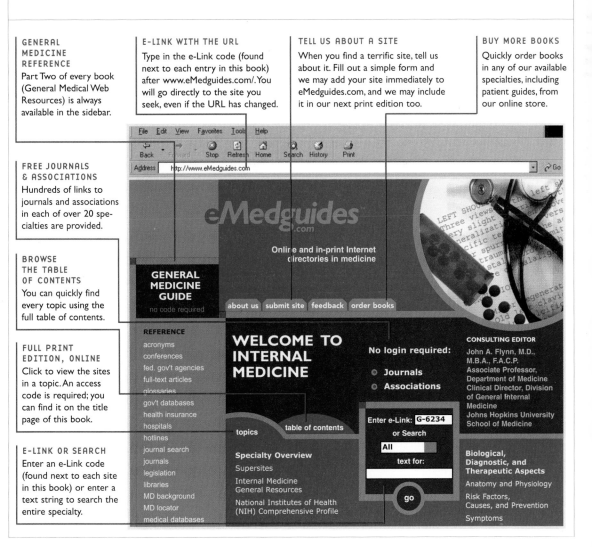

SUMMARY TABLE OF CONTENTS

TABLE OF CONTENTS

The 20th century

brought him type 2 diabetes.

The 21st gave him AVANDIA®.

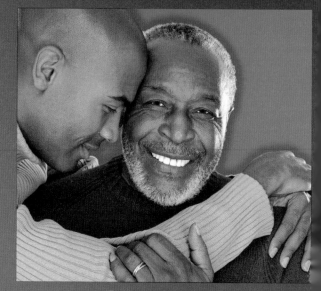

The future of type 2 diabetes therapy is now.

Insulin-sensitizing

Avandia®
rosiglitazone maleate

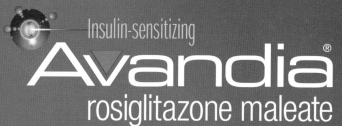

Important clinical considerations

Cardiac considerations: In clinical trials, an increased incidence of heart failure and other cardiovascular events was seen with *Avandia* in combination with insulin, including some patients not known to have prior CHF or pre-existing cardiac conditions. *Avandia* is not indicated for use in combination with insulin.

Patients with New York Heart Association (NYHA) Class 3 and 4 cardiac status were not studied during the clinical trials. *Avandia* is not recommended in these patients.

Avandia, like other thiazolidinediones, alone or in combination with other antidiabetic agents, can cause fluid retention, which may exacerbate or lead to heart failure. Patients should be observed for signs and symptoms of heart failure. *Avandia* should be discontinued if any deterioration in cardiac status occurs.

Hepatic considerations: Liver enzyme monitoring is recommended prior to initiation of *Avandia*, every 2 months for the first 12 months, and periodically thereafter. *Avandia* should not be initiated in patients with clinical evidence of active liver disease or ALT >2.5X the upper limit of normal.

Reports of hepatitis and of hepatic enzyme elevations t three or more times the upper limit of normal have bee received in postmarketing experience. Very rarely, thes reports have involved hepatic failure with and without fatal outcome, although causality has not been established.

Please see brief summary of prescribing information in Appendix A

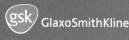 GlaxoSmithKline

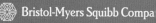 Bristol-Myers Squibb Compa

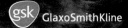

ENDURING PERFORMANCE

In Respiratory Tract Infections

Bronchitis (AECB)† and Sinusitis (ABRS)‡

BID AUGMENTIN
amoxicillin/clavulanate potassium

Efficacy and safety 17 years strong

Augmentin is contraindicated in patients with a history of allergic reactions to any penicillin or cholestatic jaundice/hepatic dysfunction associated with *Augmentin*.

* For susceptible strains of indicated organisms. *Augmentin* is appropriate initial therapy when β-lactamase–producing pathogens are suspected.
† Acute exacerbations of chronic bronchitis.
‡ Acute bacterial rhinosinusitis.

gsk GlaxoSmithKline

Please see brief summary of prescribing information in Appendix B at the end of the book for contraindications, warnings, precautions, adverse reactions, and dose and administration.

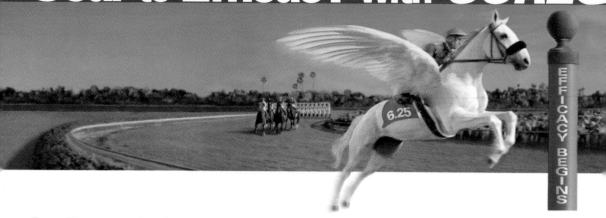

When adding a β-blocking agent for your patients with mild or moderate heart failure
Soar to Efficacy with *COREG*

Benefits across the dosage range, beginning at 6.25 mg bid

Efficacy begins at 6.25 mg bid and continues across the dosage range, from 6.25 to 25 mg bid[1]

Comprehensive triple adrenergic blockade

Coreg blocks all three adrenergic receptors (β_1, β_2, and α_1) that contribute to disease progression in heart failure*

Proven patient tolerability

In clinical trials, withdrawals from *Coreg* were no more frequent than from placebo when added to ACE-based therapy[2]

Add *Coreg* early to ACE-based therapy and discover dosing that delivers at 6.25 mg bid and across the dosage range

Easy dosing for your mild or moderate heart failure patients

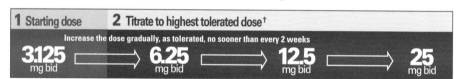

1 Starting dose	**2** Titrate to highest tolerated dose[†]		
Increase the dose gradually, as tolerated, no sooner than every 2 weeks			
3.125 mg bid →	**6.25** mg bid →	**12.5** mg bid →	**25** mg bid

Important Safety Information

The most common side effects (dizziness, symptoms of worsening heart failure, and bradycardia) of *Coreg* are predictable of an agent with vasodilating or β-blocking properties. Side effects are usually ameliorated by temporarily adjusting concomitant medications and/or *Coreg*, or by slowing the rate of titration (see Dosage and Administration section in the brief summary of the full prescribing information).

As with most agents with β-blockade, *Coreg* is contraindicated in NYHA Class IV decompensated heart failure requiring intravenous inotropic therapy, bronchial asthma, or related bronchospastic conditions, second- or third-degree AV block, sick sinus syndrome (unless a permanent pacemaker is in place), cardiogenic shock, severe bradycardia, or patients with clinically manifest hepatic impairment.

*The basis (mechanism of action) for the beneficial effects of *Coreg* in congestive heart failure has not been established.

† A maximum of 25 mg bid for patients ≤187 lb or 85 kg, or 50 mg bid for patients >187 lb or 85 kg.

References: 1. Bristow MR, Gilbert EM, Abraham WT, et al. Carvedilol produces dose-related improvements in left ventricular function and survival in subjects with chronic heart failure. *Circulation.* 1996;94: 2807-2816. **2.** Data on file, SmithKline Beecham Pharmaceuticals.

Please see brief summary of full prescribing information at the back of this book, appendix C.

C01343

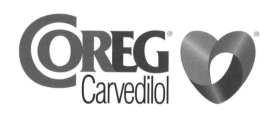

COREG® ®
Carvedilol

Let the Benefits Begin

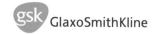

gsk GlaxoSmithKline

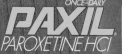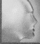

PREFACE

It has been estimated by various sources that more than half of America's physicians use the Internet and that this trend is increasing on a yearly basis. Although much use may be attributed to electronic mail and literature research, the clinical uses of the World Wide Web cannot be ignored. The Internet facilitates communication among professionals, ease of examination of numerous medical journals, focused topical research, and patient education. And, in the very near future (if not already), we will do our clinical transactions over the Internet.

This new annual directory entitled *Internal Medicine: An Internet Resource Guide* is one in a series of more than ten similar volumes that cover the various fields of medicine in great depth. Designed for clinicians, researchers, medical students, and allied healthcare professionals, these books put the user in touch with extensive screened resources on the Internet, organized in the fashion of a medical textbook.

For internists, there are daily news sites, conference schedules, clinical trials information, and new drug data appearing in a section called "Quick Reference." More than eighty journals are available where article abstracts for current issues may be consulted.

In the clinical sections, dozens of symptoms, diagnostic techniques, procedures, and pharmacological therapeutics are referenced, with links to applicable Web sites, followed by an exploration into many clinical and educational topics. An extensive chapter is devoted to hundreds of diseases and disorders, categorized according to specialty and subspecialty.

The last section of the book is devoted to general medical information resources covering a wide range of topics, from general reference to patient education and planning.

I invite colleagues and students to use this volume as a starting point for explorations into the many medical resources of the Internet. As a result of my own work with this book, I have found a number of great opportunities to enhance not only my professional education, but also to provide accurate information for my patients.

Please do not hesitate to correspond with us regarding your comments or suggested revisions.

John A. Flynn, M.D., M.B.A., F.A.C.P.
Associate Professor, Department of Medicine
Clinical Director, Division of General Internal Medicine
Johns Hopkins University

1

INTRODUCTION

1.1 WELCOME TO eMEDGUIDES

Welcome to eMedguides and to the first edition of *Internal Medicine: An Internet Resource Guide*. As a user of this book, you have a gateway to an extraordinary amount of information to help you find every useful resource in your field, from electronic journals to selected Web sites on dozens of common and uncommon diseases and disorders.

Over the past year, eMedguides have reached hundreds of thousands of physicians, healthcare professionals, researchers, and medical students. We have published guides to arthritis and rheumatology, cardiology, dermatology, endocrinology and metabolism, infectious diseases and immunology, neurology and neuroscience, psychiatry, oncology and hematology, urology and nephrology, and respiratory and pulmonary medicine. Several additional important specialties are on the way.

This volume is built upon a comprehensive table of contents in order to provide a broad overview of topics and issues in the field.

We would like to thank our Consulting Medical Editor, John A. Flynn, M.D., M.B.A, Clinical Director, Division of General Internal Medicine, Johns Hopkins University School of Medicine, for his contributions to the preparation of this volume. In addition, we appreciate the assistance and guidance from our Consulting Medical Librarian, Karen M. Albert, Director of Library Services for the Fox Chase Cancer Center.

How to Benefit Most from this Book

The most efficient method for finding information in this volume is to scan the table of contents. Our aim has been to organize the material logically, topic by topic, giving descriptions of Web sites that we feel our readers will want to visit. Part One focuses just on the fields of internal medicine, including biological, diagnostic, and therapeutic aspects, as well as recent books, CME sites, disorder resources, journal access, organization sites, and other topical information. Part Two concentrates on the broad fields of medicine reference, clinical practice, and patient education. This includes online databases, sources of current news and legislation, library access sites, government agencies, pharmaceutical data, student resources, and patient planning information.

A very extensive index is also included, covering all included topics and Web site titles, to make the fact-finding mission as efficient as possible.

Physicians and researchers will find that a wide array of material exists in the field. In addition to "supersites," many individual diseases, diagnoses, and therapies have dedicated Web sites intended for professional audiences. We have provided a comprehensive list of journal Web sites which provide access to thousands of articles and abstracts every month. A further exploration can lead to content-rich government sites, hospital and school departments, clinical research centers, recent drug trial results, and sites that provide quick updates on news, CME, and upcoming conferences.

Although much of the material in this book is intended for a professional medical audience, key patient Web resources are also provided. Physicians may wish to refer patients to these sites. Many patient sites include up-to-date news and research and clear descriptions of diseases and their treatments.

Finding a Site

We provide the full URL for each site in this volume, which can be typed into the address bar of your Internet browser. We also provide an identification number called an "e-Link," which will quickly take you to a specific Web site. Simply type in the eMedguides address, followed by a forward slash (/), followed by the e-Link number (found in the box next to each Web site in this book). For example, to reach the National Institutes of Health, enter www.eMedguides.com/g-0050. The e-Link number is associated with a Web site address in our database. Since we update Web addresses continually, you will always be directed to the appropriate address. This is especially important for medical Web site addresses, which change quite often as new information is added to bring sites up to date.

All of the content in this volume can also be accessed at our Web site, www.eMedguides.com, using the entry code found on the title page of this book. At our site you can explore the field by simply clicking on Web sites, as with a traditional Web directory. General medical sites are located in the sidebar, while specialty-specific information can be reached from the Internal Medicine section (use www.eMedguides.com/internal as a shortcut).

The Benefits of Both Print and Online Editions

We feel that both the print and online editions of eMedguides play an important role in the information-gathering process. The print edition is a "hands-on" tool, enabling the reader to thumb through a comprehensive directory, finding Web information and topical sources that are totally new and unexpected. Each page can provide discoveries of resources previously unknown to the reader that may never have been the subject of an online search. Without knowing what to expect, the reader can be introduced to useful Web site information just by glancing at the book, looking through the detailed table of contents, or examining the extensive index. This type of browsing is difficult to achieve online.

The online edition serves a different purpose. It provides direct links to each Web site so the user can visit the destination instantaneously, without having to type the Web address or our new e-Link identification code into a browser. In addition, there are search features in this edition that can be used to find specific information quickly, and then the user can print out only what he or she wishes to use.

The online edition also represents the most up-to-date information about our selected Web sites. We update our database throughout the year, adding new resources as they become available and editing those that change. The eMedguides Web site also provides a platform for communication—our Submit a Site feature lets you share your online discoveries with us, and hence other readers in a future update.

We hope you will find the print and online versions of this volume to be useful Internet companions, always on hand to consult.

1.2 RATINGS AND SITE SELECTION

Site Selection Criteria

Our medical research staff has carefully chosen the sites for this guide. We perform extensive searches for all of the topics listed in our table of contents and then select only the sites that meet carefully established criteria. The pertinence and depth of content, timeliness of the material, presentation, and usefulness of the site for physician and advisory purposes are taken into account.

The selection of sites in this physician guide includes detailed reference material, news, clinical data, and current research articles. We also include and appropriately identify numerous sites that may be useful for patient reference. The large majority of our Web sites are maintained by reputable academic, government-sponsored, or professional and research organizations. Additional material is derived from online textbooks or scholarly, referenced journals in the field. Sites operated by private individuals or corporations are only included if they are content-rich and useful to the physician. In these cases, we clearly identify the operator in the title or description of the site.

In addition, if a site requires a fee, some fees, or a free registration/disclosure of personal information, we indicate this information at the end of the site description.

Ratings Guide

Those sites that are identified based on the selection criteria are subsequently rated on a scale of one apple (🍎) to three apples (🍎🍎🍎). Scholarly material, aimed at a professional audience, and authoritative educational materials that are useful to both students and healthcare consumers are eligible for inclusion. The three-apple designation denotes a site that is a comprehensive source of relevant information derived from a major educational institution, government-sponsored organization, noteworthy professional or research group, or authoritative publication. The timeliness and accuracy of the material, its usefulness to users, and its depth of content are considered to be high. A one-apple site contains accurate, relevant information in a more succinct format.

Abbreviations

See "Medical Abbreviations and Acronyms" under "Reference Information and News Sources" in Part Two for Web sites that provide acronym translation. Below are a few acronyms you will find throughout this volume:

AMA   American Medical Association
CME   Continuing Medical Education
FAQ   Frequently Asked Questions
NIH   National Institutes of Health
PDQ   Physician Data Query
URL   Uniform Resource Locator (the address of a Web site on the Internet)

1.3 GETTING ONLINE

The Internet is growing at a rapid pace, but many individuals are not yet online. What is preventing people from jumping on the "information highway"? There are many factors, but the most common issue is a general confusion about what the Internet is, how it works, and how to access it.

The following few pages are designed to clear up any confusion for readers who have not yet accessed the Internet. We will look at the process of getting onto and using the Internet, step by step.

It is also helpful to consult other resources, such as the technical support department of the manufacturer or store where you bought your computer. Although assistance varies widely, most organizations provide startup assistance for new users and are experienced with guiding individuals onto the Internet. Books can also be of great assistance, as they provide a simple and clear view of how computers and the Internet work, and can be studied at your own pace.

What is the Internet?

The Internet is a large network of computers that are all connected to one another. A good analogy is to envision a neighborhood, with houses and storefronts, all connected to one another by streets and highways. Often the Internet is referred to as the "information super-highway" because of the vastness of this neighborhood.

The Internet was initially developed to allow people to share computers, that is, share part of their "house" with others. The ability to connect to so many other computers quickly and easily made this feasible. As computers proliferated and increased in computational power, people started using the Internet for sending information quickly from one computer to another.

For example, the most popular feature of the Internet is electronic mail (e-mail). Each computer has a mailbox, and an electronic letter can be sent instantly. People also use the Internet to post bulletins, or other information, for others to see. The process of sending e-mail or viewing this information is simple. A computer and a connection to the Internet are all you need to begin.

How is an Internet connection provided?

The Internet is accessed either through a "direct" connection, which is found in businesses and educational institutions, or through a phone line. Phone line connections are the most common access method for users at home, although direct connections are becoming available for home use. There are many complex options in this area; for the new user it is simplest to use an existing phone line to experience the Internet for the first time. A dual telephone jack can be purchased at many retail stores. Connect the computer to the phone jack, and then use the provided software to connect to the Internet. Your computer will dial the number of an Internet provider and ask you for a user name and password. Keep in mind that while you are using the Internet, your phone line is tied up and callers will hear a busy signal. Also, call waiting can sometimes interrupt an Internet connection and disconnect you from the Internet.

Who provides an Internet connection?

There are many providers at both the local and national levels. One of the easiest ways to get online is with America Online (AOL). They provide software and a user-friendly environment through which to access the Internet. Because AOL manages both this environment and the actual connection, they can be of great assistance when you are starting out. America Online takes you to a menu of choices when you log in, and while using their software you can read and send e-mail, view Web pages, and chat with others.

Many other similar services exist, and most of them also provide an environment using Microsoft or Netscape products. These companies, such as the Microsoft Network (MSN) and Earthlink, also provide simple, easy-to-use access to the Internet. Their environment is more standard and not limited to the choices America Online provides.

Internet connections generally run from $10-$20 per month (depending on the length of commitment) in addition to telephone costs. Most national providers have local phone numbers all over the country that should eliminate any telephone charges. The monthly provider fee is the only direct charge for accessing the Internet.

How do I get on the Internet?

Once you've signed up with an Internet provider and installed their software (often only a matter of answering basic questions), your computer will be set up to access the Internet. By simply double-clicking on an icon, your computer will dial the phone number, log you in, and present you with a Web page (a "home" page).

What are some of the Internet's features?

From the initial Web page there are almost limitless possibilities of where you can go. The address at the top of the screen (identified by an "http://" in front) tells you where you are. You can also type the address of where you would like to go next. When typing a new address, you do not need to add the "http://". The computer adds this prefix automatically after you type in an address and press return. Once you press return, the Web site will appear in the browser window.

You can also navigate the Web by "surfing" from one site to another using links on a page. A Web page might say, "Click here for weather." If you move the mouse pointer to this underlined phrase and click the mouse button, you will be taken to a different address, where weather information is provided.

The Internet has several other useful features. E-mail is an extremely popular and important service. It is free and messages are delivered instantly. Although you can access e-mail through a Web browser (AOL has this feature), many Internet services provide a separate e-mail program for reading, writing, and organizing your correspondence. These programs send and retrieve messages from the Internet.

Another area of the Internet offers chat rooms where users can hold roundtable discussions. In a chat room you can type messages and see the replies of other users around the world. There are chat rooms on virtually every topic, although the dialog certainly varies in this free-for-all forum. There are also newsgroups on the Internet, some of which we list in this book. A newsgroup is similar to a chat room but each message is a separate item and can be viewed in sequence at any time. For example, a user might post a question about Lyme disease. In the newsgroup you can read the question and then read the answers that others have provided. You can also post your own comments. This forum is usually not managed or edited, particularly in the medical field. Do not take the advice of a chat room or newsgroup source without first consulting your physician.

How can I find things on the Internet?

Surfing the Internet, from site to site, is a popular activity. But if you have a focused mission, you will want to use a search engine. A search engine can scan lists of Web sites to look for a particular site. We provide a long list of medical search engines in this book.

Because the Internet is so large and unregulated, sites are often hard to find. In the physical world it is difficult to find good services, but you can turn to the yellow pages or other resources to get a comprehensive list. Physical proximity is also a major factor. On the Internet, the whole world is at your doorstep. Finding a reliable site takes time and patience, and can require sifting through hundreds of similar, yet irrelevant, sites.

The most common way to find information on the Internet is to use a search engine. When you go to the Web page of a search engine, you will be presented with two distinct methods of searching: using links to topics, or using a keyword search. The links often represent the Web site staff's best effort to find quality sites. This method of searching is the core of the Yahoo! search engine (http://www.yahoo.com). By clicking on Healthcare, then Disorders, then Lung Cancer, you are provided with a list of sites the staff has found on the topic.

The keyword approach is definitely more daring. By typing in search terms, the engine looks through its list of Web sites for a match and returns the results. These engines typically only cover 15 percent of the Internet, so it is not a comprehensive process. They also usually return far too many choices. Typing lung cancer into a search engine box will return thousands of sites, including one entry for every site where someone used the words lung cancer on a personal Web page.

Where do eMedguides come in?

eMedguides offer organized listings of Web sites in each major medical specialty. Our team of editors continually scours the Net, searching for quality Web sites that relate to specific specialties, disorders, and research topics. Of the sites we find, we only include those that provide professional and useful content. By eliminating the many sites that are not on target or reliable, eMedguides fill a critical gap in the Internet research process. Each guide provides more than 1,000 Web sites that focus on every aspect of a single medical discipline.

Other Internet search engines rely on teams of "surfers" who can only cover a subject on its surface because they survey the entire Internet. Search engines, even medical search engines, return far too many choices, requiring hours of time and patience to sift through. eMedguides, on the other hand, focus on medical and physician sites in a specialty. With an eMedguide in hand, you can quickly identify the sites worth visiting on the Internet and jump right to them. At our site, http://www.eMedguides.com, you can access the same listings as in this book and can simply click on a site to go straight to it. In addition, we provide continual updates to the book through the site and annually in print. Our editors do the surfing for you and do it professionally, making your Internet experience efficient and fulfilling.

Our new e-Link identification code is the fastest way to surf the Internet. Simply append the code number to the eMedguides address (www.eMedguides.com/g-0050) to be taken directly to the site you are reading about in the book.

Taking medical action must involve a physician

As interesting as the Internet is, the information that you will find is both objective and subjective. Our goal is to expose our readers to Web sites on hundreds of topics for informational purposes only. If you are not a physician and become interested in the ideas, guidelines, recommendations, or experiences discussed online, bring these findings to a physician for personal evaluation. Medical needs vary considerably, and a medical approach or therapy for one individual could be entirely misguided for another. Final medical advice and a plan of action must come only from a physician.

INTERNAL MEDICINE
WEB RESOURCES

QUICK REFERENCE

2.1 MEDICAL GLOSSARIES/DICTIONARIES

M-0018

CancerWEB: Online Medical Dictionary The medical dictionary offered at this site covers numerous medical terms, accessible alphabetically, by subject area, or by typing a term into the search engine box. This site also provides information about cancer and patient management for clinicians, information for research specialists in various health areas, and patient and family information on cancer and treatment.
http://www.graylab.ac.uk/omd/index.html

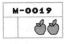
M-0019

MedicineNet.com: Medical References An extensive online medical dictionary is provided at this site by MedNet.com. Links are also provided to information files that explain diseases and conditions, procedures and tests, and medications.
http://www.medicinenet.com/Script/Main/AlphaIdx.asp?li=MNI&p=A_DICT

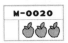
M-0020

MEDLINEplus Health Information: Dictionaries Various medical dictionaries can be accessed through this site from MEDLINEplus. Dictionaries presented include the Merriam-Webster Medical Dictionary, a multi-lingual glossary, and a list of online dictionaries compiled by Bucknell University.
http://www.nlm.nih.gov/medlineplus/dictionaries.html

2.2 MEDICAL NEWS

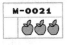
M-0021

American Medical News American Medical News features articles in the areas of government and medicine, professional issues, business, opinion, technology, and health and science. Created specifically for physicians, this site outlines current medical news arranged week by week, and offers links to news archives, regional coverage, and details about free e-mail news alerts.
http://www.ama-assn.org/public/journals/amnews/amnews.htm

M-0023

Medscape: Multispecialty News Medscape Multispecialty daily news features clinical articles, as well as articles focusing on drugs, devices, managed care, and professional news. Medscape resources highlighted at the left sidebar menu include sections on treatment updates, clinical management, practice guidelines, conference summaries and schedules, journals, patient resources, and managed care. By scrolling at the upper right corner of the site, the visitor can select news from over 25 medical specialties.

http://www.medscape.com/home/news/medscape-news.html

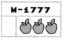 **MDLinx.com**   This Web page offers professionals more than 30 Web sites in specialties such as allergy and immunology, dermatology, family medicine, and internal medicine for the latest medical news and journal abstracts. Some full-text articles are available free of charge.

http://www.mdlinx.com

 NewsRounds: Personalized News for the Business of Medicine
NewsRounds provides visitors with daily medical news articles, as well as information on diseases and diagnostics, treatments, drug warnings, managed care and insurers, legislative and legal issues, public healthcare, economics, FDA approvals, clinical trials, vaccines, scientific research, and international issues related to health. Visitors can also access specialty news links by fields such as cardiology, family practice, internal medicine, psychiatry, and urology. This site is oriented toward healthcare professionals, and free registration is required for accessing full-text articles.

(free registration) http://www.newsrounds.com/cgi-bin/story.cgi?mode=home

 Reuters Health Medical News   Reuters Health Medical News provides daily coverage of medical news topics for healthcare professionals. Articles are divided into more than 15 categories, including clinical, economic, epidemiology, ethical, legislative, pharmaceutical, policy, and professional development topics. Over 100 medical journals are represented at this site.

http://www.reutershealth.com/frame2/med.html

2.3 Medical Conferences

A number of key Web sites that offer event calendars along with details of conference programs and locations are provided here. Although a comprehensive conference calendar is provided by the PSL Group's *Doctor's Guide* (our first listing), the other listed sites have valuable additional listings. Taken together, this group provides an overall source of conference scheduling information for the year.

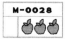 **Doctor's Guide**   The professional edition of Doctor's Guide offers this compilation of upcoming events in numerous specialties. By accessing any particular meeting, visitors are provided with specific information about the conference and details about host cities worldwide.

http://www.docguide.com

 MedicalConferences.com   Visitors to this comprehensive source for medical conference listings can search for appropriate conferences by keyword, dates, and location. The site also provides a tool for registering for conferences, links to related sites with site profiles, and answers to frequently asked questions.

http://www.medicalconferences.com

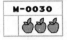

MediConf Online: Forthcoming Meetings MediConf Online provides a directory of forthcoming meetings and conferences in every major medical specialty. The menu at this site enables the visitor to select the field of choice. For each meeting, there is a listing, including the dates, contact information, and a link to the city where the visitor can learn more about accommodations. Visitors pay a fee for each medical specialty. However, the current month's listings are offered at no cost.

(some features fee-based) http://www.mediconf.com/index.html

TheScientificWorld: WorldMeet Visitors to this site will find a searchable conference database for a wide range of medical and scientific specialties, including AIDS, allergy, cancer, cardiology, dermatology, endocrinology, infectious disease, internal medicine, neurology, respiratory, and urology. The database can be searched by date, key word, or location of meeting. Results offer brief descriptions of the conference, a schedule of programs, conference location, and contact information. Some have a link to the sponsor's Web page for additional information. An e-mail alert service offers notification of new events of interest.

http://www.thescientificworld.com/WorldMeet/default.asp?uid=&bid=

2.4 DISORDER PROFILES

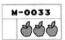

Karolinska Institutet: Alphabetical List of Specific Diseases/ Disorders Offering information to both the general public and healthcare professionals, this large collection of links offers alphabetical access to link collections across a variety of medical specialties. By clicking on any chosen disorder, visitors are brought to the appropriate Karolinska specialty page, which offers access to fact sheets, pathology pages, and general overviews for the chosen condition and related diseases.

http://www.mic.ki.se/Diseases/alphalist.html

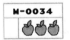

MedicineNet.com: Diseases and Conditions Index Visitors to this MedicineNet site will find brief profiles of hundreds of diseases and conditions listed in an alphabetical index. For each disorder, the visitor can obtain explanatory, diagnostic, and therapeutic information, as well as answers to important questions. Links to further resources, procedures, and medical assessments related to each disease are provided.

http://www.medicinenet.com/Script/Main/AlphaIdx.asp?li=MNI&p=A_DT

New York Online Access to Health (NOAH): Health Topics and Resources Hundreds of medical topics are searchable through the NOAH Subject Index, which offers access to coverage of specific disorders and conditions within various medical specialties. From aging and Alzheimer's to tuberculosis, visitors will find general disease information, care and treatment, and patient support pages.

http://www.noah-health.org/english/qksearch.html

Don't type in long URLs – add the site number to the eMedguides URL: www.eMedguides.com/**G-1234**.

2.5 STATISTICS

Healthcare Cost and Utilization Project: HCUPNet   Clinical information featured at this site includes evidence-based practice reports, outcomes and effectiveness, technology assessment, preventative services, and clinical practice guidelines. Visitors to this site can also access information on health conditions, prevention and wellness, quality of care, and surgery. Research findings in the areas of primary care, healthcare costs, elderly healthcare, managed care, long-term care, and rural health can be accessed.
http://www.ahcpr.gov/data/hcup/hcupnet.htm

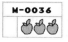

National Center for Health Statistics (NCHS)   The National Center for Health Statistics Web page provides statistics organized nationally, by state, by population group, and disease. Visitors can click on an A-to-Z listing of statistics to view data by health concern, download data spreadsheets from their data warehouse, or seek out related publications. A link entitled "FEDSTATS" provides a quick reference source for national statistics.
http://www.cdc.gov/nchs/

National Center for Health Statistics (NCHS): Fast Stats A-to-Z
Statistical data and various statistical resources for numerous health-related topics are provided by the National Center of Health Statistics. Over 200 topics are featured at this site, including asthma, cancer, diabetes, heart disease, men's health, nutrition and diet, sexually transmitted diseases, and smoking. Details regarding surveys and data collection systems represented are provided.
http://www.cdc.gov/nchs/fastats/Default.htm

2.6 CLINICAL TRIALS

CenterWatch: Clinical Trials Listing Service   Patient resources and professional sections are available at the CenterWatch home page, which offers trial listings, information about clinical research for consumer viewing, online drug directories, and an assortment of patient reports and brochures. For healthcare professionals, research center profiles, industry news, industry provider profiles, and a professional publications link are available. Industry-sponsored trial listings may be searched by specialty.
http://www.centerwatch.com/

ClinicalTrials.gov   The National Institutes of Health and the National Library of Medicine grant patients access to information about clinical trials through ClinicalTrials.gov. Visitors can search the database by entering keywords or phrases into the search engine; by using a focused search by disease, location, treatment, or sponsor; or by browsing alphabetical listings of thousands of conditions and sponsors. Links to information on studies currently recruiting offer additional details on study purpose, protocol, and researcher contact.   http://clinicaltrials.gov/ct/gui/c/b

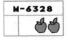

MediStudy.com: Canada's Clinical Trials   Visitors to this site will find a database of clinical trials currently in progress in Canada. Search results yield the study title, a brief trial description, and contact information. There is also a glossary of terms, along with an overview of clinical trials. Users can register for e-mail notification of future studies.
http://www.medistudy.com/clinical_trials/index.html

2.7 ONLINE TEXTS

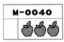

Family Practice Notebook.com   Medical notes on over 3,000 topics are available from this site of the Family Practice Notebook.com. Visitors can access hundreds of medical topics related to disorders, diagnosis, and management options. Each specialty connection offers a menu of textbook chapters, including pharmacology, pathology and laboratory medicine, and disease-related prevention, in addition to complete management outlines. Over 30 medical specialties are represented at this family medicine resource.
http://www.fpnotebook.com

Harrison's Online   Harrison's Online hosts this medical database offering members search capabilities of the 14th edition of *Harrison's Principles of Medicine.* In addition to book content, visitors have access to MEDLINE abstracts, current clinical trial data, therapeutic and clinical research breakthroughs, links to related databases and sites, and clinical tables and photographs. Visitors can receive a free trial of this service, but a subscription is necessary. (some features fee-based) http://www.harrisonsonline.com

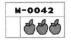

Merck Manual of Diagnosis and Therapy   The *Merck Manual of Diagnosis and Therapy* contains more than 20 chapters, covering a multitude of medical subjects. This reference book, already familiar to most physicians, features a search tool in its online version which streamlines the research process.
http://www.merck.com/pubs/mmanual

2.8 DRUG PIPELINE: APPROVED AND DEVELOPMENTAL DRUGS

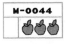

CenterWatch: Drugs Approved by the FDA (2000)   By accessing any specific approval year and specialty, visitors are returned a listing of products approved by the FDA during that time period. General information, clinical results, side effects, and mechanism of action are reviewed for each new therapy.
http://www.centerwatch.com/patient/drugs/drugls00.html

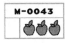

CenterWatch: Drugs in Clinical Trials Database   This online resource invites professional and consumer viewers to view information on over 1,300 new therapies in phase II and III clinical trials. Details about each new treatment, brand and generic names, sponsoring research company, and contacts for

research centers are provided. Visitors are returned results by selecting from the large variety of medical conditions listed.
http://www.centerwatch.com/patient/cwpipeline/default.asp

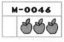

Food and Drug Administration (FDA): Center for Drug Evaluation and Research In addition to an alphabetical listing of all prescription drugs approved during the 1998-2000 time period, visitors will find links to a regularly updated, reverse chronological listing; new drugs approved for cancer indications; and the online *Orange Book,* which lists all FDA-approved prescription drugs and their generic equivalents. Major drug information pages on individual products and the Consumer Drug Information Page, which lists basic label information and provides complete package inserts, are found.
http://www.fda.gov/cder/drug/default.htm

Pharmaceutical Research and Manufacturers of America: New Medicines in Development Visitors to this site will find reports on new medicines in development for specific populations, such as children and older Americans, as well as for specific diseases, such as cancer, heart disease and stroke, AIDS, and infectious diseases. The "New Medicine in Development" database can also be accessed from the site.
http://www.phrma.org/searchcures/newmeds/

Pharmaceutical Research and Manufacturers of America: New Medicines in Development Database The "New Medicine in Development" database can be searched on this site by disease, indication, or drug name. Results yield the drug name, indications, manufacturer, and development status. http://www.phrma.org/searchcures/newmeds/webdb/

3

Journals, Articles, and Latest Books

3.1 Abstract, Citation, and Full-Text Search Tools

In addition to the PubMed search tool profiled here, several Web sites for full-text journal articles are profiled in the Reference Information and News Sources section of this book, under Full-Text Articles. (In the online version, see the home page for Full-Text Articles, under Reference.)

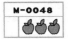

Agency for Healthcare Research and Quality (AHRQ): Search for Information The Agency for Healthcare Research and Quality offers this search tool for finding the most recent comprehensive research reports on a variety of health issues. Both a natural language query and tips for performing more precise searches are available for locating practice documents, congressional information, data sets, research programs, and news.

http://www.ahcpr.gov/query/query.htm

Aries Systems Corporation: Knowledge Finder The Knowledge Finder, presented by Aries Systems, searches medical databases and CD-ROMs to locate reference and full-text medical literature for healthcare professionals. With a membership to Knowledge Finder, publishers can access Internet and CD-ROM Electronic Publishing Services, DocuRights, Knowledge MedRef, and MedCite. ExtraLib is a feature of this service offered to libraries, hospitals, and educational institutions, providing access to a variety of indexing sources, including CINAHL, MEDLINE, Pre-MEDLINE, and the Cochrane Evidence-Based Medical Library. A free trial of this service is offered by MEDLINE, and purchase information is provided.

(some features fee-based) http://www.kfinder.com/newweb/home.html

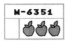

Ingenta A searchable bibliographic database—featuring more than 25,000 publications—is offered on this site for several subject areas, including medicine and nursing. Search results yield a citation with the option to purchase the full-text article. For those with a subscription to a specific journal, access to the full-text article is free. In addition, each medical specialty has links to news, conferences, clinical trials, and practice guidelines.

(some features fee-based) http://www.ingenta.com

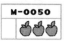

National Library of Medicine (NLM): Health Services Technology Assessment Texts (HSTAT) Approximately 20 summaries and some complete evidence-based practice reports are made available at this site from the Agency for Healthcare Research and Quality, regarding the evaluation of various treatments in a variety of specialties. Guidelines, technology assessments, preventive service documents, and NIH Consensus Development Program details are found. Several databases are included in this online literature search, including the Centers for Disease Control and Prevention Guidelines and PubMed. http://www.nlm.nih.gov/pubs/factsheets/hstat.html

National Library of Medicine (NLM): NLM Gateway By entering one or more search terms, visitors are able to scan multiple retrieval systems of the U.S. National Library of Medicine (NLM) at no charge. The Gateway searches for documents from MEDLINE, OLDMEDLINE, LOCATORPlus, AIDS Meeting, MEDLINEplus, and other online sources. Additional NLM resources may be accessed from the site, such as ClinicalTrials.gov. http://gateway.nlm.nih.gov/gw/Cmd

National Library of Medicine (NLM): PubMed A service of the National Library of Medicine, PubMed provides professionals and other interested researchers with the opportunity to access over 11-million citations from MEDLINE and additional scientific resources. Visitors may search the database by author name, journal title, or keywords and are returned connections to article abstracts and links to related literature. A journal browser is available, as are additional PubMed features, including help and answers to FAQs, clinical queries, and a service that allows visitors to store and update literature searches. Through interactive tutorials, "Coffee Break" demonstrates online bioinformatics tools available through the National Center for Biotechnology Information. http://www4.ncbi.nlm.nih.gov/pubmed/

Ovid Preview: Ovid Technologies, Inc. Ovid, software for exploring over 80 scientific, medical, and technical databases, is a useful tool for exploring MEDLINE, Current Contents, Biosis, and PsychInfo. Details about Ovid are presented at the site, along with demonstration databases and an online order form. Full-text features, full searchability, graphics, hypertext navigation, and reference links are included in the service.
(some features fee-based) http://demo.ovid.com/libpreview/index.html

TheScientificWorld: sciBase This searchable bibliographic database covers more than 19-million documents published in the scientific, technical, and medical research literature. The citations are drawn from databases created by the National Library of Medicine (MEDLINE), the British Library, BIOSIS, and PASCAL. Search results return the citation, a link for the abstract, and the cost for purchasing a full reprint of the article. The database is updated daily, and users can sign up to receive e-mail alerts for new additions in relevant areas.
(some features fee-based) http://www.thescientificworld.com/scibase/search.asp?uid=&bid=

3.2 LITERATURE DIGESTS AND REVIEWS

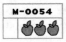
Cochrane Reviews: Abstracts Cochrane abstracts and reviews are accessible through this site, which features studies from more than 40 Collaborative Review Groups. The breast cancer, drugs and alcohol, eyes and vision, infectious disease, renal, stroke, skin, and gastrointestinal groups are just a sampling of the library, which offers new and updated reviews of the current literature. http://www.cochrane.org

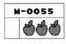
Critical Care Forum By becoming a member of the Critical Care Forum, physicians can obtain new development information in all areas of critical care. In addition, physicians can access literature reports, reviews, newspapers, free primary research articles, and Web reports. (some features fee-based)
http://ccforum.com/login.cfm?action=form&returnto=home_page.cfm

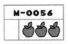
Journal Club on the Web An article search tool by subject, a reverse chronological listing of article summaries, and additional interactive features are all part of this online medical journal club. Summaries and comments from the recent medical literature are provided, and feedback from readers is recommended and appended to article summaries. Links to related sites and e-mail notification of new postings are available.
http://www.journalclub.org/#summaries

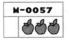
Journal of Family Practice: POEMs Editors of the *Journal of Family Practice* have compiled POEMs, otherwise known as "Patient-Oriented Evidence that Matters," a system that offers critiques of articles in over 90 journals of importance to primary care clinicians. The form at the site can be used to search for online critical appraisals that include clinical questions, study information, results, and clinical recommendations.
http://www.medicalinforetriever.com/poems/poemsearch.cfm

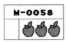
MCP Hahnemann University: Health Reviews for Primary Care Providers A listing of review topics is available at this site, which provides summaries of articles selected to serve the information needs of primary care clinicians. The collection includes Cochrane Reviews, ACP Journal Club, reviews of the *Journal of Family Practitioners, New England Journal of Medicine* abstracts, and other summary sources in primary care.
http://library.mcphu.edu/resources/reviews/revw_ind.htm

WebMedLit Plus Free citations, abstracts, and full-text articles in the areas of AIDS/virology, cancer/oncology, diabetes/endocrinology, immunology, neurology, cardiology, dermatology, gastroenterology, medical economics, and women's health are offered by WEBMEDLITPlus through this Web portal, sponsored by SilverPlatter. Visitors may enter a preferred topic at the site's search engine and are also offered a free, personalized home page.
http://webmedlit.silverplatter.com/index.html

3.3 MEDICAL JOURNAL DIRECTORIES

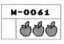

Free Medical Journals.com   Dedicated to the promotion of free information in medical practice, this site offers listings of journals that are either offered entirely free or free after a stated period of publication. In addition to the journals listed at the site, visitors are able to access more than 600 additional journals, sorted by specialty.
http://www.freemedicaljournals.com/

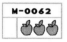

Hardin MD: Free Medical Journals   With a focus on indexed medical journals, this site of the Hardin MD database provides a selected list of free full-text electronic journals. Some are offered on a trial basis, and access to archived, current, and sample issues is provided.
http://www.lib.uiowa.edu/hardin/md/ej.html

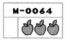

MedBioWorld: Medical Journals   Visitors can search this Internet directory by clicking on a subject area or accessing the Electric Library search form. Several broad-coverage journal home pages are available, as well as hundreds of medical journals in subjects ranging from AIDS to urology.
http://www.medbioworld.com/journals/medicine/med-bio.html

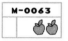

Primary Care Internet Guide: Journals in General Practice   As part of an Internet directory for primary care clinicians, this page offers listings and links to medical journals with a primary care focus. Categories of publications include general practice, public health, medical student material, and related publications, appropriate for general practice.
http://www.uib.no/isf/guide/journal.htm

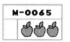

World News Network: Medical Journal   Journal sites in cardiovascular, clinical medicine, medical research, immunology, physiology, and other medical specialties are available from this link listing, which quickly identifies freely accessible publications. Database searching of MEDLINE, AIDSLINE, and other National Library of Medicine databases is also provided at the page.
http://www.medicaljournal.com/

3.4 JOURNALS ON THE INTERNET

The following journals may be accessed on the Internet. The table of information for each journal identifies content that is accessible free-of-charge or with a free registration, and also identifies publications that require a password or fee for access.

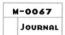

Abdominal Imaging
Publisher: Springer-Verlag **Free:** Table of Contents, Abstracts **Pay:** Articles
http://link.springer.de/link/service/journals/00261/index.htm

M-0068
JOURNAL

Academic Medicine

Publisher: Hanley & Belfus, Inc. **Free:** Table of Contents, Abstracts, Articles **Pay:** None
http://www.academicmedicine.org/

M-0069
JOURNAL

ACP Journal Club

Publisher: American College of Physicians-American Society of Internal Medicine
Free: Table of Contents, Articles **Pay:** None
http://www.acponline.org/journals/acpjc/jcmenu.htm

M-0070
JOURNAL

Age and Ageing

Publisher: Oxford University Press **Free:** Table of Contents, Abstracts, Articles **Pay:** None
http://www.ageing.oupjournals.org/

M-0071
JOURNAL

Alimentary Pharmacology and Therapeutics

Publisher: Blackwell Science **Free:** Table of Contents **Pay:** Abstracts, Articles
http://www.blackwell-science.com/~cgilib/jnlpage.bin?Journal=APT&File=APT&Page=aims

M-0072
JOURNAL

American Family Physician

Publisher: American Academy of Family Physicians **Free:** Table of Contents, Articles
Pay: None http://www.aafp.org/afp/

M-0073
JOURNAL

American Heart Journal

Publisher: Mosby, Inc. **Free:** Table of Contents, Abstracts, Articles **Pay:** None
http://www.harcourthealth.com/scripts/om.dll/
serve?action=searchDB&searchDBfor=home&id=hj

M-0074
JOURNAL

American Journal of Clinical Nutrition

Publisher: American Society for Clinical Nutrition, Inc. **Free:** Table of Contents, Abstracts,
Articles **Pay:** None http://www.ajcn.org/

M-0075
JOURNAL

American Journal of Hypertension

Publisher: Elsevier Science **Free:** Table of Contents **Pay:** Articles
http://www.elsevier.com/locate/amjhyper

M-0076
JOURNAL

American Journal of Preventive Medicine

Publisher: Elsevier Science **Free:** Table of Contents, Abstracts, Articles **Pay:** None
http://www.meddevel.com/site.mash?left=/library.exe&
m1=1&m2=1&right=/library.exe&action=home&site=AJPM&jcode=AMEPRE

M-0077
JOURNAL

American Journal of Respiratory and Critical Care Medicine

Publisher: American Lung Association **Free:** Table of Contents, Abstracts **Pay:** Articles
http://ajrccm.atsjournals.org

M-0078
JOURNAL

American Journal of Respiratory Cell and Molecular Biology

Publisher: American Lung Association **Free:** Table of Contents, Abstracts **Pay:** Articles
http://ajrcmb.atsjournals.org

M-0079 | **JOURNAL**

American Medical News
Publisher: American Medical Association **Free:** Table of Contents, Articles **Pay:** None
http://www.ama-assn.org/public/journals/amnews/amnews.htm

M-0080 | **JOURNAL**

Annals of Allergy, Asthma, and Immunology
Publisher: The American College of Allergy, Asthma & Immunology **Free:** Free registration required for Table of Contents, Abstracts **Pay:** Articles
http://allergy.edoc.com

M-0081 | **JOURNAL**

Annals of Emergency Medicine
Publisher: Mosby, Inc. **Free:** Table of Contents, Abstracts, Articles **Pay:** None
http://www.harcourthealth.com/scripts/
om.dll/serve?action=searchDB&searchDBfor=home&id=em

M-0082 | **JOURNAL**

Annals of Internal Medicine
Publisher: American Society of Internal Medicine **Free:** Table of Contents, Abstracts **Pay:** Articles http://www.acponline.org./journals/annals/annaltoc.htm

M-0083 | **JOURNAL**

Annals of Medicine
Publisher: Royal Society of Medicine Press Limited **Free:** Table of Contents, Abstracts, Articles **Pay:** None
http://www.roysocmed.ac.uk/pub/am.htm

M-0084 | **JOURNAL**

Annals of Nutrition & Metabolism
Publisher: S. Karger AG **Free:** Table of Contents, Abstracts **Pay:** Articles
http://www.karger.com/journals/anm/anm_jh.htm

M-0085 | **JOURNAL**

Annual Review of Medicine
Publisher: Annual Reviews **Free:** Table of Contents, Abstracts **Pay:** Articles
http://www.med.annualreviews.org/current/shtml

M-0086 | **JOURNAL**

Archives of Internal Medicine
Publisher: American Medical Association **Free:** Table of Contents, Abstracts **Pay:** Articles
http://archinte.ama-assn.org

M-0087 | **JOURNAL**

Arthritis Research
Publisher: BioMed Central Ltd. **Free:** Free registration required for Table of Contents, Abstracts, Articles **Pay:** Articles
http://arthritis-research.com/login.cfm?action=form&returnto=home_page.cfm

M-0088 | **JOURNAL**

Baillere's Best Practice & Research in Clinical Gastroenterology
Publisher: Harcourt Publishers Ltd. **Free:** Table of Contents, Abstracts **Pay:** Articles
http://www.harcourt-international.com/journals/bega/

M-0089 | **JOURNAL**

Blood
Publisher: American Society of Hematology **Free:** Table of Contents, Abstracts, Articles
Pay: None http://www.bloodjournal.org/.

Don't type in long URLs – add the site number to the eMedguides URL: www.eMedguides.com/**G-1234**.

M-0090
JOURNAL

British Journal of General Practice
Publisher: Royal College of General Practitioners **Free:** Table of Contents, Abstracts, Articles **Pay:** None http://www.rcgp.org.uk/rcgp/journal/index.asp

M-0091
JOURNAL

British Medical Journal
Publisher: BMJ Publishing Group **Free:** Table of Contents, Abstracts, Articles **Pay:** None http://www.bmj.com/

M-0092
JOURNAL

Canadian Respiratory Journal
Publisher: Pulsus Group Inc. **Free:** Table of Contents, Abstracts **Pay:** Articles http://www.pulsus.com/Respir/home.htm

M-0093
JOURNAL

CHEST
Publisher: American College of Chest Physicians **Free:** Table of Contents, Abstracts **Pay:** Articles http://www.chestjournal.org

M-0094
JOURNAL

Circulation
Publisher: Lippincott, Williams & Wilkins **Free:** Table of Contents, Abstracts, Articles **Pay:** None http://circ.ahajournals.org/

M-0095
JOURNAL

Clinical and Investigative Medicine
Publisher: Canadian Medical Association **Free:** Table of Contents, Abstracts, Articles **Pay:** Articles http://www.cma.ca/cim/index.htm

M-0096
JOURNAL

Clinics in Chest Medicine
Publisher: W. B. Saunders **Free:** Table of Contents **Pay:** Articles http://www.harcourthealth.com/fcgi-bin/displaypage.pl?isbn=02725231

M-0097
JOURNAL

Colorectal Disease
Publisher: Blackwell Science **Free:** Table of Contents **Pay:** Abstracts, Articles http://www.blackwell-science.com/~cgilib/jnlpage.bin?Journal=cdi&File=cdi&Page=aims

M-0098
JOURNAL

Current Medical Research and Opinion
Publisher: LibraPharm Limited **Free:** Table of Contents, Abstracts, Articles **Pay:** None http://www.librapharm.co.uk/cmro/index.htm

M-0099
JOURNAL

Current Opinion in Gastroenterology
Publisher: Lippincott, Williams & Wilkins **Free:** Table of Contents, Abstracts **Pay:** Articles http://www.biomednet.com/cgi-bin/members1/shwtoc.pl?J:gas

M-0100
JOURNAL

Current Opinion in Pulmonary Medicine
Publisher: Lippincott, Williams & Wilkins **Free:** Table of Contents, Abstracts **Pay:** Articles http://www.biomednet.com/cgi-bin/members1/shwtoc.pl?J:pul

M-0101
JOURNAL

Diabetes
Publisher: American Diabetes Association **Free:** Table of Contents, Abstracts **Pay:** Articles http://www.diabetes.org/Diabetes/

M-0102	**Diabetes Care**
JOURNAL	**Publisher:** American Diabetes Association **Free:** Table of Contents, Abstracts **Pay:** Articles

http://www.diabetes.org/DiabetesCare/default.asp

M-0103	**Digestion**
JOURNAL	**Publisher:** S. Karger AG **Free:** Table of Contents, Abstracts **Pay:** Articles

http://www.karger.ch/journals/dig/dig_jh.htm

M-0104	**Digestive Surgery**
JOURNAL	**Publisher:** S. Karger AG **Free:** Table of Contents, Abstracts **Pay:** Articles

http://www.karger.ch/journals/dsu/dsu_jh.htm

M-0105	**Diseases of the Colon and Rectum**
JOURNAL	**Publisher:** Lippincott, Williams & Wilkins **Free:** Table of Contents, Abstracts **Pay:** Articles

http://www.discolrect.com

M-0106	**Dysphagia**
JOURNAL	**Publisher:** Springer-Verlag **Free:** Table of Contents, Abstracts **Pay:** Articles

http://link.springer.de/link/service/journals/00455/index.htm

M-0107	**Emerging Infectious Diseases**
JOURNAL	**Publisher:** National Center for Infectious Diseases, Centers for Disease Control and Prevention **Free:** Table of Contents, Abstracts, Articles **Pay:** None

http://www.cdc.gov/ncidod/eid/

M-0108	**Family Practice**
JOURNAL	**Publisher:** Oxford University Press **Free:** Table of Contents, Abstracts **Pay:** Articles

http://www.fampra.oupjournals.org/

M-0109	**Family Practice Management**
JOURNAL	**Publisher:** American Academy of Family Physicians **Free:** Table of Contents, Abstracts, Articles **Pay:** None http://www.aafp.org/fpm/

M-0110	**Gastroenterology**
JOURNAL	**Publisher:** American Gastroenterological Society **Free:** Table of Contents, Abstracts **Pay:** Articles http://www.gastrojournal.org

M-0111	**Geriatrics**
JOURNAL	**Publisher:** Advanstar Communications, Inc. **Free:** Table of Contents, Abstracts, Articles **Pay:** None http://www.geri.com/journal/index.html

M-0112	**Gut**
JOURNAL	**Publisher:** BMJ Publishing Group **Free:** Table of Contents, Abstracts **Pay:** Articles

http://gut.bmjjournals.com

M-0113	**Hospital Practice**
JOURNAL	**Publisher:** McGraw-Hill Companies **Free:** Table of Contents, Abstracts, Articles **Pay:** None

http://www.hosppract.com/index.htm

Don't type in long URLs – add the site number to the eMedguides URL: www.eMedguides.com/**G-1234**.

M-0114	**Hypertension**
JOURNAL	**Publisher:** Lippincott, Williams & Wilkins **Free:** Table of Contents, Abstracts, Articles **Pay:** None http://hyper.ahajournals.org/

M-0115	**Internal Medicine Journal**
JOURNAL	**Publisher:** Blackwell Science **Free:** Table of Contents **Pay:** Articles http://www.blackwell-science.com/~cgilib/jnlpage.bin?Journal=imj&File=imj&Page=aims

M-0116	**International Journal of Colorectal Disease**
JOURNAL	**Publisher:** Springer-Verlag **Free:** Table of Contents, Abstracts **Pay:** Articles http://link.springer.de/link/service/journals/00384/index.htm

M-0117	**Journal of Alternative & Complementary Medicine**
JOURNAL	**Publisher:** Mary Ann Liebert, Inc. **Free:** Table of Contents, Abstracts, Articles **Pay:** None http://www.liebertpub.com/ACM/default1.asp

M-0118	**Journal of Cardiopulmonary Rehabilitation**
JOURNAL	**Publisher:** Lippincott, Williams & Wilkins **Free:** Table of Contents, Abstracts **Pay:** Articles http://www.ajn.org/journals/catch.cfm?id= AC9F81F0%2D1522%2D11D3%2D8EB0%2D0090276F330E

M-0119	**Journal of Clinical Investigation**
JOURNAL	**Publisher:** American Society for Clinical Investigation **Free:** Table of Contents, Abstracts, Articles **Pay:** None http://www.jci.org/

M-0120	**Journal of Gastroenterology**
JOURNAL	**Publisher:** Springer-Verlag **Free:** Table of Contents, Abstracts **Pay:** Articles http://link.springer.de/link/service/journals/00535/index.htm

M-0121	**Journal of Gastroenterology and Hepatology**
JOURNAL	**Publisher:** Blackwell Science **Free:** Table of Contents **Pay:** Abstracts, Articles http://www.blackwell-science.com/~cgilib/jnlpage.bin?Journal=XJGH&File=XJGH&Page=aims

M-0122	**Journal of General Internal Medicine**
JOURNAL	**Publisher:** Blackwell Science **Free:** Table of Contents **Pay:** Abstracts, Articles http://www.blackwell-science.com/~cgilib/jnlpage.bin?Journal=XJGIM&File=XJGIM&Page=aims

M-0123	**Journal of Human Hypertension**
JOURNAL	**Publisher:** Nature Publishing Group **Free:** Table of Contents **Pay:** Abstracts, Articles http://www.stockton-press.co.uk/jhh/

M-0124	**Journal of Hypertension**
JOURNAL	**Publisher:** Lippincott, Williams & Wilkins **Free:** Table of Contents, Abstracts **Pay:** Articles http://www.jhypertension.com/

M-0125
JOURNAL

Journal of Internal Medicine
Publisher: Blackwell Science **Free:** Table of Contents **Pay:** Abstracts, Articles
http://www.blackwell-science.com/~cgilib/jnlpage.bin?Journal=JINT&File=JINT&Page=aims

M-0126
JOURNAL

Journal of Medical Practice Management
Publisher: Greenbranch Publishing, LLC **Free:** Table of Contents, Abstracts, Articles
Pay: None http://www.managedcare.medscape.com/JMPM/public/JMPM-journal.html

M-0127
JOURNAL

Journal of Medicine
Publisher: The National Medical Society **Free:** Table of Contents **Pay:** Abstracts, Articles
http://www.ccspublishing.com/i_med.htm

M-0128
JOURNAL

Journal of Occupational and Environmental Medicine
Publisher: Lippincott, Williams & Wilkins **Free:** Table of Contents **Pay:** None
http://www.joem.org/

M-0129
JOURNAL

Journal of the American Board of Family Practice
Publisher: Cadmus Journal Services **Free:** Table of Contents, Abstracts, Articles
Pay: None http://www.abfp.org/journal.htm

M-0130
JOURNAL

Journal of the American Dietetic Association
Publisher: The American Dietetic Association **Free:** Table of Contents **Pay:** Abstracts, Articles http://www.eatright.org/journal/

M-0131
JOURNAL

Journal of the American Medical Association
Publisher: American Medical Association **Free:** Table of Contents, Abstracts **Pay:** Articles
http://www.jama.ama-assn.org/

M-0132
JOURNAL

Journal of the National Cancer Institute
Publisher: Oxford University Press **Free:** Table of Contents, Abstracts, Articles **Pay:** None
http://jnci.oupjournals.org/

M-0133
JOURNAL

Lung
Publisher: Springer-Verlag **Free:** Table of Contents, Abstracts **Pay:** Articles
http://link.springer.de/link/service/journals/00408/index.htm

M-0134
JOURNAL

Medical Decision Making
Publisher: Hanley & Belfus, Inc. **Free:** Table of Contents, Abstracts **Pay:** Articles
http://www2.hanleyandbelfus.com/

M-0135
JOURNAL

Medical Practice Communicator
Publisher: Healthcare Media International, Inc. **Free:** Table of Contents, Abstracts, Articles
Pay: None
http://www.medscape.com/HMI/MPCommunicator/public/journal.MPCommunicator.html

M-0136
JOURNAL

Medical Principles and Practice
Publisher: S. Karger AG **Free:** Table of Contents, Abstracts **Pay:** Articles
http://www.karger.com/journals/mpp/mpp_jh.htm

M-0137
JOURNAL

Medical Tribune: Internist and Cardiologist
Publisher: Medscape **Free:** Table of Contents, Abstracts, Articles **Pay:** None
http://www.medscape.com/jobson/MedTrib/interncard/public/journal.IC.html

M-0138
JOURNAL

Medicine
Publisher: Lippincott, Williams & Wilkins **Free:** Table of Contents, Abstracts **Pay:** Articles
http://www.md-journal.com/

M-0139
JOURNAL

Nature Medicine
Publisher: Macmillan Publishers Ltd. **Free:** Table of Contents, Abstracts **Pay:** Articles
http://www.nature.com/nm/

M-0140
JOURNAL

Neurogastroenterology and Motility
Publisher: Blackwell Science **Free:** Table of Contents **Pay:** Abstracts, Articles
http://www.blackwell-
science.com/~cgilib/jnlpage.bin?Journal=NGEM&File=NGEM&Page=aims

M-0141
JOURNAL

New England Journal of Medicine
Publisher: Massachusetts Medical Society **Free:** Table of Contents, Abstracts **Pay:** Articles
http://content.nejm.org

M-0142
JOURNAL

Postgraduate Medical Journal
Publisher: BMJ Publishing Group **Free:** Table of Contents, Abstracts, Articles **Pay:** None
http://www.postgradmedj.com/

M-0143
JOURNAL

Postgraduate Medicine
Publisher: McGraw-Hill Companies **Free:** Table of Contents, Abstacts, Articles **Pay:** None
http://www.postgradmed.com/journal.htm

M-0144
JOURNAL

Pulmonary Pharmacology and Therapeutics
Publisher: Academic Press **Free:** Table of Contents, Abstracts **Pay:** Articles
http://www.academicpress.com/ppt

M-0145
JOURNAL

Respiration
Publisher: S. Karger AG **Free:** Table of Contents, Abstracts **Pay:** Articles
http://www.karger.ch/journals/res/res_jh.htm

M-0146
JOURNAL

Respiration Physiology
Publisher: Elsevier Science **Free:** Table of Contents, Abstracts **Pay:** Articles
http://www.elsevier.com/locate/resphysiol

M-0147
JOURNAL

Respiratory Medicine
Publisher: W. B. Saunders **Free:** Table of Contents, Abstracts **Pay:** Articles
http://journals.harcourt-international.com/wbs/rem

M-0148
JOURNAL

Rheumatology
Publisher: Oxford University Press **Free:** Table of Contents, Abstracts, Articles **Pay:** None
http://rheumatology.oupjournals.org/

M-0149	**Southern Medical Journal**
JOURNAL	**Publisher:** Southern Medical Association **Free:** Table of Contents, Abstracts, Articles **Pay:** None http://www.sma.org/smj/

M-0150	**The American Journal of Gastroenterology**
JOURNAL	**Publisher:** Elsevier Science **Free:** Table of Contents, Abstracts **Pay:** Articles http://www-east.elsevier.com/ajg

M-0151	**The American Journal of Medicine**
JOURNAL	**Publisher:** Elsevier Science **Free:** Table of Contents, Abstacts **Pay:** Articles http://www.amjmed.org/

M-0152	**The Journal of Family Practice**
JOURNAL	**Publisher:** Dowden Publishing Company, Inc. **Free:** Table of Contents, Abstracts, Articles **Pay:** None http://www.jfampract.com/

M-0154	**The Lancet**
JOURNAL	**Publisher:** The Lancet Publishing Group **Free:** Table of Contents, Abstracts **Pay:** Articles http://www.thelancet.com/

M-0156	**Thorax**
JOURNAL	**Publisher:** BMJ Publishing Group **Free:** Table of Contents, Abstracts **Pay:** Articles http://thorax.bmjjournals.com

M-0155	**Western Journal of Medicine**
JOURNAL	**Publisher:** BMJ Publishing Group **Free:** Table of Contents, Abstracts, Articles **Pay:** None http://www.ewjm.com/

3.5 LATEST BOOKS ON INTERNAL MEDICINE

The following listing contains books published during the past 12 months in the field of internal medicine. The books are categorized under major topics, although many books contain material that extends beyond the highlighted subject. All of these books may be purchased through Amazon at http://www.amazon.com.

The following topics appear below:

Internal Medicine	Diabetes	Immunization
AIDS/HIV	Diagnostics	Informatics
Allergies	Epidemiology	Injury Control
Antibiotics	Evidence-Based Medicine	Medical Students
Arthritis and Rheumatology	Family Medicine	Medications/Drug Therapy
Cardiology	Gastroenterology	Mental Health
Clinical Medicine	General Medicine	Neurology
Complementary Medicine	Genetics	Occupational Medicine
Consumer Health	Geriatrics	Oncology
Critical Care	Hospital Medicine	Ophthalmology

Otolaryngology	Pulmonology	Surgery in Primary Care
Pediatrics	Reproductive Medicine	Toxicology
Preventive Medicine	SexuallyTransmitted Diseases	Wellness
Primary Care	Sports Medicine	Women's Health

INTERNAL MEDICINE

Advances in Internal Medicine (Advances in Internal Medicine, Vol. 46) Robert W. Schrier (Editor), John D. Baxter (Editor), Victor J. Dzau (Editor). Mosby-Year Book, 2000, ISBN: 0815128185.

Cecil Review of General Internal Medicine, J. Allen D. Cooper, M.D., Peter G. Pappas. W. B. Saunders Co., 2000, ISBN: 0721677894.

Cleveland Clinic Intensive Review of Internal Medicine, James K. Stoller (Editor), Muzaffar Ahmad (Editor), David L. Longworth. Lippincott Williams & Wilkins Publishers, 2000, ISBN: 0781722241.

Core Textbook of Internal Medicine, Jay H. Stein. Mosby-Year Book, 2001, ISBN: 0815129246.

Field Guide to Internal Medicine, David S. Smith, M.D. (Editor). Lippincott Williams & Wilkins Publishers, 2001, ISBN: 0781728282.

Frontrunners Internal Medicine Board Review Syllabus, Bradley D. Mittman, M.D. Frontrunners Board Review, 2000, ISBN: 0967702518.

Harrison's Principles of Internal Medicine, Eugene Braunwald, M.D., Anthony S. Fauci, M.D., Dennis L. Kasper, M.D., Stephen L. Hauser, M.D., Dan L. Longo M.D., J. Larry Jameson, M.D. McGraw-Hill Professional Publishing, 2001, ISBN: 0070072728.

ICD-9 CM Easy Coder: Internal Medicine, 2001, Paul K. Tanaka. Unicor Medical, Inc., 2000, ISBN: 1567811345.

Internal Medicine Certification Exam Version 5, Individual Version (CD-ROM) Exam Master Corporation, 2001, ISBN: 1581290802.

Internal Medicine: Handbook for Clinicians, Resident Survival Guide, Elbert Huang, Wilson Tang, David Lee, Carey Conley Thompson, Melissa A. Fischer. Scrub Hill Press, Inc. 2000, ISBN: 0964546752.

Internal Medicine Pearls, John E. Heffner, M.D., Steven A. Sahn, M.D. Hanley & Belfus, 2001, ISBN: 1560534044.

Internal Medicine: Pearls of Wisdom, Michael Zevitz, Scott H. Plantz, Jonathan Adler. Boston Medical Pub. Inc., 2000, ISBN: 1584090391.

Internal Medicine: The Essential Facts, Nicholas J. Talley, Brad Frankum, David Currow. , ISBN: 0632056134.

Kelley's Essentials of Internal Medicine, H. David Humes, M.D. (Editor), William N. Kelley. Lippincott Williams & Wilkins Publishers, 2001, ISBN: 0781719372.

Kelley's Textbook of Internal Medicine, H. David Humes (Editor). Lippincott Williams & Wilkins Publishers, 2000, ISBN: 0781717876.

Mayo Internal Medicine Board Review, 2000-2001, Udaya B. S. Prakash (Editor), Thomas M. Habermann (Editor). Raven Press, 2000, ISBN: 0781723930.

Nail the Boards!: The Ultimate Internal Medicine Review for Board Exams, Bradley D. Mittman, M.D. Frontrunners Board Review, 2000, ISBN: 0967702526.

Rapid Access Guide to Internal Medicine: Companion to Kelley's Textbook of Internal Medicine, Paul L. Fine, M.D. Lippincott Williams & Wilkins Publishers, 2000, ISBN: 0781723574.

Review of Internal Medicine: For Use with the 4th Edition of Kelley's Textbook of Internal Medicine, David R. Schlossberg. Lippincott Williams & Wilkins Publishers, 2000, ISBN: 0781719674.

Tarascon Internal Medicine & Critical Care Pocketbook, Robert J. Lederman. Tarascon Press, 2000, ISBN: 1882742206.

Textbook of Internal Medicine, Lippincott Williams & Wilkins Publishers, 2000. ISBN: 0781717868.

Textbook of Internal Medicine, Stein. Elsevier Science Ltd, 2000, ISBN: 0444006001.

The Internal Medicine Casebook: Real Patients, Real Answers, Robert W. Schrier (Editor). Lippincott Williams & Wilkins Publishers, 2000, ISBN: 078172029X.

AIDS/HIV

After the Cure: Managing AIDS and Other Public Health Crises (Studies in Government and Public Policy), Martin A. Levin, Mary Bryna Sanger. Univ. Press of Kansas, 2000, ISBN: 0700610227.

Handbook of HIV Prevention, John L. Peterson (Editor), Ralph J. Diclemente (Editor). Kluwer Academic Publishers, 2000, ISBN: 0306462230.

Outpatient Management of HIV Infection, Joseph R. Masci. CRC Press, 2001, ISBN: 0849323193.

Working With Families in the Era of HIV, Willo Pequegnat (Editor), Jose Szapocznik (Editor). Sage Publications, 2000, ISBN: 0761922164.

ALLERGIES

Allergy in Primary Care, Leonard C. Altman, Jonathan W. Becker, Paul V. Williams. W. B. Saunders Co., 2000, ISBN: 0721681662.

Allergy Relief and Prevention: A Doctor's Guide to Treatment & Self-Care, Jacqueline Krohn, M.D. Frances Taylor, Erla Mae Larson. Hartley & Marks, 2000, ISBN: 0881791946.

ANTIBIOTICS

Biological Cost of Resistance to Antibiotics (Comprehensive Summaries of Uppsala Dissertations from the Faculty of Science and Technology, 539), Johanna Bjorkman. Uppsala Universitet, 2000, ISBN: 9155447201.

Magic Bullets, Lost Horizons: The Rise and Fall of Antibiotics, Sebastian G.B. Amyes. Harwood Academic Pub, 2001, ISBN: 905702442X.

ARTHRITIS AND RHEUMATOLOGY

Managing Osteoarthritis in Primary Care, Gillian Hosie, John Dickson. Blackwell Science Inc, 2000, ISBN: 0632053534.

The Arthritis Action Program: An Integrated Plan of Traditional and

Complementary Therapies, Michael E. Weinblatt. Simon & Schuster, 2000, ISBN: 0684868024.

CARDIOLOGY

Acute Myocardial Infarction (Contemporary Management in Internal Medicine Ser Vol, 2 No. 2), David MacCall (Editor). Churchill Livingstone, 2000, ISBN: 0443088381.

An Atlas of Heart Rhythms, Roy Pittman. Roy Pittman Publishing, 2000, ISBN: 0971051607.

Cardiac Arrhythmias, 1999, Volume 1: Proceedings of the 6th International Workshop on Cardiac Arrhythmias (Venice, October 5-8, 1999), Antonio Raviele, International Workshop on Springer-Verlag, 2000, ISBN: 8847000718.

Cardiology in Primary Care, William T. Branch (Editor), R. Wayne Alexander (Editor), Robert C. Schlant (Editor). McGraw-Hill Professional Publishing, 2000, ISBN: 0070071624.

Diagnosis and Management of Hypertension, Mancia. Churchill Livingstone, 2001, ISBN: 0443061955.

Primary Care Management of Heart Disease, George Jesse Taylor (Editor), Sc Charleston. Mosby-Year Book, 2000, ISBN: 0323002560.

Primary Care Provider's Guide to Cardiology, Glenn N. Levine, Douglas L. Mann. Lippincott Williams & Wilkins Publishers, 2000, ISBN: 068330688X.

CLINICAL MEDICINE

A Clinical Approach to Medicine, Ong Yong Yau (Editor), Woo Keng Thye (Editor), Ng Han Seong (Editor), Tang Ong Teng (Editor). World Scientific Pub. Co, 2001, ISBN: 9810243723 .

An Introduction to the Symptoms and Signs in Clinical Medicine: A Hands on Guide to Developing Core Skills, Peter Toghill (Editor), David Gray (Editor). Edward Arnold, 2001, ISBN: 0340732075.

Clinical History Taking and Examination, Welsby. Churchill Livingstone, 2001, ISBN: 0443070881.

Conn's Current Therapy, 2001: Latest Approved Methods of Treatment for the Practicing Physician, Robert E. Rakel, Edward T. Bope. W. B. Saunders Co., 2001, ISBN: 0721687431.

Current Clinical Strategies, Treatment Guidelines for Medicine and Primary Care, 2002 (CD-ROM for Windows & Macintosh), Paul D. Chan, Margaret T. Johnson. Current Clinical Strategies, 2000, ISBN: 1929622015.

Current Medical Diagnosis and Treatment 2001, Lawrence M. Tierney (Editor), Stephen J. McPhee (Editor), Maxine A. Papadakis. McGraw-Hill Professional Publishing, 2000, ISBN: 0071364668.

Disease: Identification, Prevention, and Control, Barbara P. Hamann, Ph.D. Mosby Great Performance, 2000, ISBN: 0074091387.

Diseases of the Human Body, Carol D. Tamparo, Marcia A. Lewis. F. A. Davis Co, 2000, ISBN: 0803605641.

Essentials of Human Diseases and Conditions, Margaret Schell Frazier, Jeanette Drzymkowski, Sandra J. Doty. W. B. Saunders Co., 2000, ISBN: 0721684750.

Ferri's Clinical Advisor 2000: Instant Diagnosis and Treatment, Fred F. Ferri, M.D. ASIN: 0323009719.

Final MB: A Guide to Success in Clinical Medicine, H. R. Dalton (Editor). Churchill Livingstone, 2001, ISBN: 0443070067.

Griffith's 5 Minute Clinical Consult, 2001 9E + The 5-Minute Patient Advisor, 1E (2 Book Package), Mark R. Dambro, M.D. (Editor). Lippincott Williams & Wilkins Publishers, 2001, ISBN: 078173083X.

High-Yield Clinical Science Set (Includes: Psychiatry, Internal Medicine, Acid Base, Surgery, and Biostatistics, 2E), Lippincott. Lippincott Williams & Wilkins Publishers, 2001, ISBN: 0781735173.

Hutchison's Clinical Methods, Michael Swash (Editor). W. B. Saunders Co., 2001, ISBN: 0702025305.

McLeod's Clinical Examination, John F. Munro (Editor), Ian W. Campbell (Editor). Churchill Livingstone, ISBN: 0443061726.

McQs in Clinical Medicine, Ragavendra R. Baliga. W. B. Saunders Co., 2000, ISBN: 0702022969.

Practical Guide to the Care of the Medical Patient, Fred F. Ferri (Editor). Mosby, Inc., 2001, ISBN: 0323012841.

Professional Guide to Diseases. Springhouse Pub. Co, 2001, ISBN: 1582550735.

The Book of Symptoms and Treatments: A Comprehensive Guide to the Safety and Effectiveness of Alternative and Complementary Medicine for Common Ailments Roland Bettschard (Editor), Gerd Glaeske, Kurt Langbein, Saller. Harper Collins - UK, 2000, SBN: 1862041717.

COMPLEMENTARY MEDICINE

ABC of Complementary Medicine, Catherine Zollman, Andrew J. Vickers. B M J Books, 2000, ISBN: 0727912372.

Clinician's Complete Reference to Complementary/Alternative Medicine, Donald W. Novey. Mosby-Year Book, 2000, ISBN: 0323007554.

Complementary and Alternative Medicine: Challenge and Change, Merrijoy Kelner (Editor), Beverly Wellman (Editor). Harwood Academic Pub, 2000, ISBN: 9058230996.

Complementary and Alternative Medicine & Psychiatry _vol 19#1, Philip R., M.D. Muskin (Editor). Amer. Psychiatric Press, 2000, ISBN: 0880481749.

Healing with Complementary and Alternative Therapies, Lynn Keegan, Kip Summerlin. Delmar Publishers, 2000, ISBN: 076681890X.

Mosby's Complementary & Alternative Medicine: A Research-Based Approach, Lyn W. Freeman, Ph.D., G. Frank Lawlis, Ph.D. Mosby-Year Book, 2000, ISBN: 0323006973.

Nurses' Handbook of Complementary Therapies, Denise Rankin-Box. Churchill Livingstone, 2000, ISBN: 0443064849.

Orthodox and Complementary Medicine: An Alliance for a Changing World, William Kirkaldy-Willis, Aubrey A. Swartz. North Atlantic Books, 2000, ISBN: 1556433557.

The Clinical Practice of Complementary, Alternative, and Western Medicine, W. John Diamond. CRC Press, 2000, ISBN: 0849313996.

The Directory of Complementary & Alternative Medicine, High P. Greeley (Editor), Hugh P. Greeley, Anne M. Banas. Opus Communications, 2000, ISBN: 1578390656.

CONSUMER HEALTH

Consumer Health Information Source Book: Sixth Edition, Alan M. Rees (Editor). Oryx Press, 2000, ISBN: 1573561231.

Health and Ethnicity, Helen M. MacBeth (Editor), Prakash S. Shetty (Editor), Shetty Prakash. Taylor & Francis, 2001, ISBN: 0415241669.

Healthy People 2010 (2 Volume Set), International Medical Publishing, Inc., 2000. ISBN: 1883205751.

Your Family Medical Record: An Interactive Guide to Getting the Best Care, A. Maria Hester, M.D., Melrose Blackett, M.D., Carolyn Whitney, M.D. John Wiley & Sons, 2000, ISBN: 0471347922.

CRITICAL CARE

Acute Emergencies and Critical Care of the Geriatric Patient, Thomas T. Yoshikawa (Editor), Dean C. Norman (Editor). Marcel Dekker, 2000, ISBN: 0824703456.

Office Urgencies and Emergencies (AAFP): The Academy Collection—Quick Reference Guides for Family Physicians, Richard B. Birrer (Editor). Lippincott Williams & Wilkins Publishers, 2001, ISBN: 0781720559.

DIABETES

Alternative and Complementary Diabetes Care: How to Combine Natural and

Traditional Therapies, Diana W. Guthrie, Richard Guthrie, M.D. John Wiley & Sons, 2000, ISBN: 0471347841.

Churchill's Pocketbook of Diabetes, Andrew J. Krentz. W. B. Saunders Co., 2000, ISBN: 0443061181.

Diabetic Adolescents and Their Families: Stress, Coping, and Adaptation, Inge Seiffge-Krenke. Cambridge Univ. Press (Short), 2001, ISBN: 0521792002.

Drug Treatment of Type 2 Diabetes, Andrew J. Krentz (Editor). Adis International, Ltd., 2000, ISBN: 0864710852.

DIAGNOSTICS

A Pocket Manual of Differential Diagnosis, Stephen N. Adler (Editor), Dianne B. Gasbarra (Editor), Debra Adler-Klein (Editor). Lippincott Williams & Wilkins Publishers, 2000, ISBN: 0781719437.

EPIDEMIOLOGY

Ending Neglect: The Elimination of Tuberculosis in the United States, Lawrence Geiter (Editor), Committee on Tuberculosis Elimination in the United States, Institute of Medicine. National Academy Press, 2000, ISBN: 0309070287.

Public Health Systems and Emerging Infections: Assessing the Capabilities of the Public, Jonathan R. Davis (Editor), Joshua Lederberg (Editor). National Academy Press, 2000, ISBN: 0309068290.

The Global Epidemiology of Noncommunicable Diseases: The Epidemiology and Burdens of Cancers, Cardiovascular Diseases, Diabetes Mellitus, Respiratory, Christopher J. L. Murray (Editor), Alan D. Lopez (Editor). Harvard Univ. Press, 2001, ISBN: 0674354478.

EVIDENCE-BASED MEDICINE

Best Evidence 4: Linking Medical Research to Practice (CD-ROM for Windows & Macintosh), Richard Lee (Editor), Frank Davidoff (Editor), American College of Physicians, American Society of Internal Medicine. Amer. College of Physicians, 2000, ISBN: 0943126967.

Best Evidence 5: Linking Medical Research to Practice (CD-ROM for Windows & Macintosh), American College of Physicians, American Society of Internal Medicine. Amer. College of Physicians, 2001, ISBN: 1930513135.

Evidence Based Acute Medicine, Sharon Straus, Stephen Hsu, Christopher Ball, Robert Phillips. Churchill Livingstone, 2001, ISBN: 0443064113.

Evidence-Based Clinical Pearls in Internal Medicine, Todd B. Ellerin, Luis A. Diaz. Lippincott Williams & Wilkins Publishers, 2001, ISBN: 0781732808.

Evidence-Based Clinical Practice: Concepts and Approaches, John P. Geyman (Editor), Richard A. Deyo (Editor), Scott D. Ramsey (Editor)Butterworth-Heinemann Medical, 2000. , ISBN: 0750670975.

Evidence-Based Medicine: How to Practice and Teach EBM (Book with CD-ROM), David L. Sackett, Sharon E. Straus, W. Scott Richardson, Rosenberg. Wolfe Pub Ltd, 2000, ISBN: 0443062404.

Evidence-Based Treatment for Lower Respiratory Tract Infections: Countermeasures to Guard Against the Emergence of Resistance (Chemotherapy. M.B. Siasoco (Editor). S. Karger Publishing, 2000, ISBN: 3805570856.

Handbook of Evidence-Based Critical Care, Paul Ellis, M.D. MarikSaC. Springer-Verlag, 2001, ISBN: 0387951539.

Intervention Mapping: Designing Theory and Evidence Based Health Promotion Programs, L. Kay Bartholomew (Editor). Mayfield Publishing Company, 2000, ISBN: 0767412788.

Statistical Questions in Evidence-Based Medicine, Martin Bland, Janet Peacock. Oxford Univ. Press, 2000, ISBN: 0192629921.

FAMILY MEDICINE

A Textbook of Family Medicine Companion Handbook, John W. Saultz (Editor). McGraw-Hill Professional Publishing, 2000, ISBN: 0070579776.

Current Clinical Strategies: Family Medicine, 2000 Edition, Paul D. Chan. Current Clinical Strategies, 2000, ISBN: 1881528790.

Family Medical Advisor: The Complete Guide to Alternative & Conventional Treatments. Time Life, 2001, ISBN: 078350909X.

Family Medicine, Paul D. Chan. Current Clinical Strategies, 2001, ISBN: 1929622147.

Family Medicine for Handheld and Desktop PCs, Paul D. Chan. Current Clinical Strategies, 2001, ISBN: 1929622155.

Family Practice Sourcebook 2001, Kenneth G. Marshall. Mosby, Inc., 2000, ISBN: 1556644698.

Guide to the Family Medicine Clerkship, Susan L. Montauk, M.D. Lippincott

Williams & Wilkins Publishers, 2001, ISBN: 0781723493.

Manual of Family Practice, Robert Taylor (Editor). Lippincott Williams & Wilkins Publishers, 2001, ISBN: 0781726522.

Mosby's Family Practice Sourcebook: Evidence-Based Emphasis, Kenneth G. Marshall, M.D. Mosby-Year Book, 2000, ISBN: 155664468X.

Swanson's Family Practice Review: A Problem-Oriented Approach, Alfred F. Tallia (Editor), Dennis A. Cardone, David F. Howarth (Editor). Mosby-Year Book, 2000, ISBN: 032300914X.

Textbook of Family Practice, Robert E. Rakel (Editor). W. B. Saunders Co., 2001, ISBN: 0721680011.

The Family Practice Handbook, Mark Graber. Mosby, Inc., 2001, ISBN: 0323012094.

The Hamlyn Encyclopedia of Family Health, Michael Apple, M.D. Hamlyn (UK), 2000, ISBN: 0600592545.

GASTROENTEROLOGY

Gastroenterology in Primary Care: An Evidence-Based Guide to Management, Pali Hungin (Editor), Greg Rubin (Editor). Blackwell Science Inc, 2000, ISBN: 0632051914.

GENERAL MEDICINE

Cecil Essentials of Medicine, Thomas E. Andreoli (Editor), Charles C.J. Carpenter (Editor), Robert C. Griggs, Joseph Loscalzo. W. B. Saunders Co., 2000, ISBN: 0721681794.

Cecil Textbook of Medicine (Single-Volume), Russell L. Cecil (Editor), J. Claude Bennett (Editor), Lee Goldman (Editor). W. B. Saunders Co., 2000, ISBN: 072167996X.

Concise Oxford Textbook of Medicine, J. G. G. Ledingham (Editor), David A. Warrell (Editor). Oxford Univ. Press, 2000, ISBN: 0192628704.

Harrison's Manual of Medicine, Eugene Braunwald, M.D., Anthony S. Fauci, M.D., Dennis L. Kasper, M.D., Stephen L. Hauser, M.D., Dan L. Longo, M.D., J. Larry Jameson, M.D.. McGraw-Hill Professional Publishing, 2001, ISBN: 0071373772.

Integrative Medicine: The Patient's Essential Guide to Conventional and Complementary Treatments for More Than 300 Common Disorders, Alan H. Pressman (Editor), Donna Shelley, M.D. (Editor), Alan Pressman, Ph.D. St Martins Press (Trade), 2000, ISBN: 0312253796.

Pocket Companion to Cecil Textbook of Medicine (21st ed.), Lee Goldman, J. Claude Bennett. W. B. Saunders Co., 2000, ISBN: 0721689728.

Saint-Frances Guide to Outpatient Medicine, Craig Frances, M.D., Stephen, Bent, M.D., Sanjay Saint, M.D. Lippincott Williams & Wilkins Publishers, 2000, ISBN: 0781726123.

Saunders Manual of Medical Practice, Robert E. Rakel, Ray Kersey (Editor). W. B. Saunders Co., 2000, ISBN: 072168002X.

Textbook of Rural Medicine, John P. Geyman (Editor), Thomas E. Norris (Editor), L. Gary Hart (Editor). McGraw-Hill Professional Publishing, 2000, ISBN: 007134540X.

The Official ABMS Directory of Board Certified Medical Specialists 2001 (Official ABMS Directory of Board Certified Medical Specialists, 33rd Ed) Marquis Who's Who, 2000, ISBN: 0837905710.

Tutorials in General Practice, Michael Mead, Henry Patterson. Churchill Livingstone, 2000, ISBN: 0443061971.

GENETICS

Clinical Genetics: A Short Course, Golder Wilson. John Wiley & Sons, 2000, ISBN: 0471298069.

Genetics and Public Health in the 21st Century: Using Genetic Information to Improve Health and Prevent Disease, Muin J. Khoury (Editor), Wylie Burke (Editor), Elizabeth Thomson (Editor). Oxford Univ. Press, 2000, ISBN: 0195128303.

GERIATRICS

Improving Care for the End of Life: A Sourcebook for Health Care Managers and Clinicians, Joanne Lynn, Janice Lynch Schuster, Center to Improve Care of the Dying, Andrea Kabcenell, Institute for Healthcare Improvement. Oxford Univ. Press, 2000, ISBN: 0195116615.

Oxford Textbook of Geriatric Medicine (Oxford Medical Publications), J. Grimely Evans, T. Franklin Williams (Editor). ASIN: 0192615904.

Primary Care for Older People (Oxford General Practice Series, No. 43), Steve Iliffe, Vari Drennan. Oxford Univ. Press, 2000, ISBN: 0192629514.

Senior's Guide to Pain-Free Living: All-Natural Drug-Free Relief for Everything That Hurt!, Doug Dollemore (Editor). Rodale Pr, 2000, ISBN: 1579542956.

HOSPITAL MEDICINE

Hospital Medicine, Robert M. Wachter (Editor), Lee Goldman (Editor), Harry Hollander (Editor). Lippincott, Williams & Wilkins, 2000, ISBN: 0683304828.

Infections in the ICU: Implications for the Clinician (Topics in Anaesthesia and Critical Care), G. Sganga, L. Silvestri, H. K. F. Van Saene, A. Gullo (Editor). Springer-Verlag, 2001, ISBN: 8847001382.

IMMUNIZATION

Calling the Shots: Immunization Finance, Policy & Practice, Committee on Immunization Finance Policies, Institute of Medicine, Practices. National Academy Press, 2000, ISBN: 0309070295.

Pocket Immunofacts: Vaccines & Immunologics, John D. Grabenstein, Laurie A. Grabenstein. Facts & Comparisons, 2000, ISBN: 1574390619.

The Immunization Resource Guide: Where to Find Answers to All Your Questions about Childhood Vaccinations, Diane Rozario. Patter Publications, 2000, ISBN: 0964336650.

INFORMATICS

Information Technologies in Medicine, Volume 1, Medical Simulation and Education, Metin Akay (Editor), Andy Marsh (Editor). John Wiley & Sons, 2001, ISBN: 0471388637.

INJURY CONTROL

Injury Control: Research and Program Evaluation, Frederick P. Rivara (Editor), Thomas Koepsell (Editor), Ronald V. Maier (Editor). Cambridge Univ. Press (Short), 2000, ISBN: 0521661528.

MEDICAL STUDENTS

Medical Short Cases for Medical Students, R. E. J. Ryder, M. A. Mir, E. A. Freeman. Blackwell Science Inc, 2001, ISBN: 0632057297.

MEDICATIONS/ DRUG THERAPY

A Caregiver's Guide to Giving Medicines, Carol Heerema. Prentice Hall, 2000, ISBN: 0835953882.

Challenger/PDR Drug Therapy, Steven Permut, Department of Family Medicine: Temple University. Challenger Corporation, 2000, ISBN: 1580160832.

Clinician's Handbook of Prescription Drugs, Seymour Ehrenpreis, Ph.D., Eli Ehrenpreis, M.D. McGraw-Hill Professional Publishing, 2001, ISBN: 0071343857.

Pharmacology for the Primary Care Provider, Marilyn Winterton Edmunds, Maren Stewart Mayhew. Mosby, Inc, 2000, ISBN: 0815130929.

The PDR Family Guide to Natural Medicines and Healing Therapies, Ballantine Books, 2000. ISBN: 0345433777.

The Pharmacotherapy of Common Functional Syndromes: Evidence-Based

Guidelines for Primary Care Practice, Peter Manu, M.D., FACP (Editor). Haworth Press, 2000, ISBN: 0789005883.

MENTAL HEALTH

Brief Mental Health Interventions for the Family Physician, M. V. Bloom, D. A. Smith. Springer-Verlag, 2001, ISBN: 0387952357.

Dealing With Depression Naturally: Complementary and Alternative Therapies for Restoring Emotional Health, Syd Baumel. NTC/Contemporary Publishing Co., 2000, ISBN: 0658002910.

Geriatric Mental Health Care, Gary J. Kennedy. Guilford Press, 2000, ISBN: 1572305924.

Handbook of Psychological Assessment in Primary Care Settings, Mark E. Maruish (Editor). Lawrence Erlbaum Assoc, 2000, ISBN: 0805829997.

Survivors Recovering from Sexual Abuse, Addictions, and Compulsive Behaviors: 'Numb' Survivors, Sandy Knauer. Haworth Press, 2001, ISBN: 0789014572.

The Encyclopedia of Phobias, Fears, and Anxieties, Dr. Ronald M. Doctor, Ada P. Kahn, Isaac M. Marks. Facts on File, Inc, 2000, ISBN: 0816039895.

The Primary Care Physician's Guide to Common Psychiatric and Neurologic Problems: Advice on Evaluation and Treatment from Johns Hopkins, Phillip R. Slavney, M.D. (Editor), Orest Hurko (Editor). Johns Hopkins Univ. Press, 2001, ISBN: 0801865549.

NEUROLOGY

Primary Neurologic Care, Jeannine Millette Petit. Mosby, Inc., 2000, ISBN: 081515304X.

OCCUPATIONAL MEDICINE

Hunter's Diseases of Occupations, Donald Hunter (Editor), Peter H. Adams (Editor). Edward Arnold, 2000, ISBN: 0340677503.

Occupational Medicine (AAFP): The Academy Collection—Quick Reference Guides for Family Physicians, James D. Lomax, Eckhardt Johanning. Lippincott Williams & Wilkins Publishers, 2001, ISBN: 0781720532.

ONCOLOGY

Cancer Medicine Review, Richard M. Stone, Arno J. Mundt, Richard Essner. B C Decker, 2000, ISBN: 1550091387.

Cancer & Nutrition: Prevention & Treatment (Nestle Nutrition Workshop Series: Clinic Series), J. Mason, Gerard Nitenberg. S. Karger Publishing, 2000, ISBN: 3805570813.

Complementary Cancer Therapies: Combining Traditional and Alternative Approaches for the Best Possible Outcome, Dan Labriola. Prima Publishing, 2000, ISBN: 076151922X.

Expert Guide to Oncology, Jacob D. Bitran, M.D. Amer. College of Physicians, 2000, ISBN: 0943126886.

OPHTHALMOLOGY

The Eye in Clinical Practice, Peggy Frith. Blackwell Science Inc, 2001, ISBN: 0632058951.

OTOLARYNGOLOGY

Ear, Nose & Throat Disorders for Primary Care Providers, Gayle E. Woodson. W. B. Saunders Co., 2000, ISBN: 0721674313.

PEDIATRICS

Healthy Child, Whole Child: Integrating the Best of Conventional and Alternative Medicine to Keep Your Kids Healthy, Stuart H. Ditchek, M.D., Russell H. Greenfield, M.D., Andrew Weil, M.D. Harper Resource, 2001, ISBN: 0062737457.

Ritalin-Free Kids: Safe and Effective Homeopathic Medicine for ADHD and Other Behavioral and Learning Problems, Judyth Reichenberg-Ullman, Robert Ullman, Edward M. Hallowell, Edward H. Chapman (Preface). Prima Publishing, 2000, ISBN: 0761527699.

PREVENTIVE MEDICINE

20 Common Problems in Preventive Health Care, Doug Campos-Outcalt. McGraw-Hill, 2000, ISBN: 0070120447.

20 Common Problems: Surgical Problems And Procedures In Primary Care, Dana Lynge, Barry D. Weiss. McGraw-Hill Professional Publishing, 2001, ISBN: 0071360026.

2000 National Fee Analyzer. Medicode Inc, 2000, ISBN: 1563373327.

50 Ways to Prevent Colon Cancer, M. Sara Rosenthal. Lowell House, 2000, ISBN: 0737304596.

Practice Tips, John Murtagh. McGraw-Hill Higher Education, 2001, ISBN: 0074708872.

Prevention and Cure, Lise Wilkinson, Anne Hardy, London School of Hygiene and Tropical Medicine. Kegan Paul Intl, 2000, ISBN: 0710306245.

Prevention of Disease Progression Throughout the Cardiovascular Continuum: The Role of Adrenergic B-Blockade, L. Ryden (Editor). Springer-Verlag, 2001, ISBN: 3540415033.

Preventive Medicine & Public Health: PreTest Self-Assessment and Review, Sylvie Ratelle. McGraw-Hill Professional Publishing, 2000, ISBN: 0071359621.

Primary and Secondary Preventive Nutrition: Primary and Secondary Prevention (Nutrition and Health), Adrianne Bendich, Ph.D. (Editor), Richard J. Deckelbaum, M.D. (Editor). Humana Press, 2000, ISBN: 0896037584.

PRIMARY CARE

Adult Primary Care, Pamela Vesta Meredith, Nancy Mathes Horan. W. B. Saunders Co. 2000, ISBN: 0721660371.

Ambulatory Medicine: Primary Care Families, Mark B. Mengel (Editor), L. Peter Schwiebert. McGraw-Hill Professional Publishing, 2000, ISBN: 083850387X.

Current Clinical Strategies Outpatient and Primary Care Medicine, 2001 Edition, Elizabeth Stanford, M.D., Paul D. Chan, M.D., Eric W. McKinley, M.D., David M.

Thomas. Current Clinical Strategies, 2000, ISBN: 1881528898.

Mosby's Primary Care Procedures CD-ROM, Wigton, Tape. Mosby, Inc., 2001, ISBN: 1556645465.

Nursing, Medicine and Primary Care, Anne Williams. Open Univ. Press, 2000, ISBN: 0335201679.

Patient Presentations in General Practice: A Comprehensive Guide to Diagnosis and Management, Ian D. Steven. McGraw Hill Text, 2000, ISBN: 0074708236.

Practice Guidelines in Primary Care, Ralph Gonzales, M.D., Jean S. Jutner, M.D. McGraw-Hill Professional Publishing, 2000, ISBN: 0838534171.

Practice Parameters in Medicine and Primary Care, Year 2000 Edition, Paul D. Chan. Current Clinical Strategies, 2000, ISBN: 1881528359.

Primary Care Medicine (CD-ROM), John Noble. Mosby-Year Book, 2001, ISBN: 032300833X.

Primary Care Medicine: Office Evaluation and Management of the Adult Patient, Allan H. Goroll, M.D., Albert G. Mulley, Jr., Lawrence A. May. Lippincott Williams & Wilkins Publishers, 2000, ISBN: 0781712483.

Procedures for Primary Care Providers, Denise L. Robinson, Cheryl McKenzie. Lippincott Williams & Wilkins Publishers, 2000, ISBN: 0781719682.

Resuscitation in Primary Care, Michael Colquhoun, Philip Jevon. Butterworth-Heinemann, 2001, ISBN: 0750642491.

Telephone Medicine: Triage and Training for Primary Care, Harvey P. Katz M.D. F A Davis Co, 2001, ISBN: 0803604351.

Textbook of Primary Care Medicine, John Noble, M.D. (Editor), Harry L. Greene, M.D. (Editor), W. Levinson. Mosby, Inc., 2000, ISBN: 0323008283.

PULMONOLOGY

Primary Pediatric Pulmonology, David L. Hayes, Margaret A. Lloyd, Paul A. Friedman. Futura Pub. Co. 2001, ISBN: 0879934646.

REPRODUCTIVE MEDICINE

Complex Adoption and Assisted Reproductive Technology, Vivian B. Shapiro, Janet R. Shapiro, Isabel H. Paret. Guilford Press, 2001, ISBN: 1572306289.

Encyclopedia of Birth Control, Vern L. Bullough (Editor). Abc-Clio, 2001, ISBN: 1576071812.

Experiencing Infertility: An Essential Resource, Debby Peoples, Harriette Rovner Ferguson. W.W. Norton & Company, 2000, ISBN: 0393320006.

Handbook of Family Planning and Reproductive Healthcare, Anna Glasier (Editor), Ailsa Gebbie (Editor), Nancy Loudon. Churchill Livingstone, 2000, ISBN: 0443064504.

Infertility in the Modern World: Present and Future Prospects (Biosocial Society Symposium, 12), Gillian R. Bentley, C. G. N. Mascie-Taylor (Editor). Cambridge Univ. Press (Short), 2001, ISBN: 0521643643.

SEXUALLY-TRANSMITTED DISEASES

Sexually Transmitted Diseases: Vaccines, Prevention and Control, David I. Bernstein (Editor), Lawrence R. Stanberry. Academic Press, 2000, ISBN: 0126633304.

SPORTS MEDICINE

Principles and Practice of Primary Care Sports Medicine, William E. Garrett, Jr., M.D., Ph.D. (Editor), Donald T. Kirkendall, Ph.D. Lippincott Williams & Wilkins Publishers, 2000, ISBN: 0781729564.

Sports Medicine in Primary Care, Rob Johnson (Editor). W. B. Saunders Co. 2000, ISBN: 0721678718.

SURGERY IN PRIMARY CARE

General Surgery: A Step-by-Step Guide to Minor and Intermediate Surgery, Shukri K. Shami, Delilah A. Hassanally, Caroline Munklinde (Illustrator). Springer-Verlag, 2000, ISBN: 1852331313.

TOXICOLOGY

Poisonous Plants of Paradise: First Aid and Medical Treatment of Injuries from Hawaii's Plants, Susan Scott, Craig Thomas, M.D. Univ. of Hawaii Press, 2000, ISBN: 082482251X.

WELLNESS

Promoting Human Wellness: New Frontiers for Research, Practice, and Policy, Margaret Schneider Jamner (Editor), Daniel Stokols (Editor). Univ. California Press, 2000, ISBN: 0520226097.

Talking About Health and Wellness with Patients: Integrating Health Promotion and Disease Prevention Into Your Practice, Steven Jonas. Springer-Verlag Berlin and Heidelberg GmbH & Co. KG, 2000, ISBN: 0826113389.

WOMEN'S HEALTH

The Planned Parenthood Women's Health Encyclopedia, ASIN: 0517888238.

Women's Health: Prevention Is the Best Medicine (Pennington Center Nutrition Series, Vol 11), George A. Bray, M.D. (Editor), Donna H. Ryan, M.D. (Editor. Louisiana State Univ. Press, 2000, ISBN: 0807126543.

4

Internal Medicine Overview Sites

4.1 General Resources

American Board of Internal Medicine (ABIM) Dedicated to the field of internal medicine, this site offers information on ABIM's training requirements, policies, pass rate data, exam data, as well as on the number of diplomates certified, organized by state and by country. Other resources include information on recertification, current and back issues of the board's newsletters in internal medicine and its subspecialties, a directory of diplomates, and a physician's personal stories on caring for the dying. Links to ABIM subspecialty pages, as well as to related resources, are provided.

http://www.abim.org/home.htm

American College of Physicians-American Society of Internal Medicine (ACP-ASIM): Patient Care Resources This ACP-ASIM Web page offers resources related to patient care. There are clinical practice guidelines, conference proceedings, information on immunization efforts, and updates on managed care. Members can access a clinical practice discussion group. Links to the college's journals are also provided, along with related resources and online CME activities. A catalog of books, videos, and related products is also featured.

http://www.acponline.org/patcare/?hpnav

American Family Physician: Health Information for the Whole Family Directed toward consumers, this site provides a collection of fact sheets on a variety of conditions that can be searched by keyword, population group, or region of the body. The fact sheets can also be browsed alphabetically under the "Health Information Handouts" section. Advice on topics such as lowering cholesterol, preventing flus and colds, and relief for lower back pain can be found under the AAFP family health facts section. Self-care flowcharts for health concerns covering symptoms, diagnosis, self-care, and when to see a doctor are also provided. In addition, there are databases for conventional drug information, herbal and alternative drugs, and drug interactions that explain proper use, side effects, and reactions. A national directory of family doctors is available, and the site can be translated into Spanish.

http://www.familydoctor.org/

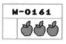

Harrison's Online   Directed to physicians, this Web page features the online text of *Harrison's Principles of Medicine*. Each chapter includes information such as diagnosis, prevalence, pathogenesis, clinical features, treatment, complications, and a bibliography. Links are also provided on each topic for related sites, updates, clinical trial information, and self-assessment quizzes. (fee-based) http://www.harrisonsonline.com/

Internal Medicine on the Web   Visitors to this Web site will find a consortium of Web pages devoted to the improvement of medical education. The Web pages include the Association of Professors of Medicine, the Association of Program Directors in Internal Medicine, the Association of Subspecialty Professors, the General Internal Medicine Faculty Development program, Clerkship Directors in Internal Medicine, and Administrators of Internal Medicine. There is also a link to an academic internal medicine job bank. http://www.im.org/

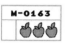

Journal of Internal Medicine   A description of the *Journal of Internal Medicine* is provided on this Web page, including a listing of instructions for authors and tables of contents dating back to 1997. Related links are provided. http://www.blackwell-science.com/~cgilib/jnlpage.bin?Journal=jint&File=jint&Page=aims

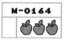

Medscape: Internal Medicine   Directed to physicians, this Web page offers a broad array of resources related to internal medicine. Visitors will find news stories, full-text articles, conference proceedings, tools and articles for the Palm OS, and CME online activities. Resource centers offer information specific to topics such as geriatric care, sepsis, and weight management. In addition, there are case studies, practice guidelines, links to journals, and related resources. http://internalmedicine.medscape.com/
Home/Topics/InternalMedicine/InternalMedicine.html

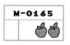

Medscout: Internal Medicine   A directory of more than 15 links related to internal medicine is provided on this site. The links are organized into categories such as associations, residency programs, journals, education and training, and Web resources. http://www.medscout.com/specialties/internal_medicine/

National Guideline Clearinghouse (NGC)   The National Guideline Clearinghouse is a comprehensive database of evidence-based clinical practice guidelines and related documents produced by the Agency for Healthcare Research and Quality, in partnership with the American Medical Association and the American Association of Health Plans. The guidelines can be searched by keyword or browsed by category such as disease/condition, treatment/intervention, and issuing organization. Each guideline has a brief summary and information for obtaining the full text. The "Compare Guidelines" feature allows users to add guidelines on a specific topic to their collection and produce customized reports. In addition, multidisciplinary guidelines are included. http://www.guidelines.gov/index.asp

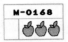

National Library of Medicine (NLM) The U.S. National Library of Medicine, the world's largest medical library, collects materials in all areas of biomedicine and healthcare and focuses on biomedical aspects of technology, the humanities, and the physical, life, and social sciences. This site contains links to government medical databases, including MEDLINE and MEDLINE-plus; information on funding opportunities at the National Library of Medicine and other federal agencies; and details of services, training, and outreach programs offered by NLM. Users can access NLM's catalog of resources (LOCA-TORplus), as well as NLM publications, including fact sheets, published reports, and staff publications. NLM research programs discussed at the site include topics in computational molecular biology, medical informatics, and other related subjects. The Web site features 15 searchable databases, covering journal searches via MEDLINE; AIDS information via AIDSLINE, AIDSDRUGS, and AIDSTRIALS; bioethics via BIOETHICSLINE; and numerous other important topics. The NLM Gateway—a master search engine—searches MEDLINE using the user-friendly retrieval engine called PubMed. There are over 11-million citations in MEDLINE and PreMEDLINE and the other related databases. Additionally, the NLM provides sources of health statistics, serials programs, and services maintained through a system called SERHOLD.
http://www.nlm.nih.gov/

National Study of Graduate Education in Internal Medicine This organization works each year to gather information for a national survey on the size and composition of the internal medicine resident physician workforce. Their Web page offers data and key findings of recent surveys, along with a summary of workforce trends. Summary data and graphs are provided for residents and fellows. In addition, more than 20 publications related to the national surveys are available.
http://www.nasgim.org/nasgim.htm

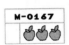

The Med Engine! This comprehensive site offers a directory of links related to medicine. The links are organized under topics such as drugs, news, products and services, publications, medical dictionaries and online texts, medical libraries, and hospitals. Additional categories include disease, consumer health, education, associations, reference, and government agencies.
http://www.themedengine.com/

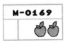

U.S. News & World Report: Graduate Schools for Internal Medicine A ranking of the best graduate schools for internal medicine is provided on this Web site, courtesy of *U.S. News & World Report*. Hyperlinks are provided to each school's Web page.
http://www.usnews.com/usnews/edu/beyond/gradrank/gbmedsp3.htm

Virtual Hospital: Internal Medicine Dedicated to internal medicine, this Web page offers more than 40 resources, categorized as multimedia textbooks, multimedia teaching files, patient simulations, lectures, CME materials, and

clinical practice guidelines. Topics covered include travel medicine, lung anatomy, adult critical care, gastrointestinal endoscopy, hypertension, and asthma.
http://www.vh.org/Providers/ProviderDept/InfoByDept.IntMed.html

5

Medical Specialty Supersites

5.1 General Supersites

American Medical Association (AMA) The AMA develops and promotes standards in medical practice, research, and education; acts as advocate on behalf of patients and physicians; and provides discourse on matters important to public health in America. General information is available at the site about the organization; journals and newsletters; policy, advocacy, activities, and ethics; education; and accreditation services. AMA news and consumer health information are also found at the site. Resources for physicians include membership details; information on the AMA's current procedural terminology (CPT)information services, the resource-based relative value scale (RBRVS), and electronic medical systems; information on the AMA Alliance (a national organization of physicians' spouses); descriptions of additional AMA products and services; a discussion of legal issues for physicians; and information on AMA's global activities. Information for consumers includes medical news; a link to the Medem Web page for detailed information on a wide range of conditions; a hospital locator; and a directory of physicians. Specific pages are devoted to comprehensive resources related to adolescent health, alchohol, and smoking cessation.
http://www.ama-assn.org/

Doctor's Guide: Global Edition Featured sections of Doctor's Guide-Global Edition include news, daily Webcast links, and interesting case presentations. A scroll-down menu located at the upper-right portion of the page allows visitors to "Select a Channel" and retrieve focused news and resources on hundreds of individual disorders. Other features require a registration.
(some features fee-based) http://www.docguide.com/dgc.nsf/ge/Unregistered.User.545434

Familydoctor.org Health information materials from the American Academy of Family Physicians (AAFP) regarding numerous health topics are accessible through this useful patient site. AAFP family health facts are presented along with self-care flowcharts for 45 health conditions. Information on drugs is accessible, including the brand names, category, medication descriptions, cautions, and possible side effects. A search engine at this page allows visitors to visit information on a specific topic of interest.
http://familydoctor.org

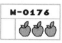

Hardin MD: Meta-Directory of Internet Health Sources The Hardin Meta Directory leads the visitor to extensive resources in over 40 areas of specialty, including cancer, emergency medicine, hematology, orthopedics, psychiatry/mental health, and public health and preventive medicine. Resources for each area of concentration are accessible from this site and include links to additional major resources, such as the Virtual Hospital, MedWebPlus, About.com, the National Cancer Institute, and MedMark. Visitors can access selected online medical journals.
http://www.lib.uiowa.edu/hardin/md

HealthWeb HealthWeb provides information covering more than 60 medical disciplines and related health areas, including hematology, substance abuse, diabetes, and alternative medicine. Each topic is a link to further connections, including academic institutions, clinical resources, consumer health resources, online publications, organizations, and clinical practice guidelines for each field represented. User guides are offered to assist physicians and consumers in the evaluation of Internet resources, searching the Internet, and document delivery.
http://www.healthweb.org

Karolinska Institutet: Diseases, Disorders, and Related Topics The Karolinska Institutet, geared toward a variety of audiences, offers search tools for accessing information on hundreds of disorders. Visitors can choose from an alphabetical list of diseases and conditions, use the search engine, or visit medical specialty sections. Information is provided from numerous resources, including MEDLINE and databases, electronic journals, biomedical links, and other authoritative sources. A substantial online CME section is also available.
http://micf.mic.ki.se/Diseases

MD Consult MD Consult provides online medical texts, offers medical journal articles, and tracks current medical developments. Over 600 clinical practice guidelines, approximately 3,000 patient education summaries, and clinical topic tours are offered to its members. The most current health news, medical conferences information, and the latest updates regarding drug approvals are provided, as well as general information on over 30,000 medications. A free 10-day trial of this service is offered to visitors.
(some features fee-based) http://home.mdconsult.com/bin/login?Tag=/&URI=

MedConnect MedConnect, an online resource for medical professionals, offers news features, health policy updates, a CME center, and Internet research tools at its site. Health management tools include online calculators, interactive discussion forums, and a daily assortment of articles from the *Interactive Journal of Primary Care*. Illustrative case presentations, new therapies, and patient guides are provided. Offering a complete online resource for professionals, this site supplies details regarding upcoming conferences and a variety of teaching materials. http://www.medconnect.com/

Medical Matrix Medical Matrix features special areas dedicated to providing physicians, medical students, and other healthcare professionals with disease management information. Daily medical headlines are listed with direct links to the articles. Through the site map link, visitors will find Medscape.com content, which includes articles, case reports and interactive material, conference schedules and summaries, journals, resource centers, clinical practice guidelines, and treatment updates. Separate medical specialties can be accessed, providing links to extensive information in each field.

(free registration) http://www.medmatrix.org

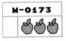

MEDLINEplus Health Information Sponsored by the world's largest medical library, the National Library of Medicine, and the National Institutes of Health, this site provides reliable up-to-date healthcare information. Resources on this Web page cover an array of health information for professionals and consumers. The "Health Topics" section offers access to more than 30 broad topics that contain links to information on clinical trials, diagnosis and symptoms, specific conditions, policy, organizations, statistics. The site also features drug information, with a guide to more than 9,000 prescription and over-the-counter medications from the United States Pharmacopeia (USP) and the USP Drug Information (USPDI) and Advice for the Patient. There are several medical dictionaries, along with directories of physicians and hospitals. Information found under the "Other Resources" section includes organizations, libraries, publications, databases, and access to MEDLINE.

http://www.medlineplus.gov/

MedMark: Medical Bookmarks All principal medical specialties are represented categorically at this site, hosted by MedMark. The more than 30 fields include preventive medicine, psychiatry, plastic surgery, rheumatology, and cardiology, and medical resources for each concentration include links to medical school departments, medical groups and clinics, centers and hospitals, professional societies, journals, news/publications, research, navigational guides, and primary care/emergency. Resources that offer information on specific disorders and diseases in the selected field are found.

http://members.kr.inter.net/medmark

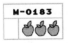

Medscape Today The professional resources available at this Web site include access to over 25,000 full-text articles, case reports, practice guidelines, and a drug database with over 200,000 listed medications. The site also boasts the Web's largest offering of CME modules. Upon completion of certain CME activities, instant CME certificates are available online. Other useful resources include conference summaries and schedules and a patient resources page.

(free registration) http://www.medscape.com/Home/Topics/multispecialty/multispecialty.html

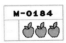

Medscout From aging to travel medicine, Medscape offers links to information across a variety of medical specialties. CME resources, an A-to-Z disease resource listing, medical journal access, and a host of additional material can be accessed from this vast medical information portal. Links are classified in several additional categories, including organizations, telemedicine, and pharmacy information. Medscout offers fee-based services for healthcare professionals, including electronic insurance processing, referrals, and answers to medical questions. (some features fee-based) http://www.medscout.com/

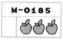

Physicians' Online   After a free registration process, visitors have access to an online community of physicians and healthcare professionals at Physicians' Online, which was created to provide a community for private and secure communication. The site contains links to comprehensive medical resources, associations, health plans, and healthcare organizations.
(free registration) http://www.po.com/

Virtual Hospital   Physicians can access educational materials assembled by the University of Iowa derived from multimedia textbooks, teaching files, and patient simulations. In addition, visitors can view lectures, practice guidelines, and clinical references through this Virtual Hospital page. A section dedicated to healthcare providers offers information categorized by common problems and provides custom views by specialty, and information by organ systems. Extensive patient resources regarding a large number of conditions and diseases are presented. Several, additional medical resources are accessible from the site, including health agencies, professional health societies, non-profit consumer organizations, health sciences libraries, and departments of the University of Iowa Health Sciences Center.
http://www.vh.org

5.2 ADDICTION MEDICINE

American Society of Addiction Medicine   Dedicated to educating physicians and improving treatment of individuals with addictions, the American Society of Addiction Medicine offers a broad array of resources for professionals on their Web page. Clinical practice guidelines related to AIDS and addiction, as well as to alcohol withdrawal, are featured, and access is provided to current and back issues of their newsletter, abstracts and tables of contents from the *Journal of Addictive Diseases,* and certification information. Other resources include information on nicotine, AIDS and addiction, and pain management; a schedule of conferences and meetings; a discussion board; fellowship information; policy statements; and news stories related to managed care. Related resources are provided.
http://www.asam.org/Frames.htm

MEDLINEplus Health Information: Substance Abuse   More than 35 topics related to substance abuse are featured on this Web page, including alcoholism, club drugs, cocaine abuse, fetal alcohol syndrome, heroin abuse, marijuana abuse, and smoking. Each topic offers resources such as the latest news, overviews, clinical trials, prevention, research, and treatment. Many topics have information specific to seniors, teenagers, and women. Some resources are available in Spanish.
http://www.nlm.nih.gov/medlineplus/substanceabuse.html

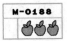

Medscape: Addiction   Created to provide information about addiction, this Web page offers the latest news, full-text articles, conference summaries, MEDLINE abstracts collections, and abstracts from journal articles. In addition, there are clinical practice guidelines and related links.
http://www.medscape.com/Medscape/features/
ResourceCenter/addiction/public/RC-index-addiction.html

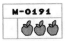

Prevention Online   Sponsored by the National Clearinghouse for Alcohol and Drug Information Division of the Substance Abuse and Mental Health Service, this Web site features prevention information. The site can be searched by keyword or browsed through a drop-down menu related to drugs of abuse, specific populations, or series publications. Fact sheets, articles, reports, videos, conferences, and Web resources are provided for drugs such as alcohol and cocaine, as well as for specific populations such as African-Americans and Native Americans. Series publications include *Prevention Alerts, Tips for Teens,* and *Treatment Improvement Protocols.* In addition, the site offers Webcasts of conferences, downloadable electronic books, audio and video clips, and live Web chats. Several bibliographic databases are available on the site including MEDLINE and SMOKING. Research briefs, funding information, discussion boards, and related links are also provided.
http://www.health.org/

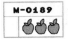

Web of Addiction   A comprehensive directory of resources on addiction is featured on this Web site. The site features alcohol and drug prevention information, self-help information, self-help and recovery newsgroups, and e-mail discussion groups. There is also information related to tobacco, AIDS, brief therapy, mental health, and related organizations. A brief description of each site is provided.
http://www.well.com/user/woa/aodsites.htm

5.3 ALLERGY MEDICINE

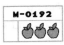

Allernet   Sponsored by the National Pollen Network, this Web page offers national allergy forecasts for tree, weed, and grass pollen, as well as mold spores. It also presents a fact sheet on allergies, along with allergy prevention tips. Other resources include a newsletter, FAQs, and an aeroallergen photolibrary containing photographs and electron microscopy images of common allergens. Video clips of dust mites and links to related resources are also provided.   http://www.allernet.com/

American College of Allergy, Asthma & Immunology (ACAAI)   The American College of Allergy, Asthma, and Immunology offers physicians practice resources, such as annual meeting proceedings, guidelines for asthma management, patient questionnaires on treatment outcome, and information on immunotherapy. Practice parameters for a variety of conditions are also provided such as asthma, eczema, and sinusitis. There is also information on annual meetings, as well as an online store featuring audio, video, and CD-ROM materials. Members can access the *Annals of Allergy, Asthma, & Immunology* and related discussion boards.

(some features fee-based) http://www.acaai.org/index.shtml

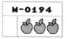

AllAllergy.net Described as a "gateway to all asthma, allergy, and intolerance information on the Web," this Web page offers a directory of links organized under categories such as articles, organizations, publications, events, products, and databases. Visitors have access to MEDLINE, as well as numerous search tools. A discussion board and related news stories are also available.

http://allallergy.net/

Allergy Internet Resources A comprehensive directory of allergy Internet resources is featured on this site. The links are organized under categories such as general allergy information, asthma, food allergies, childrens' allergies, latex allergy, and hay fever. Additional categories include skin allergies, insect stings, e-mail lists, and newsgroups.

http://www.immune.com/allergy/allabc.html

Allergy, Asthma & Immunology Online Sponsored by the American College of Allergy, Asthma, and Immunology, this site offers professionals information on CME courses, allergy practice parameters, and an asthma disease management resource manual. Patients will find fact sheets, FAQs, and screening information. There is also an allergist directory, as well as asthma quizzes for adults and children.

http://allergy.mcg.edu/

5.4 ANATOMY AND PHYSIOLOGY

Anatomy and Physiology Links Compiled by North Harris College, Texas, this site offers a directory of more than 100 links related to anatomy and physiology. Topics covered include chemistry, cells, cellular respiration, nucleic acids and protein synthesis, and histology. There are also links related to joints, the muscular system, the nervous system, the brain, the spinal cord, and endocrinology. http://students.nhmccd.edu/academics/info/divisions/nsci/biol/ap1.html

Anatomy of the Human Body The fulltext of Henry Gray's *Anatomy of the Human Body* is provided on this site. Chapters in the book cover embryology, osteology, syndesmology, myology, angiology, the arteries, the veins, neurology, the lymphatic system, organs of the senses and the common integument, and splanchnology. Surface anatomy of specific regions of the body is also featured. More than 1,200 full-color illustrations complement the text. A detailed bibliography is provided.

http://www.bartleby.com/107/

Human Anatomy and Physiology Society The Human Anatomy and Physiology Society was created to promote communication among teachers of human anatomy and physiology. Visitors to the site will find a resource section with position statements, course guidelines, grant and scholarship information, and laboratory activities for teaching anatomy and physiology concepts. The site also contains information on annual and regional conferences, job openings, and related resources.

http://www.hapsweb.org/

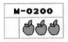

Martindale's Health Science Guide: Anatomy and Histology Created by Jim Martindale, this site features a directory of links related to anatomy and histology. The links are organized into categories such as overviews, dictionaries and glossaries, metabolic pathways and genetic maps, and literature. For anatomy there are atlases, courses, and teaching files, as well as anatomy exams. There are also histology atlases, courses, databases, exams, and laboratory protocols. Brief descriptions of each site are provided.

http://www-sci.lib.uci.edu/HSG/MedicalAnatomy.html

National Library of Medicine (NLM): Visible Human Project The Visible Human Project is a complete three-dimensional digital representation of the normal male and female bodies. Made up of images from CT, MRI, and physical sections of cadavers, this extensive dataset is available through a licensing agreement with the National Library of Medicine. On the Web site, visitors will find sample images, as well as links for software applications for viewing the dataset, sources of images and animation from other related projects, and tools for use with the dataset.

(some features fee-based) http://www.nlm.nih.gov/research/visible/visible_human.html

5.5 ANESTHESIOLOGY

American Society of Anesthesiologists Dedicated to anesthesiology, this comprehensive Web page offers professionals the latest news, ASA position statements, practice guidelines, a newsletter, and a publications catalog. Abstracts and some full-text articles from the current issue of the society's journal, *Anesthesiology*, are available on the site, along with continuing education resources. Members can request a free quarterly placement bulletin containing job announcements. Patients will find several patient education brochures and fact sheets related to anesthesiology, along with related links.

http://www.asahq.org/homepageie.html

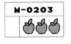

Anesthesia, Critical Care, and Emergency Medicine on the Internet A comprehensive directory of Web resources related to anesthesia, critical care, and emergency medicine is featured on this site, created by Bruno Grenier. Resources are offered for anesthesia departments, societies, medical images, journals, libraries, research, statistics, and patient information. Principles of anesthesia are also covered, including its effects on the cardiovascular system, transfusion and fluid replacements, and pharmacology. Information on anesthesia in

a variety of applications is also provided. Shorter lists of links are provided for critical care and emergency medicine.
http://www.invivo.net/bg/index2.html

Karolinska Institutet: Anesthesia and Analgesia More than 75 links related to anesthesia and analgesia are provided on this Web page. The sites are drawn from around the world and include associations, clinical management, principles of anesthesiology, and related information.
http://www.mic.ki.se/Diseases/e3.html

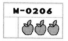

Virtual Anaesthesia Textbook Sponsored by Datex Ohmeda, this site strives to collect all anesthesia Web resources in one place in the form of a text-book. Intended for professionals, the textbook contains hundreds of sites organized into chapters on general information, such as FAQs, journals, and societies; professional issues, such as statistics and research, legal and ethical issues, and history; and basic sciences, including anatomy, principles of pharmacology, and respiration. Sections of the book are also dedicated to anesthesia equipment, patient care, and specific applications.
http://www.virtual-anaesthesia-textbook.com/

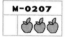

WWW Virtual Library: Anesthesiology This online library of anesthesiology information offers more than 150 links to academic, commercial, and educational sites, as well as to organizations and other related resources. Each site has a brief description, along with a notation for the number of visits it has received from users of this Web page.
http://www.gasnet.org/vl/vl.php

5.6 ARTHRITIS AND RHEUMATOLOGY

American College of Rheumatology The Home Page of the American College of Rheumatology (ACR) contains links to a variety of sites within the ACR. Readers will find abstracts from recent ACR annual scientific meetings; educational programs offered; news on legislative affairs for arthritis advocates; and a schedule of upcoming ACR meetings and conferences.
http://www.rheumatology.org/index.asp

Hardin MD: Meta-Directory of Rheumatology & Arthritis The *Hardin Meta Directory of Internet Health Sources* provides this overview of rheumatology and arthritis Web sites. It consists of a master list of 15 sites that list other sites that contain useful information in the field of rheumatology and arthritis. Sites listed include the New York Online Access to Health (NOAH) page for Arthritis and Rheumatic Disease, the Arthritis page from Healthfinder, and an online directory from the U.S. Department of Health and Human Services.
http://www.lib.uiowa.edu/hardin/md/rheum.html

Karolinska Institutet: Musculoskeletal Diseases A collection of links to sites related to musculoskeletal diseases is found at this domain, provided by

Karolinska Institutet. Links are organized by topic and subtopic, with most major diseases in the field represented. Visitors will find an assortment of fact sheets, case presentations, pathology databases, and online textbook pages in the field of rheumatology.
http://www.mic.ki.se/Diseases/c5.html

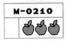 **Medscape: Rheumatology** A comprehensive listing of links on rheumatology is offered on this Web page. Sections on news, journal articles, conference proceedings, and practice guidelines are provided, as well as a CME center, event schedules, an exam room, and further rheumatology links.
(free registration)
http://rheumatology.medscape.com/Home/Topics/Rheumatology/Rheumatology.html

5.7 CARDIOLOGY

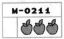 **American College of Cardiology (ACC)** The American College of Cardiology provides rigorous criteria to improve the quality of healthcare delivered by its professional members. As the premier organization for authoritative information in the field, this site offers a large database of professional publications, position papers, clinical information, conference details, and patient-education opportunities. http://www.acc.org

 American Heart Association (AHA) The AHA, a preeminent source of information in the field, is devoted to providing the public with authoritative information on the treatment of heart disease and stroke. Visitors will find an assortment of resources, including interactive risk assessment tools, fact sheets, local chapter information, conference and meeting details, scientific statements and guidelines, and the AHA Pharmaceutical Roundtable. Other professional education opportunities, clinical health news, and a particulary effective search engine are included.
http://www.americanheart.org

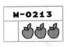 **Global Cardiology Network** Offering a search engine for cardiology professionals, this site provides detailed instructions for first-time users. Search categories include journals, practice guidelines, clinical trials, and CME information. Direct links to member organizations, such as the American College of Cardiology, are provided.
http://www.globalcardiology.org

 Hardin MD: Meta Directory of Cardiology and Heart Diseases This site provides a list of links to other large sources of cardiology information and includes connections to MEDLINEplus, Healthfinder, HealthWeb, and MedMark's listings of Internet specialty pages. The Hardin Meta Directories catalogue the best sites on the Web and offer a strategic advantage in Internet research. http://www.lib.uiowa.edu/hardin/md/cardio.html

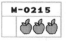

HealthWeb: Cardiology   Divided into three resource categories, this site offers links to pages for consumers, educators, and healthcare professionals. Professional resources include associations, journals, headlines, and discussion groups, and consumer-oriented links to the *Harvard Heart Letter* and a "Congenital Heart Disease Resource Page" are found. Students and educators will discover useful cardiology atlases and the "Cardiovascular Pathology Index."
http://bones.med.ohio-state.edu/hw/cardiology/index.html

5.8 COMPLEMENTARY AND ALTERNATIVE MEDICINE

Acupuncture.com   Dedicated to traditional Chinese medicine, this site offers FAQs, fact sheets, and articles on acupuncture, herbal medicine, Tui Na (massage), and dietetics. Each section is divided into separate areas for consumers, students, and practitioners. There is also information on diagnosis, theory, and clinical point selections. College programs, patient stories, and an acupuncturist referral service are also provided.
http://www.acupuncture.com/

American Holistic Medical Association   The American Holistic Medical Association is open to medical and osteopathic doctors who have an interest in holistic medicine. Professional resources on the site include a members-only discussion board, FAQs about holistic medicine, information on American Board of Holistic Medicine examinations, and conference information. There are also current and back issues of the association's newsletter and a brief list of related resources.   http://www.holisticmedicine.org/

NaturalHealthWeb   A directory containing hundreds of sites related to natural health is featured on this Web page. The sites are organized into broad categories such as body work, counseling, exercise, food and nutrition, healing, health maintenance and recovery, home environment, and spiritual practices. Each topic offers online articles, as well as links to related nonprofit and commercial organizations.
http://www.naturalhealthweb.com/

New York Online Access to Health (NOAH): Alternative and Complementary Medicine   Resources related to alternative and complementary medicine are provided in this directory of more than 100 Web links. The sites cover therapies such as acupuncture, herbal medicine, homeopathy, and reflexology. Resources related to alternative medicine include education, online journals, and research centers. The use of alternative therapies for specific diseases and conditions is also covered, including treatment for arthritis, cancer, and menopause.   http://www.noah-health.org/english/alternative/alternative.html

WholeHealthMD   Dedicated to complementary and alternative health, this Web page contains a broad array of consumer information. The "Healing Centers" section offers healing paths for a variety of conditions. Recipes, fact sheets, and supplement recommendations are included. A "Reference Library" offers

fact sheets and articles on alternative therapies, supplements, foods, and drugs. Visitors will also find the "Expert Opinions" columns, news stories, and an index of healthy recipes. A link is provided to an online store for supplements.
http://www.wholehealthmd.com/

5.9 CRITICAL CARE MEDICINE

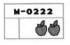

Anesthesia, Critical Care, and Emergency Medicine on the Internet
Although most of the sites in this directory are related to anesthesia, there are still more than 150 links related to critical care. Compiled by Bruno Grenier, topics covered include sepsis, trauma, pediatric critical care, and hyperbarics.
http://www.invivo.net/bg/index2.html

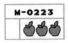

Critical Care Web   Created by a critical care nurse, this site offers more than 20 links to Web sites related to critical care. Intended for professionals, the links cover associations, clinical information, and LISTSERVs. A brief description of each site is provided.
http://w3.one.net/~gloriamc/critcare.html

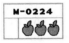

MEDLINEplus Health Information: Critical Care   Of interest to professionals and consumers, this Web page offers resources related to critical care. There is information on respirators, intensive care unit psychosis, critical care nursing, and respiratory failure. Additional topics covered include endotracheal intubation and the neonatal intensive care unit. There are also links to related organizations and a glossary.
http://www.nlm.nih.gov/medlineplus/criticalcare.html

Pediatric Critical Care Medicine (PCCM)   Supported in part by the American Academy of Pediatrics, the Society of Critical Care Medicine, and the Pediatric Critical Care Colloquium, the PCCM Web page offers professionals information on the new journal, *Pediatric Critical Care Medicine,* along with information on meetings, job opportunities, and related links. A "Clinical Resources" section offers an online textbook, abstracts and full-text articles, case reports, e-mail discussion lists, and information for pediatric critical care nursing. In addition, a "Clinical Research" section offers reviews of evidence-based journal articles, clinical trials, and grant resources.
http://pedsccm.wustl.edu/

Society of Critical Care Medicine   Professionals will find information on the society's activities, educational events, and grants. General information on the journals *Critical Care Medicine* and *Pediatric Critical Care* is provided. Consumers can access FAQs, as well as fact sheets on critical care and end-of-life decisions. A glossary is also available.
http://www.sccm.org/home/sccm_home_set.html

M-0221

M-0222

M-0223

M-0224

M-0225

5.10 DERMATOLOGY

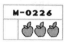

American Academy of Dermatology (AAD) The AAD is the largest of all dermatological associations, representing over 11,000 dermatologists in the U.S. and Canada. Their site offers a wealth of information, including patient and professional information sections, online resources for acne and melanoma, a dermatologist locator, and access to abstracts from the *Journal of the American Academy of Dermatology*.
http://www.aad.org

Hardin MD: Dermatology and Skin Diseases The Hardin Meta Directory includes this compilation of sites related specifically to the field of dermatology. Top Internet sources in the field are included, with large and medium-sized lists of sites of interest to dermatologists and other healthcare professionals. Disease-specific topical links, cases, treatment information, and tutorials on some of the more common dermatologic diagnoses are found.
http://www.lib.uiowa.edu/hardin/md/derm.html

Karolinska Institutet: Skin and Connective Tissue Diseases This major Internet database provides extensive resources on skin and connective tissue diseases, with several all-inclusive dermatology links, as well as patient education pages, online textbooks, and dermatology case presentations. The Cutaneous Drug Reaction Database, sites reviewing cutaneous anatomy and physiology, and an A-to-Z listing of skin disease connections are provided.
http://www.mic.ki.se/Diseases/c17.html

Medscape: Dermatology Various areas within the field of dermatology are explored at this site from Medscape, including treatment updates, practice guidelines, and information for patients on several conditions of the skin. Access to an archive of recent dermatology articles, medical journals, and links to government sites, DermWeb, Matrix Dermatology Resources, and Skinema.com are found. A free registration process is required to access various resources and information. (free registration)
http://dermatology.medscape.com/Home/Topics/Dermatology/Dermatology.html

5.11 EMERGENCY MEDICINE

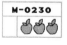

American College of Emergency Physicians Resources at this site include information about membership and activities of the college, as well as a schedule of meetings, their newsletter, and tables of contents to the *Annals of Emergency Medicine*. Members can access several news magazines published by the college, such as *EM Today*. In addition, there are policy statements, position papers on practice management, legislative and regulatory information, and a comprehensive listing of related resources. In the "Research and Academics" section, there is a list of approved residencies, along with funding information from the Emergency Medicine Foundation. For the public, there is an extensive collection of fact sheets, brochures, and articles related to topics such as adult immunization, bicycle helmets, and acting in an emergency. Medical forms, such as pediatric consent to treatment, are also provided.

(some features fee-based) http://www.acep.org/

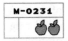

Medic8.com: Emergency Medicine   Resources for general information on emergency medicine are provided on this site, along with links to organizations, journals, textbooks, and databases.

http://www.medic8.com/EmergencyMedicine.htm

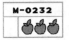

MedWeb: Emergency Medicine   Maintained by Emory University, this site offers a comprehensive directory of links related to emergency medicine. Links are provided for categories such as discussion groups, clinical information, educational resources, medical libraries, and associations.

http://www.medweb.emory.edu/MedWeb/FMPro?-DB=secondaries.FP3&-Format=
Secondary.htm&-Lay=Web&-Max=1000&-Op=eq&Index==Emergency_Medicine:*&-
Sortfield=Sec&-Token=Emergency_Medicine:&-Find

Merginet: Emergency Services Resource Center   More than 1,800 links related to emergency services are featured in this extensive collection. Categories include air medical, associations, companies, conferences, directories of Web links, and emergency medical services. There are also categories for education, government resources, and publications.

http://www.merginet.com/index-disp.htm

Virtual ER   Created by a physician, this Web page offers professionals links to emergency medicine tutorials, case studies, clinical images, and a library containing links to medical informatics sites, journals, newsletters, and drug information. The "Professional Network" section offers links to organizations, forums, job listings, e-mail lists, newsgroups, and CME opportunities. There is also residency and fellowship information.

http://www.virtualer.com/

5.12   ENDOCRINOLOGY AND METABOLISM

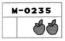

EndocrineWeb   EndocrineWeb provides a searchable patient education site about endocrine disorders and endocrine surgery. Articles on the specialty areas of endocrinology, endocrine surgery, thyroid and parathyroid glands, adrenal glands, diabetes, and osteoporosis are provided, with colorful illustrations at each site, and links to diagnosis and treatment details for both consumer and professional reference.

http://www.endocrineweb.com

Hardin MD: Meta Directory of Endocrinology and Diabetes   The Hardin Meta Directory offers professionals and other interested visitors access to some of the largest link listings in endocrinology on the Internet. New York's Online Access to Health, diabetic-only link listings, MEDLINEplus Health Information, and Emory University's MedWeb links in endocrinology are just a

formation, and Emory University's MedWeb links in endocrinology are just a handful of the large number of listings provided, offering visitors starting points for research in each medical specialty.
http://www.lib.uiowa.edu/hardin/md/endocrin.html

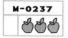

Karolinska Institutet: Endocrine Diseases A wide range of general resources, such as case studies and tutorials in endocrinology and site listings devoted to specific endocrine disorders, can be found through this comprehensive Internet directory. Each group of disorder connections includes an assortment of general disease information, fact sheets from disorder-specific organizations, clinical guidelines for practitioners, and pathology and case studies.
http://www.mic.ki.se/Diseases/c19.html

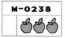

Medscape: Diabetes and Endocrinology Interesting connections include a Web-enabled documentation tool for clinicians, a CME center, a journal room, treatment updates, and a listing of expertly authored reports from key meetings in endocrinology. Today's diabetes and endocrinology news, case studies, and a general information library are all found, providing diagnostic, nutritional, statistical, and other disease management information. An upcoming conference listing and state-of-the-art treatment strategies in endocrinology are provided.
http://endocrine.medscape.com/Home/Topics/endocrinology/endocrinology.html

5.13 FAMILY MEDICINE

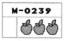

American Academy of Family Physicians (AAFP) Primarily for professionals, this site offers a broad array of information relevant to family medicine. The "Family Practice" section provides data on family physicians, information on legislative and policy issues, and resources for international family medicine. The "Clinical Information" section offers grant and funding opportunities, policy statements, treatment guidelines, updates on specific diseases, and full-text articles from the journal *American Family Physician*. In addition, the site offers CME opportunities, practice management tools and software information, job opportunities, and directories of residencies, fellowships, and clerkships in family medicine.
http://www.aafp.org/

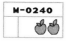

Canadian Library of Family Medicine: Resources Sites of interest to family physicians are featured on this Web page, including associations and organizations, journals and newsletters, CME information, and medical education. In addition, there is clinical information, guidelines, consumer health, and libraries. http://www.uwo.ca/fammed/clfm/sites.html

FamilyPractice.com Designed as a resource for family physicians, this Web page offers CME activities, a CME credit tracker, a guide to maintaining medical records, and links to medical suppliers. Interactive case studies are featured, and users can conduct patient interviews in determining their diagnosis. In addi-

tion, full-text articles from the *Journal of the American Board of Family Practice* are provided for current and back issues. Related links are found.
http://www.familypractice.com/index.htm

MedMark: Family Medicine Dedicated to family medicine, this comprehensive directory offers hundreds of links. Categories include associations; institutes, centers, and laboratories; departments; education; consumer information; general information; and guidelines. In addition, there are journals, programs, and organizations. http://medmark.org/family/fam2.html

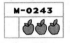

Primary Care Resources Selector Created by professionals at Virginia Commonwealth University, this site offers hundreds of Internet resources for primary care physicians. There are links for CME opportunities, educational sites for students, job opportunities, evidence-based medicine, and government agencies. Additional topics covered include managed care, e-mail discussion groups, medical schools, medical organizations, journals, and research grants.
http://views.vcu.edu/dimlist/

5.14 GASTROENTEROLOGY

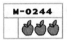

American Gastroenterological Association Both physician/scientist and public sections are offered at the American Gastroenterological Association site, with a "Digestive Health Resource Center," "Patient Wellness Brochures," an "Online Digestive Health and Nutrition Magazine," message boards, news, and a "Gastroenterologist Locator Service." Professional position statements and practice guidelines are available at no cost, as well as postgraduate course information and conference details. An up to date "Topic of the Month" and membership information are provided.
(free registration) http://www.gastro.org/

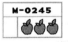

Hardin MD: Meta Directory of Gastroenterology and Intestinal Diseases Hardin MD offers visitors a convenient starting point for research at this site, devoted exclusively to gastroenterology resources. Providing links to the Karolinska Disorder sites, "MEDLINEplus Digestive Diseases," "New York Online Access to Health (NOAH)," "Stomach and Intestinal Disorders," and a variety of additional large, medium, and small lists of Internet site directories, all interested visitors can gain access to the best of the Web in the field of gastroenterology. http://www.lib.uiowa.edu/hardin/md/gastro.html

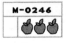

MedMark: Gastroenterology Medmark hosts an extensive source of gastroenterology resources, including associations/societies, centers/institutes/laboratories, clinics and hospitals, departments and divisions, education and training resources, and the online "Virtual Hospital." A consumer resource section; links to guidelines, images, and pediatric databases; and numerous journals are provided, including *Cancer News on the Net, Digestive Diseases,* and the *New England Journal of Medicine.*
http://www.medmark.org/gastro

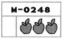

Medscape: Gastroenterology Medscape offers numerous sources of information on gastroenterology to its visitors. Current and archived news and journal articles in the field of gastroenterology are accessible, as well as CME conference summaries, clinical practice guidelines, medical images, numerous medical journals, patient resources, and related links. This site is an extensive source of information for a very broad audience.
http://gastroenterology.medscape.com/
Home/Topics/gastroenterology/gastroenterology.html

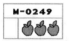

National Institute of Diabetes and Digestive and Kidney Diseases (NIDDK): Health Information: Digestive Diseases Online publications are provided by the National Institutes of Diabetes and Digestive and Kidney diseases, covering over 50 conditions in the field. Digestive disease statistics are presented, along with links to the "National Digestive Diseases Information Clearinghouse" and a directory of digestive disease organizations for patients.
http://www.niddk.nih.gov/health/digest/digest.htm

5.15 GERIATRICS AND GERONTOLOGY

Administration on Aging (AOA) Dedicated to providing information on older persons and services for the elderly, the Administration on Aging (AOA) offers a broad array of resources. Information on the site is divided into sections for older persons and their families, healthcare professionals, and researchers and students. The older persons section offers a comprehensive listing of Internet resources including an AOA guide for caregivers, an eldercare locator, booklets on health topics, and fact sheets on issues such as age discrimination, longevity, and pensions. Professional resources include information on legal issues, general resources, statistics, and specific program resources such as managed care. A section entitled the "Aging Network" offers a list of general resources, and a research section emphasizes statistics.
http://www.aoa.dhhs.gov/

Administration on Aging (AOA): Resources Directed to professionals, this directory of resources on the aging offers general information, referral resources, and related Web pages. Each site has a brief description.
http://www.aoa.dhhs.gov/practice.html

American Geriatrics Society (AGS) A national nonprofit association of geriatrics health professionals, research scientists, and other concerned individuals, the American Geriatrics Society (AGS) is dedicated to "improving the health, independence, and quality of life for all older people." The site offers a description of the society, adult immunization information, AGS news, conference and other events notices, legislation news, career opportunities, directories of geriatrics healthcare services in managed care, position statements, practice guidelines, awards information, and other professional education resources. Patient education resources, a selected bibliography in geriatrics, links to related organizations and government sites, and surveys, are also found at this address. (some features fee-based) http://www.americangeriatrics.org/

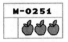

GeroWeb Hosted by Wayne State University, GeroWeb offers hundreds of links related to gerontology. The directory can be searched by keyword or browsed by topic, such as gerontology, medicine, Alzheimer's disease, genetics, and legal issues. Brief descriptions of each site are provided.
http://www.iog.wayne.edu/medlinks.html

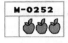

National Institute on Aging (NIA) Primarily of interest to professionals, this Web page offers information related to geriatrics, such as the latest news, conferences, training opportunities, and information on research programs and funding opportunities. Other resources include a comprehensive list of publications, a resource directory for older people, information on Alzheimer's disease, and links to related government sites.
http://www.nih.gov/nia/

5.16 HEMATOLOGY

American Society of Hematology Clinicians will find numerous educational materials that can be accessed by year or by topic, as well as abstracts from the organization's annual meeting and outlines of curriculum for the hematology/oncology training programs. Press releases, current and archived issues of the *Blood* journal, patient advocacy group links, and recent issues of the organization's newsletter, are offered as well.
(some features fee-based) http://www.hematology.org/

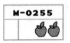

HealthWeb: Hematology General resource Web sites, clinical connections, disease resources, and educational opportunities in the field of hematology are all accessible from this hematology-only page. Pathology tutorials and blood morphology links, online publications, and hematology research program information can be accessed.
http://healthweb.org/browse.cfm?subjectid=46

Karolinska Institutet: Hemic and Lymphatic Diseases Hundreds of reputable resources provide coverage of various topics in the area of hemic and lymphatic diseases. Educational presentations include an interactive hematology atlas, blood count interpretation, fact sheets about blood and blood disorders, and consensus statements and guidelines from authoritative sources. Pathology pages, online textbook chapters, and patient care information on anemias, myeloproliferative disorders, and lymphatic conditions are offered.
http://www.mic.ki.se/Diseases/c15.html

MedMark: Hematology Connections at this assortment of Internet resources in hematology include links in over 10 category listings. Both professionals and consumers will find associations, laboratories, education, and

online atlas connections. Journals and news, a department geared specifically toward consumers, and a list of related resources and Internet directories are provided, making this site a top-rated Internet guide for the field.
http://www.medmark.org/hem

5.17 IMMUNOLOGY

 American College of Allergy, Asthma & Immunology (ACAAI) The American College of Allergy, Asthma, and Immunology offers physicians practice resources, such as annual meeting proceedings, guidelines for asthma management, patient questionnaires on treatment outcome, and information on immunotherapy. Practice parameters for a variety of conditions are also provided such as asthma, eczema, and sinusitis. There is also information on annual meetings, as well as an online store featuring audio, video, and CD-ROM materials. Members can access the *Annals of Allergy, Asthma, & Immunology* and discussion boards. (some features fee-based) http://www.acaai.org/index.shtml

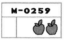 **Centers for Disease Control and Prevention (CDC): National Immunization Program** The CDC's National Immunization Program site offers news releases concerning vaccines on the market and current vaccine research. Childhood and adult immunization schedules are available, as well as information on vaccine safety. Vaccine Information Statements can be downloaded from this site.
http://www.cdc.gov/nip/

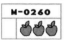 **Immune Deficiency Disorders** Part of the Open Directory Project, this site offers a directory of links on immune deficiency disorders, along with a link for another comprehensive directory of AIDS information.
http://dmoz.org/Health/Conditions_and_
Diseases/Immune_Disorders/Immune_Deficiency_Disorders/

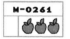 **MedMark: Immunology** MedMark provides links to immunology-related sites, including associations, research and educational institutes, consumer and patient organizations, information resources, and publications. The listing provides visitors with tools to find topics on the Web concerning general immunology, allergies, and asthma.
http://www.medmark.org/imm

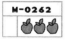 **World Health Organization (WHO): Vaccines, Immunization, and Biologicals** The World Health Organization offers a broad array of immunization information on this Web site, available in English, French, or Spanish. Fact sheets, articles, and publications are organized by health topic, including infectious diseases, tropical diseases, vaccine-preventable diseases, and the environment. There are also graphics and statistics on global disease information, as well as on specific diseases such as hepatitis, measles, polio, and yellow fever. The "Documents" section offers articles, conference proceedings, and guidelines

on disease control, immunization systems, and innovation. Research information, along with related links, is found.
http://www.who.int/vaccines/

5.18 INFECTIOUS DISEASE

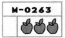

Centers for Disease Control and Prevention (CDC): Health Topics A-to-Z This site from the CDC and Prevention provides visitors with an alphabetical index to the CDC online database, covering 100's of infectious diseases. Each medical disorder connection is a link to further information on numerous health-related topics, including air pollution, birth defects, blindness, cancer, Lyme disease, rabies, suicide, syphilis, women's health, and vaccine safety.
http://www.cdc.gov/health/diseases.htm

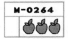

Infectious Disease WebLink Continuously updated, this supersite in infectious disease offers breaking news in the field, a "Site of the Month" connection, current reports from reputable research centers, and a top-10 resource site listing. Also accessible from this page are lecture and conference highlights, microbiology Web links, university sites, related journal connections, and a CME site listing.
http://pages.prodigy.net/pdeziel/

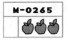

National Institute of Allergy and Infectious Diseases (NIAID) Research divisions accessible from this governmental connection include the microbiology, AIDS-related, and vaccine research centers. Information on clinical trials of the division, grants, and strategic health plans of the organization are, additionally, provided. In addition to information on major areas of investigation in the field, visitors to the site will discover updated treatment guidelines, prevention research, and the latest news and publications in infectious disease.
http://www.niaid.nih.gov/default.htm

5.19 NEPHROLOGY

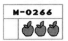

Medical Matrix: Nephrology Medical Matrix offers a directory of links to nephrology-related sites that provide news, journals, multimedia resources, major nephrology sites, practice guidelines, case studies, continuing medical education, patient education materials, and other directories of Internet resources. Related organization links, employment listings, and nephrology communication forums are available.
(free registration) http://www.medmatrix.org/_SPages/Nephrology.asp

MedMark: Nephrology This site serves as a comprehensive directory of Internet resources in the field of nephrology. Links are available to associations and societies, research institutes, academic departments, education and training resources, consumer resources, nephrology images, disease and research information sources, journals, and news sources. Visitors can also search the site by keyword. http://www.medmark.org/neph

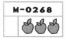

Nephrology   This extensive collection of links contains current news about nephrology issues, a calendar of events, a discussion forum, opportunities to earn CME credits, and an online bookstore to find various resources and services. Connections to a wealth of government and institutional resources, a listing of job opportunities, and international nephrology news are provided.
http://www.medicalnews.com/nephrology/index.html

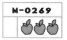

RENALNET   The RENALNET Web site describes itself as a kidney information clearinghouse. Among its features are links to nephrology and healthcare resources, information about End Stage Renal Disease, a link to the Integrated Dialysis Data Management home page, online discussion forums, a dialysis unit search engine, and the RENALNET search engine.
http://www.renalnet.org

5.20 NEUROLOGY

American Academy of Neurology (AAN)   The American Academy of Neurology contains weekly news stories at its home page and connections to clinical and practice information, education and CME, publications and product information, and consumer-oriented material. Annual meetings details and information on other neurology-related events can be obtained at the site. Portions of the site are restricted to members.
(some features fee-based) http://www.aan.com/

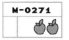

American Neurological Association (ANA)   This professional organization of neurologists and neuroscientists offers information on its annual meeting, a members-only database, fellowship-and- funding resources, and educational material for medical students. Information about the association's journal, *Annals of Neurology,* is found, as well as links to academic neurology programs. (some features fee-based) http://www.aneuroa.org

Medscape: Neurology   Medscape provides today's news in the field of neurology, as well as archived news articles, treatment updates, practice guidelines, conference summaries, and resource centers for Alzheimer's, multiple sclerosis, migraines, and pain management. Consumer resources for information on neurological diseases are presented, as well as links to government agencies, journals, and additional Internet resources.
http://www.medscape.com/Home/Topics/neurology/neurology.html

National Institute of Neurological Disorders and Stroke (NINDS)
Information on neuroscientific studies, laboratory research details, and studies seeking patients are provided at this governmental division of the National Institutes of Health. Visitors have access to quick disorder links that offer disease information; current, related research of the division; and links to associated

disorder organizations. Funding; news and events; and departments of technology, genetics, and neural environment research are offered.
http://www.ninds.nih.gov

Neuroland Neuroland's main directory offers a professional and reliable tool for accessing information in neurology, neuroscience, and psychiatry. Internet guides, free online textbooks, full-text medical journals, and neurological disease-management information are available. Case studies and practice guidelines are offered, as well as coverage of a wide range of topics in neuropharmacology, neuroanatomy, and neurohistology.   http://neuroland.com/default_old.htm

5.21 OBSTETRICS AND GYNECOLOGY

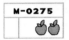

American College of Obstetricians and Gynecologists (ACOG)
Meetings and events, governmental affairs, and ACOG news releases and recommendations are provided at this completely public section of the ACOG. Additional features of the site include the "ACOG Bookstore," which allows visitors to order educational materials online, and an ACOG "Physician Directory." Visitors may perform a patient-education-pamphlet search by entering keywords or phrases. A portion of the site is restricted to ACOG members.
(some features fee-based) http://www.acog.org/

Karolinska Institutet: Female Genital Diseases and Pregnancy Complications   A large variety of Internet resources in obstetrics and gynecology may be accessed from this disorder-oriented site, including textbook chapters, Cochrane reviews, fact sheets, and other information on pathophysiology, diagnosis, and disease treatment. Topical coverage includes everything from sexually transmitted diseases to complications of pregnancy.
http://www.mic.ki.se/Diseases/c13.html

MedMark: Obstetrics and Gynecology   Hundreds of links are found at this supersite for obstetrics and gynecology, including associations, research institutions, an A-to-Z listing of academic departments, and an abundance of information for consumer viewing. This one-stop site in obstetrics and gynecology provides visitors with lists of links that include online gynecologic handbooks and textbook chapters, as well as interactive and educational information on disorders, self-care, and disease prevention. Journals and news in the field, consensus statements, and gynecologic/obstetric organizations are accessible.
http://medmark.org/obgy/obgy2.html

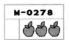

OBGYN.net   In addition to a site-specific search engine, this page allows visitors access to a complete physician-reviewed network for healthcare professionals, consumers, and the medical industry. Featured sections include attention to a variety of gynecologic disorders, surgical procedures, and diagnostic technologies. Announcements and press releases, upcoming events, online images and videos, and OBGYN.net discussion forums are provided.
http://www.obgyn.net/

5.22 OCCUPATIONAL AND ENVIRONMENTAL MEDICINE

M-0279

Agency for Toxic Substances and Disease Registry Dedicated to preventing exposure and health effects from hazardous substances, the agency offers comprehensive information on their site, of interest to professional and consumers. There are ToxFAQs, offering fact sheets on the health effects of a broad array of hazardous substances, as well as information on the top 20 hazardous substances and on minimal risk levels allowed per substance. Visitors can also search the HazDat database for information on hazardous substances released from Superfund sites or emergency events and their health effects. An "Interactive Map Server" offers maps of hazardous waste sites by region, state, city, and zip code. There are also reports and articles drawn from the National Exposure Registry, a registry of people who have been exposed to hazardous substances. In addition, there are grant funding opportunities, a newsletter, and related links.
http://atsdr1.atsdr.cdc.gov/

M-0280

American College of Occupational and Environmental Medicine Described as the "world's largest organization of occupational and environmental physicians," the American College of Occupational and Environmental Medicine offers information on conferences, courses, online seminars, and abstracts of recent articles from the *Journal of Occupational and Environmental Medicine.* There are also position statements, treatment guidelines, and a detailed list of recommended library and Internet resources. A list of core competencies, a link for job opportunities, and related resources are provided.
http://www.acoem.org/

M-0281

Environmental Health Information Service Provided as a service of the National Institute of Environmental Health Sciences and the National Toxicology Program, this site offers abstracts and tables of contents from the journal, *Environmental Health Perspectives,* as well as National Toxicology Program reports, full-text news articles from *EnviroNews,* and articles on the health effects of global warming. Physicians can access "Grand Rounds in Environmental Medicine" to view case studies. There are also reports from the National Toxicology Program, along with a report on carcinogens. Several databases can be accessed through the site, including information on chemicals from the Center for the Evaluation of Risks to Human Reproduction and "Rodent Historical Control Data" for a variety of toxic substances.
http://ehis.niehs.nih.gov/

M-0282

Karolinska Institutet: Occupational and Environmental Diseases More than 30 links related to occupational and environmental diseases are featured on this Web page. The links are drawn primarily from universities, government agencies, and nonprofit organizations around the world.
http://www.mic.ki.se/Diseases/c21.html#occdis

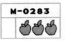

MEDLINEplus Health Information: Occupational Health Resources on occupational health are offered on this Web site, of interest to professionals and consumers. News stories, prevention, research, and specific conditions, such as eye protection in the workplace, are covered. There is also information specific to women and teenagers. Links to statistics, related organizations, and Spanish language publications are provided.
http://www.nlm.nih.gov/medlineplus/occupationalhealth.html

5.23 ONCOLOGY

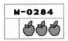

American Cancer Society By selecting a cancer type, visitors are directed to individual resource centers that contain newsletters, treatment guidelines, free brochures, related Web sites, cancer drug information, detection fact sheets, and Spanish-language publications, in addition to printer-friendly versions of general information. Prevention and awareness literature, and research, media, conference, and journal details are provided for professional viewers.
http://www.cancer.org

CancerNet A component of the National Cancer Institute (NCI), CancerNet offers the most comprehensive and accurate information needed for those interested in cancer types, treatment options, clinical trials, risk factors, diagnosis, support resources, and cancer literature. The Physician Data Query (PDQ) service offers the latest in cancer management guidelines, with both professional and consumer documents provided. An A-to-Z listing of all cancer types offers visitors a starting point for exploring this vast and comprehensive resource.
http://cancernet.nci.nih.gov/

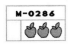

National Cancer Institute (NCI) From general cancer information to resources for scientists, the National Cancer Institute (NCI) provides a one-stop resource for learning about the latest in cancer types, research, and statistics. Clinical trial information, publications on risk factors, treatment discussions, and the latest news on funding and discoveries are part of this NCI site.
http://www.nci.nih.gov

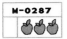

OncoLink Sponsored by the University of Pennsylvania, OncoLink offers professional and patient visitors ample opportunity to find the latest in cancer news, diagnosis, and management. Disease-oriented menus, medical specialty oriented pages, psychosocial support resources, and connections to cancer causes, screening, and prevention are found. Global resources for cancer information, including national and international organizations, and answers to FAQs about all types of cancerous illness are provided at this reputable Internet domain. http://www.oncolink.upenn.edu

5.24 OPHTHALMOLOGY

American Academy of Ophthalmology The American Academy of Ophthalmology sponsors the EyeNet Web site, which features a downloadable version of the *Washington Report;* an online education center with links to journals, clinical updates, CME, and self-assessment area; information on federal affairs; ophthalmic practice, services, and products; and publication information. Members are entitled to the "Eye M.D. Practice Center," as well as Academy publications.
(some features fee-based) http://www.aao.org

EyeWorld Providing in-print and online information, this Internet location offers news in the world of ophthalmology, refractive surgery, practice management, and cutting-edge advancements in the field. Registration for upcoming conferences in emerging treatments and online presentations in current and future applications in surgical procedures are provided. Expert interview transcripts and online discussion forums are, additionally, included.
http://www.eyeworld.org

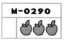

MedMark: Ophthalmology Links to over 50 associations and societies, centers and clinics, hospitals, academic departments, and over 100 resources geared toward consumers are offered. Journals and other publications, including the *American Journal of Ophthalmology,* are offered.
http://www.medmark.org/oph

Medscape: Ophthalmology The Medscape Ophthalmology site offers daily news articles in the field of ophthalmology, along with featured and archived journal articles, conference summaries, clinical management strategies, patient resources, and practice guidelines. Ophthalmology links to various journals, societies, foundations, national and international institutes, and government agencies are also provided.
http://www.medscape.com/Home/Topics/Ophthalmology/Ophthalmology.html

5.25 ORTHOPEDICS AND SPORTS MEDICINE

American Academy of Orthopaedic Surgeons This orthopedic specialty site contains general information about orthopedics, information for Spanish visitors, and a host of useful tools for gathering details regarding common orthopedic ailments. By linking to orthopedic problems related to any one of several anatomical locations, visitors are offered fact sheets, patient education brochures, and online patient education booklets. A "Find a Surgeon" connection and the "Orthopaedic Connection Search" complete this medical supersite.
http://www.aaos.org/

American College of Sports Medicine Integrating scientific research, education, and practical applications in the field, this medical supersite contains access to meetings and continuing education opportunities, as well as membership details and access to a wide selection of informational publications and multimedia material.

(some features fee-based) http://www.acsm.org/

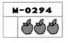

MedMark: Orthopedic Surgery   Listings of associations, academic divisions, consumer information links, journals, news headlines, and related resources in the field of orthopedics are all accessible at this collection of over 100 orthopedic sites. The list of related links includes everything from information on occupational-related injuries to musculoskeletal cases and teaching files.

http://www.medmark.org/os

Medscape: Orthopaedics   "Today's Orthopaedic News," conference coverage, and the latest developments in the field can be accessed at this medical specialty supersite of Medscape. Orthopaedics resources available at the site include treatment updates, practice guidelines, a CME center, and journal room. A multimedia library and patient- resource sections are included, as well as expert opinions and case reports.

http://orthopedics.medscape.com/Home/Topics/orthopedics/orthopedics.html

Physician and Sports Medicine   Locating information on the evaluation and treatment of sports-related injuries has never been easier with this McGraw-Hill division's top-rated site. Primary care issues in the field are addressed, including helpful links to online CME; a resource center of clinic, groups, and fellowship listings; and articles for consumers on exercise, injury prevention, and rehabilitation.

http://www.physsportsmed.com/

5.26 OTOLARYNGOLOGY

American Academy of Otolaryngology - Head and Neck Surgery, Inc.   The American Academy of Otolaryngology-Head and Neck Surgery, Inc., hosts this page, featuring daily news articles, online coverage of the annual meeting, an online bookstore, highlights from the Academy's bulletin, and a special Web site service for members. Visitors will find links to information on clinical indicators, educational materials, clinical research, and the Academy's journal, as well as patient information focusing on allergy, balance, hearing, sinuses, snoring, as well as tobacco and cancer.

(some features fee-based) http://www.entnet.org

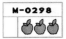

HealthWeb: Otolaryngology   In addition to academic institutions, visitors will find links to listings of sites in the categories of clinical resources, conferences, consumer health, education, journals, and organizations related to otolaryngology. HealthWeb, of the Medical College of Wisconsin, offers visitors the opportunity to view simple link listings or connect to a long display, which provides descriptions of each recommended site.

http://healthweb.org/browse.cfm?subjectid=69

MEDLINEplus Health Information: Ear, Nose, and Throat Topics

Resources on the anatomy and physiology, clinical trials, symptoms, treatments, specialized organizations, and treatments for more than 25 conditions dealing with the ear, nose, and throat can be accessed through this site. Conditions presented include canker sores, ear infections, tinnitus, and cancers of the mouth, throat, head, and neck.

http://www.nlm.nih.gov/medlineplus/earnoseandthroat.html

MedMark: Otorhinolaryngology

Hundreds of hotlinks to otorhinolaryngology associations and societies are provided by MedMark at this site. Visitors can access the Web domains of numerous research centers, over 150 divisions and departments, extensive educational and consumer resources, clinical and consumer guidelines, images and databases, and journals and other publications, including the *American Journal of Otorhinolaryngology, ARO News,* and the *Hearing Journal.*

http://www.medmark.org/orl

5.27 PAIN MANAGEMENT

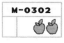

American Academy of Pain Management

This site provides information about the academy and its activities, resources for finding a professional program in pain management, accreditation and CME resources, and a membership directory for locating a pain management professional. It also provides general information on pain management and a listing of relevant links. Access to the National Pain Data Bank is available at the site, containing statistics on various pain management therapies based on an outcomes measurement system. The site is divided into two sections with information tailored to the needs of both patients and healthcare professionals.

http://www.aapainmanage.org/

Pain Central

Intended for patients with chronic pain and their families, this Web page offers a directory of Internet resources for several conditions, including arthritis, cancer, and diabetes. There are also discussion boards, chat rooms, and an online marketplace.

http://www.paincentral.com/

Pain Net

Pain Net was created to provide educational and support services to physicians in pain management. Physicians will find job opportunities, online CME activities, and related links. There are also current and back issues of the Pain Net newsletter. For the public, there are fact sheets on pain, a patient's bill of rights, and a directory of professionals interested in pain management.

http://www.painnet.com/

Pain.com

This site is a comprehensive resource for information on pain and pain management, with separate sections available for health professionals and consumers. For clinicians, information on meetings, free online CME courses, pain management standards, and full-text articles from pain journals are provided. Pages specifically addressing perioperative pain, cancer pain, interventional pain management, migraine and headache pain, and regional anesthesia are found and include information on related CME and discussion forums. Consumers can locate both a list of support groups and a directory of pain clinics. http://www.pain.com/

Partners Against Pain   Both professionals and patients may find this Web page of interest for information on pain management. Professionals will find articles on topics such as cancer pain, postoperative pain, and the use of opioids. Other resources include information on regulatory issues, CME opportunities, case studies, and pain assessment scales for a variety of conditions. For patients, there are news stories, articles on pain control, a list of recommended books, personal stories, and support group information. There is also a physician directory. http://www.partnersagainstpain.com/

5.28 PEDIATRICS

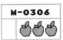

American Academy of Pediatrics (AAP)   "AAP News Online," a CME calendar, research information, and various resources dealing with professional education are offered at the premier organization for pediatric medical practice. The AAP offers access to policy reference guides, new AAP publications, and nearly 10 parenting books. An advocacy section presents federal and government affairs updates and campaign details.
http://www.aap.org

HealthWeb: Pediatrics: General Resources   Connecting visitors to some of the best healthcare information on the Web, this collection includes general resources, clinical guidelines, educational material, online publications, and organizations in the field of pediatrics. Visitors may view the site's pages via a brief display or long display listing, which provides both Web site links and descriptions. http://healthweb.org/browse.cfm?subjectid=71

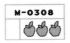

MedMark: Pediatrics   Pediatric associations, links to numerous research centers and academic departments, journals and other publications, and resources by subspecialty are provided at this supersite of pediatric Internet material. The site contains hundreds of links, including sites dedicated exclusively to genetic and metabolic disease, neonatology, and pediatric nephrology.
http://www.medmark.org/ped

5.29 PHYSICAL MEDICINE AND REHABILITATION

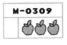

American Academy of Physical Medicine and Rehabilitation   Healthcare professionals will find information on membership to the academy, along with practice guidelines, online CME activities, legislative issues, and related resources. For medical students, resources include information on the field, a di-

rectory of training programs, and related links. Patients will find a physician directory, a directory of sports organizations for athletes with disabilities, and articles on a variety of topics such as stroke, arthritis, and cancer rehabilitation.
http://www.aapmr.org/

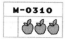

MEDLINEplus Health Information: Rehabilitation Both professionals and consumers may find rehabilitation resources of interest on this site. The information provided includes the latest news, clinical trials, policy, children's issues, and related organizations. Specific situations are also addressed, such as making the transition back to work, ergonomics, and tying one's shoes.
http://www.nlm.nih.gov/medlineplus/rehabilitation.html

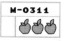

MedMark: Physical Medicine and Rehabilitation This comprehensive directory of more than 100 links on physical medicine and rehabilitation covers topics such as biomechanics, research resources, government resources, journals, and consumer health. Major conditions covered include arthritis, stroke, neuromuscular disease, and spinal cord injury.
http://www.medmark.org/pmr/

National Rehabilitation Information Center Funded by the National Institute on Disability and Rehabilitation Research, the center is dedicated to disseminating disability-related results from federally funded projects. More than 60,000 bibliographic records are contained within the center's databases of literature, organizations, and research. The center will photocopy documents of interest to users.
http://www.naric.com/

rehabNET Hosted by the Northeast Rehabilitation Health Network, this Web page offers articles related to topics such as sports medicine, prevention of back injuries, adaptive equipment, and the use of animal-facilitated therapy. A comprehensive list of related links is provided.
http://www.rehabnet.com/

5.30 PREVENTIVE MEDICINE

American College of Preventive Medicine In addition to membership information, this Web page offers information on policy issues, the annual meeting, and core competencies for residents. Information on residency training programs, along with some full-text articles from the *American Journal of Preventive Medicine,* is provided. There are also some related links.
http://www.acpm.org/

Centers for Disease Control and Prevention (CDC): National Prevention Information Network Designed to provide information on HIV/AIDS, sexually transmitted diseases, and tuberculosis, the CDC's National Prevention Information Network site offers resources for the healthcare professional and consumer. A bulletin board, distance learning information, FAQs, mortality/morbidity reports, and related links are provided for each of the disease categories covered. The reader will also find a large list of publications, along with a database of organizations. Information on the CDC's prevention research is also available, with links to numerous reports and journal articles. http://www.cdcnpin.org/

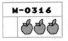

Centers for Disease Control and Prevention (CDC): Prevention Guidelines Database   Created and maintained by the CDC, this site features a database of more than 400 prevention guidelines. Topics covered include AIDS, adolescent health, diabetes, hospital infections, measles, and viral diseases.   http://aepo-xdv-www.epo.cdc.gov/wonder/PrevGuid/prevguid.shtml

Office of Disease Prevention and Health Promotion   Part of the U.S. Department of Health and Human Services, the Office of Disease Prevention and Health Promotion offers a variety of publications on their Web page, such as the *Clinician's Handbook of Preventive Services,* and *Nutrition and Your Health: Dietary Guidelines for Americans.* Links to related resources are also featured.   http://odphp.osophs.dhhs.gov/default.htm

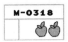

Preventive Medicine Research Institute   This nonprofit organization, run by Dr. Dean Ornish, offers information on programs, such as the Ornish program and lifestyle modification retreats, as well as a bibliography of the institute's publications, related links, and the latest prevention news. http://www.pmri.org/home.htm

5.31 PSYCHIATRY

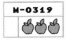

American Psychiatric Association (APA)   This international association of psychiatric physicians provides updates, public policy, and advocacy information at its site, as well as clinical and research-oriented resources for practitioners. Medical education, related organizations, and psychiatric news can be accessed.   http://www.psych.org

Internet Mental Health   A free encyclopedia of mental health information is available from this start page, funded by Phillip Long, M.D. Anyone with an interest in mental illness may freely access mental disorder information, treatment, research, and online information booklets from professional organizations and support groups. Related magazine articles from national publications and newsletters and an online diagnostic program are offered. In addition, viewers will discover profiles of the most commonly prescribed psychiatric medications, access to *Mental Health Magazine,* and numerous recommended links.   http://www.mentalhealth.com/

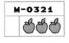

Medscape: Psychiatry and Mental Health   Medscape's psychiatry division includes extensive links and information on treatment updates, conferences, news, practice guidelines, journals, books, patient resources, and addi-

tional links related to the field of psychiatry. (free registration)
http://psychiatry.medscape.com/home/misc/redirHost.cfm?/psychiatry.medscape.com

 National Institute of Mental Health (NIMH) The primary biomedical and behavioral research agency of the National Institutes of Health offers breaking news, clinical trials, and mental disorder information departments at its home page. Current stories on research endeavors of the division, material in Spanish, outreach and education program information, and special pages dedicated separately to the public and practitioners are provided.
http://www.nimh.nih.gov/

5.32 PUBLIC HEALTH

 American Public Health Association Intended for professionals, this site offers the latest public health news, as well as abstracts from the *American Journal of Public Health* and the full text of the online version of the association's monthly newspaper, *The Nation's Health*. A publications catalog, continuing education oppportunities, job opportunities, and information on the annual meeting, legislative issues, grants, and activities of the association are also featured. There are links to state public health association resources, as well as international resources and related health resources.
http://www.apha.org/

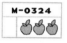 **HealthWeb: Public Health Statistics** Provided by the National Center for Health Statistics, this site offers numerous reports on vital statistics, life expectancy, and national health statistics. There are also links to related resources from other U.S. organizations, and to international sources of statistics.
http://www.lib.umich.edu/hw/public.health/health.stats.html

 Martindale's Health Science Guide: Public Health Created by Jim Martindale, the "Virtual Public Health Center" offers resources such as overviews, travel warnings, immunization information, journals, and bibliographic databases. Additional information on the site includes statistics, CME opportunities, and epidemiology.
http://www-sci.lib.uci.edu/HSG/PHealth.html

 Public Health Foundation The foundation's Web page offers information on applied public health research, assistance to state agencies for complying with the U.S. Department of Health and Human Services' "Healthy People 2010" project, and full-text reports on a variety of topics such as environmental health and community health. Readers will find tools and resources for assistance in public health planning, an online bookstore, and an extensive listing of links that include government agencies, nonprofit organizations, and related information sources.
http://www.phf.org/

University of California Berkeley: Public Health Resources A comprehensive directory of public health resources is featured on this Web page. The directory is organized into categories such as topics, indexes and publications, and organizations. Topics include alternative medicine, environmental health, nutrition, and reproductive health. Short site descriptions are provided. http://www.lib.berkeley.edu/PUBL/internet.html

5.33 RADIOLOGY AND NUCLEAR MEDICINE

American College of Nuclear Medicine In addition to membership information, this site offers current and back issues of the *ACNM Report,* as well as information on their annual meeting. http://www.acnucmed.org/

American College of Radiology Intended for professionals, this comprehensive Web page offers the latest radiology news, current standards, information on accreditation programs, and a database of mammography data. There are also publications on coding, a list of accredited facilities, and information on economics and health policy, residency and training, job opportunities, and CME activities. http://www.acr.org/

HealthWeb: Nuclear Medicine Hosted by the Northwestern University Health Sciences Library, this Web page offers an annotated list of nuclear medicine Web sites. The sites are categorized as educational resources, academic programs, organizations, electronic publications, and discussion groups. There are also conferences and events, job opportunities, and related information resources. http://healthweb.org/browse.cfm?subjectid=59

MedWeb: Radiology and Imaging Hosted by Emory University, this site offers more than 300 Internet resources for radiology and imaging. Resources include organizations, academic departments, online image libraries, and related information.
http://www.medweb.emory.edu/MedWeb/FMPro?-DB=Records.FP3&-Format=kw_records.htm&-lay=Web&-error=search_kwerror.htm&-Max=25&-op=eq&subject==*;
Radiology_and_Imaging*&-Token=Radiology_and_Imaging:&-SortField=Lnk_txt&-Find

5.34 RESPIRATORY AND PULMONARY MEDICINE

American College of Chest Physicians CHESTNET is a comprehensive resource for healthcare professionals, offering CME, links to relevant publications, advocacy activity information, consensus statements and guidelines online. The site contains a regularly updated "Highlight" section, which offers the latest from Capitol Hill, the current *CHEST* issue, new patient education guides, and special information on upcoming events. http://www.chestnet.org

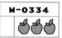

American Lung Association (ALA)   At the forefront of the nation's fight against lung disease, the ALA site is devoted to providing education, advocacy, and research resources. An A-to-Z disease listing, documents related to tobacco control, lung disease statistical information, and extensive listings of association-sponsored events, publications, and reports are found at this address.
http://www.lungusa.org

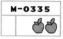

American Thoracic Society   Seeking to establish standards for the prevention and management of respiratory disease, the American Thoracic Society (ATS) site provides ample information on educational programs, conferences, publications, and clinical research in the field. News updates, advocacy and public policy initiatives, and membership information are provided, as well as leads to local ATS chapters and an online store.
(some features fee-based) http://www.thoracic.org/

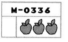

MedMark: Respiration Medicine   This exceptional directory of Internet links contains hundreds of site listings, including associations, research institutes, and academic divisions in the field of respiratory medicine. Clinical practice, journals and news, and an extensive list of online patient educational material are accessible.
http://www.medmark.org/rm

5.35 SURGERY

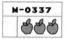

American College of Surgeons   A broad array of information on surgery is featured on this Web page. Professionals can sign up for a weekly e-mail newsletter, as well as access the *Bulletin of the American College of Surgeons,* tables of contents and abstracts to the *Journal of the American College of Surgeons,* meeting information, and CME opportunities. There is also information on fellowships, scholarships, job opportunities, and an electronic library of publications. Medical students will find information on choosing a residency. Patient education brochures explain procedures such as tonsillectomy, Cesarean section, and hernia repair. Links to the National Cancer Database, the National Trauma Databank, and the National Trauma Registry System are provided.
http://www.facs.org/

Karolinska Institutet: Surgical Procedures   In addition to resources on general surgical information, this site offers more than 100 links related to specific surgical procedures. The procedures include neurosurgical procedures, vascular, thoracic, orthopedic, digestive, and transplantation.
http://www.mic.ki.se/Diseases/e4.html

Martindale's Health Science Guide: Anesthesiology and Surgery
Resources on anesthesiology and surgery are provided in this directory of links, created by Jim Martindale. Visitors will find links to journals, bibliographic databases, conferences, blood banks, courses, and tutorials. There is also information for specific kinds of surgery, such as cardiovascular and arthroscopic pro-

cedures. Infection control, trauma and shock, and emergency medicine are also covered. http://www-sci.lib.uci.edu/HSG/MedicalSurgery.html

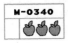

MEDLINEplus Health Information: Surgery Visitors to this site will find resources related to surgery. The latest news stories, overviews, statistics, and related organizations are found. In addition, specific conditions are addressed such as laser surgery, ambulatory surgery, and pain control after surgery. Information specific to children and seniors is also provided.
http://www.nlm.nih.gov/medlineplus/surgery.html

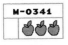

Medscape: Surgery Directed to healthcare professionals, this Web page offers information on surgery. The latest news, conference proceedings, journal highlights, and treatment updates are featured. In addition, there are online CME opportunities, full-text articles, and an online library.
(free registration) http://surgery.medscape.com/Home/Topics/surgery/surgery.html

5.36 TOXICOLOGY

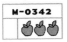

American College of Medical Toxicology For those interested in medical toxicology, this site offers information on membership to the college, a listing of fellowship training programs, and position statements. Full-text articles are available from the *Internet Journal of Medical Toxicology*. Other resources include a discussion group, grant information, and related Web resources.
http://www.acmt.net/

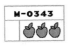

Karolinska Institutet: Pharmacology and Toxicology More than 40 links related to pharmacology and toxicology are provided on this Web page. The sites are drawn from universities, government agencies, and nonprofit organizations around the world. http://www.mic.ki.se/PharmTox.html

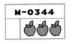

MEDLINEplus Health Information: Poisoning, Toxicology, and Environmental Health A variety of topics related to poisoning, toxicology, and environmental health are featured on this Web page. Topics include asbestos, carbon monoxide poisoning, pesticides, and radon. Each topic contains additional information such as the latest news, overviews, symptoms, diagnosis, treatment, and related organizations. Some offer information specific to children, seniors, and women.
http://medlineplus.nlm.nih.gov/medlineplus/poisoningtoxicologyenvironmentalhealth.html

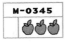

MedWeb: Toxicology Maintained by Emory University, this site offers a directory of Web resources for toxicology. Topics covered include academic departments, databases, discussion groups, guidelines, and organizations. There is also information specific to environmental health, occupational health, public health, and radiation.
http://www.medweb.emory.edu/MedWeb/FMPro?-DB=secondaries.FP3&-
Format=Secondary.htm&-Lay=Web&-Max=1000&-Op=eq&Index==Toxicology:*&-
Sortfield=Sec&-Token=Toxicology:&-Find

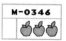

National Toxicology Program The National Toxicology Program is a collaborative effort among the National Institute of Environmental Health Sciences, the National Institute of Occupational Safety and Health, and the National Center for Toxicological Research. The site offers information on federally funded studies of toxicology, grant information, and a health and safety database containing data on more than 2,000 chemicals. Visitors will also find an extensive citation database of studies on a variety of topics.
http://ntp-server.niehs.nih.gov/

5.37 UROLOGY

American Urological Association The home page of the American Urological Association contains information about the association, along with membership details. Members can access publications, including the *Journal of Urology*, clinical practice guidelines, and best-practice policies, as well as information on practice management, government affairs, and the latest reports on conditions. A student section offers research opportunities, residency programs, program vacancies, and educational opportunities.
(some features fee-based) http://www.auanet.org/index_hi.cfm

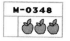

MedMark: Urology Both consumers and healthcare professionals seeking information in urology will find many resources, including a catalogue of organizations in the fields of general urology, andrology, endourology, incontinence, voiding dysfunction, oncology, pediatric urology, and prostate disease. In addition, journals such as the *American Journal of Kidney Disease* and the *Journal of Urology;* academic divisions; and information and guidelines in all the fields listed by organization as well as research on infectious disease and urinary stones are offered. http://www.medmark.org/uro

Medscape: Urology Numerous resources dealing with urology are made available at this site, including news and journal articles, clinical practice guidelines, treatment updates, CME conference summaries and schedules, interactive cases, clinical calculators, disease information for patients, and access to numerous medical journals. Links to related sites, including the "National Guidelines Clearinghouse" and the *Digital Urology Journal*, are offered.
http://urology.medscape.com/Home/Topics/urology/urology.html

National Institute of Diabetes and Digestive and Kidney Diseases (NIDDK): Urologic Diseases More than 20 online publications on topics such as bladder control for women, cystocele, incontinence, kidney stones, and vesicoureteral reflux are provided at this page of the institute. Spanish-language material, statistics, and links to other resources are found, including the "National Kidney and Urologic Diseases Information Clearinghouse." Links to national organizations concerned exclusively with urologic disease are provided, as well as bibliographic searches in the field.
http://www.niddk.nih.gov/health/urolog/urolog.htm

5.38 WOMEN'S HEALTH

American College of Obstetricians and Gynecologists (ACOG)
Primarily for professionals, this site offers information and resources specific to adolescent care, underserved women, and violence against women. There is also information on residencies, legislative and policy issues, the annual meeting and events, and a directory of physicians. Tables of contents from the journal *Obstetrics & Gynecology* are featured, as well as a publications catalog of educational materials for patients and professionals.
(some features fee-based) http://www.acog.com/

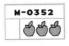

Feminist Majority Foundation: Women's Health   Internet resources related to women's health are provided on this Web page. The sites are organized into categories such as general women's health, cancer, women and body image, and general health. Each site is briefly described.
http://www.feminist.org/gateway/h_exec2.html

MEDLINEplus Health Information: Women's Health   A broad array of women's health topics is featured on this Web page, including contraception, breast cancer, endometriosis, menopause, and sexually transmitted diseases. Each topic has a link to further information and resources, such as the latest news, research, clinical trials, treatment, and overviews. Some resources are available in Spanish.
http://www.nlm.nih.gov/medlineplus/womenshealth.html

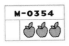

Medscape: Women's Health   Professionals interested in women's health will find the latest news, conference proceedings, practice guidelines, online CME activities, and full-text articles on this Web page of interest. There are also resource centers with information on specific topics such as breast cancer, urinary tract infections, and menopause. Clinical software tools and articles can be downloaded to Palm OS devices.   (free registration)
http://womenshealth.medscape.com/Home/Topics/WomensHealth/womenshealth.html

Women's Health Information Center   Hosted by the *Journal of the American Medical Association,* this site offers an electronic library of commentaries on women's health articles, along with abstracts from the original studies on a variety of topics such as arthritis, contraception, and eating disorders. An "STD Information Center" and "Contraception Information Center" offer abstracts of major articles, some full-text articles, and recommended Web resources.   http://www.ama-assn.org/special/womh/womh.htm

6

CONTINUING MEDICAL
EDUCATION

6.1 CME RESOURCES

Accreditation Council for Continuing Medical Education (ACCME)
This organization, providing accreditation to voluntary providers, describes its
mission and standards of development at this site. Recognition of accredited
providers can be found at the page, which lists nearly 200 healthcare education
networks by state or alphabetical listing.
http://www.accme.org/

**American College of Physicians-American Society of Internal
Medicine Online: Clinical Problem-Solving Cases** "Clinical Problem-
Solving Cases," a special program offered by the American College of Physicians-American Society of Internal Medicine, provides physicians with the opportunity to earn CME credit online by managing a selection of over 40 interactive cases in various subspecialties in internal medicine. Complimentary demonstration of clinically-based patient care scenarios are available for those interested in learning more about this service, available for a reasonable fee.
(some features fee-based) http://cpsc.acponline.org/

**American College of Physicians-American Society of Internal
Medicine Online: CME** The American College of Physicians-American Society of Internal Medicine sponsors information about live events, such as the
ACP-ASIM Annual Session; postgraduate course details; regional scientific
meetings; and in-print and electronic educational product information at this
subsite. Information on effective medical practice, a national residency database, and a curriculum development guide in internal medicine are available at
the site's connections.
http://www.acponline.org/cme/

American Family Physician: CME Presented by the American Academy of
Family Physicians (AAFP), the home page of this online article collection guides
visitors to the current issue and those released within the last 12 months. Identi-
cal to the journal version, these articles offer continuing medical education
credit online to AAFP members. Content includes online cases, an index to
management algorithms, and clinical briefs and practice guidelines.
http://home.aafp.org/afp/

American Medical Association (AMA): CME Select AMA CME offers an assortment of online programs, a CME information locator, and the opportunity to participate in live activities and complimentary courses. Featured CME courses include case studies in diabetes management and osteoporosis detection and clinical issues. Visitors can access multimedia professional programs or view a list of current CME meetings, conferences, and in-print self-study material. http://www.ama-assn.org/ama/pub/category/2797.html

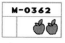

Cleveland Clinic: Center for Continuing Education Online CME, clinical practice guidelines, and new features, including "Pharmacotherapy Update" and the "Cleveland Clinic One-minute Consult," offer important new information to practitioners on therapies, treatment protocols, and other disease management issues. Visitors will find this continuously updated site to be a major source of live and online CME courses sponsored by the Cleveland Clinic in numerous medical specialties. More than 15 broad topic areas are available in the core series of online presentations.
(some features fee-based) http://www.clevelandclinicmeded.com/

CMEInc.com Both mental health and medical continuing education opportunity links are available at this page, including MedInfoSource, the CMEInfoStore, and the Mental Health InfoSource. Visitors may access pages of materials to order, CME registrations, and the latest in live conference education. http://www.cmeinc.com/home.html

CMEInfo.com Providing multimedia home study programs, CMEinfo.com is an indispensable resource for authoritative educational material in over 30 medical specialties. Course selections may be chosen for purchase at the sidebar menu of concentrations, which also provides links to video information and free audio samples. New releases, upcoming programs, and special offers are found. http://www.cmeinfo.com/

CMESearch.com By clicking on the U.S. map at this site, visitors can search the site's CME database of live events nationwide. Alternatively, viewers can access information on live and online programs through a search by medical specialty or by entering select keywords. A CME calendar of events is available, as well as "CD-ROM Core Curriculum" in adult primary care programs. http://www.cmesearch.com/

CMEWeb Over 1,300 credit hours in over 20 specialty areas are represented at this major online CME provider. Visitors may choose to take a tour of the site; display courses by specialty or topic; or display listings of other CME Internet resources, such as PDR.net Online Education. CMEWeb members can also discover state requirements for certification and purchase bulk-testing options.
(some features fee-based) http://www.cmeweb.com/

Doctor's Guide: Global Edition: CME-Related Sites A listing of over 70 CME-related Internet sites are collected at this Doctor's Guide page. CeWeb, CME Unlimited, and Cyberounds are just a few of the medical education and

training-related resources provided. Virtual Hospital's continuing education courses and "Conference Calendar," "Medical Studies Seminar," and the CExpress series for physicians are all accessible.
http://www.pslgroup.com/dg/cmesites.htm

Medical Computing Today: Electronic CME   Created and maintained by Marjorie Lazoff, M.D., this very large collection offers visitors online CME and software resource listings and information. Numerous links to sites with multiple specialties, general internal medicine and family medicine resources, and connections to CME Internet locations in over 30 medical specialties are offered at this comprehensive directory.
http://www.medicalcomputingtoday.com/0listcme.html

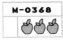

Mypatient.com   Offering a case-based approach to learning, Mypatient.com provides visitors with a virtual experience in medical education. Opportunities are available to update clinical skills and develop new approaches through interactive presentations in over 25 medical concentrations that are peer-reviewed and offered as a method of obtaining CME credit. A sample case and trial membership are provided for those interested in subscribing to this unique, online learning experience.
(some features fee-based) http://www.mypatient.com:8000/publicsite/home/home.jsp

Online CME Sites   Assembled by Bernard Sklar, M.D., this compilation of Web sites offers Accreditation Council for Continuing Medical Education (ACCME)-accredited CME programs. From presentations of the American Academy of Family Physicians to Virtual Lecture Hall courses, visitors are sure to find medical content appropriate to their chosen needs.
http://www.netcantina.com/bernardsklar/cmelist.html

7

ORGANIZATIONS AND INSTITUTIONS

7.1 ASSOCIATIONS

DIRECTORIES

Council of Academic Societies: AAMC Member Academic and Professional Societies Located within the Association of American Medical Colleges Web page, this site features a comprehensive A-to-Z listing of more than 90 members of the Council of Academic Societies. Most listings contain hyperlinks leading to members' home pages.
http://www.aamc.org/hlthcare/academ/asalpha.htm

Healthcare Foundations and Nonprofit Organizations A list of 40 foundations and nonprofit organizations is featured on this Web page, courtesy of the American Hospital Association.
http://www.aha.org/resource/links.asp#5

Indiana University: Medical and Nursing Organizations The Indiana University School of Medicine maintains this large listing of links to helpful medical sites. By clicking on "Medical and Nursing Organizations" at the top of the page, visitors will be taken directly to more than 100 hyperlinks for organizations. http://www.medlib.iupui.edu/ref/bookmarks.html#Organizations

MedBioWorld: Medical Associations A comprehensive directory of more than 3,500 associations in more than 80 medical specialties, including internal medicine, family and primary care medicine, complementary and alternative medicine, and infectious diseases, is featured on this Web site. The associations are drawn from domestic and international sources.
http://www.medbioworld.com/home/lists/medassoc.html

WebMDHealth: Medical Associations Index Containing both contact information and hyperlinks to a variety of reputable medical organizations, this compilation of sites offers visitors an A-to-Z listing of more than 75 associations across a variety of medical specialties.
http://my.webmd.com/medcast_toc/medical_associations

INDIVIDUAL ASSOCIATIONS

Below are profiles of more than 50 associations and societies relevant to the field of Internal Medicine. Those organizations that have a specific focus appear a second time in this volume under particular diseases and disorders or under an appropriate topical heading.

Alzheimer's Association The Alzheimer's Association offers information and support on issues related to the disease. Patients and caregivers can access general facts about Alzheimer's disease as well as detailed discussions of diagnosis, expected lifestyle changes, treatment options, and planning for the future. Resources for investigators include lists of grant opportunities and information on the Reagan Institute. The association also offers publications and information on advocacy activities.
http://www.alz.org

American Academy of Allergy, Asthma, and Immunology (AAAAI) The academy is focused on the study and treatment of allergic diseases through education, research, and cooperation. The site is divided into patient, medical/professional, and media/resource areas. A physician referral directory is offered at the site. The patient-targeted section provides clear definitions and explanations of topics specific to allergy and asthma, and the physician-targeted area includes journals, online reference materials, patient/public education materials, research grant details, and training program information. The National Allergy Bureau, a division of the academy, includes current and historic pollen counts recorded at stations located throughout the continental United States.
http://www.aaaai.org

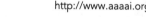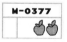

American Academy of Child and Adolescent Psychiatry A comprehensive site, the American Academy of Child and Adult Psychiatry (AACAP) Web site is designed to serve both AACAP members and other audiences. Information is provided on adult and child psychiatry, current research and practice guidelines, legislative updates, and awards and fellowships. Access to the *Journal of the American Academy of Child and Adolescent Psychiatry* is also available. In addition, there are fact sheets for parents and caregivers, job listings, and links to related sites. Visitors to the site can track legislation related to adult or child psychiatry or contact a member of Congress.
http://www.aacap.org/web/aacap

American Academy of Cosmetic Surgery The academy, with a membership representing several different medical specialties, offers departments at its site for the education and advancement of knowledge in cosmetic surgical procedures. The "Surgeons' Center" provides registration opportunities for educational courses and liposuction guidelines. By visiting the "Media Center," press releases, statistical information, and answers to FAQs regarding cosmetic procedures are accessible. Patient information found at the site may assist consumers in making informed decisions.
http://www.cosmeticsurgery.org

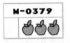 **American Academy of Dermatology (AAD)**   The AAD site includes patient information, a referral service, and a link to the society's official journal. There is a link to a special physician and patient education section providing information about melanoma. A professional section offers a virtual exhibit hall, meetings information, residents' news, and a marketplace.
http://www.aad.org

 American Academy of Family Physicians (AAFP)   Primarily for family physicians, the AAFP offers this site containing clinical information, CME courses, practice management tips, and publications. Highlights of the clinical information section include research grants, a drug database, and access to the online version of the *American Family Physician* journal.
http://www.aafp.org

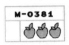 **American Academy of Neurology (AAN)**   This site provides a keyword search of publicly available and members-only documents, courtesy of the AAN. There are also links to the Excite search engine and the PubMed search engine and an extensively detailed site map with links to information on neurological conditions, awards, educational programs, and CME.
http://www.aan.com

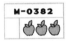 **American Academy of Ophthalmology**   The Home Page of EyeNet is the official Web site of the American Academy of Ophthalmology (AAO). Resources for ophthalmology professionals include the AAO's new online *Ophthalmology Journal,* online clinical education courses, news reports, and information on legal and advocacy issues. Resources for consumers are also provided such as eye anatomy and health information, eye safety tips, fact sheets on eye diseases, and a searchable worldwide database of ophthalmologists.
(some features fee-based) http://www.aao.org

 American Academy of Orthopaedic Surgeons   The Web site of the American Academy of Orthopaedic Surgeons offers information on CME courses and online exams, research funding, and a publication catalog. Policy statements, legislative updates, and a list of related resources are available in addition to patient education materials.
(some features fee-based) http://www.aaos.org

 American Academy of Otolaryngology - Head and Neck Surgery, Inc.   The professional resources available on this site include clinical indicators for a variety of otolaryngological procedures, CME information, research grant information, and guidelines for participating in humanitarian service efforts. A separate link is designated for patient information that includes many online fact sheets and a "find an otolaryngologist" service.
(some features fee-based) http://www.entnet.org

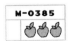 **American Academy of Pain Management**   The American Academy of Pain Management provides numerous resources for information on pain management at its Web site. Professionals are presented with links to the National

Pain Data Bank, along with links to information about pain program accreditation, CME, and announcements and opportunities. Also featured at this site are the Patient's Bill of Rights, and separately-listed FAQs for patients and for doctors. http://www.aapainmanage.org/

American Academy of Pain Medicine   This continually updated site offers answers to FAQs about pain, annual meeting details, and access to online publications and products. Position and consensus statements on treatment, basic ethical principles for the practice of pain medicine, and end of life care are available. *Pain Medicine Network,* a quarterly newsletter and its archives, are also accessible from the site.
http://www.painmed.org/

American Academy of Pediatrics (AAP)   Intended for pediatricians, the American Academy of Pediatrics site provides information on research monies, CME programs, advocacy, and a comprehensive list of publications. Patients can be directed to the "You and Your Family" section of the site for parent publications and brochures on child care.
(some features fee-based) http://www.aap.org

American Academy of Physical Medicine and Rehabilitation   Portions of this site are dedicated specifically to member physicians, other medical professionals, students, and public audiences. Online case reviews, CME, practice guidelines and outcomes, and a resource link make this site, dedicated to the field of physiatry, complete. Fact sheets on the variety of conditions treated by those who specialize in physical medicine and rehabilitation are offered.
(some features fee-based) http://www.aapmr.org

American Association for the Study of Liver Diseases   Provided by the American Association for the Study of Liver Diseases (AASLD), this Web page offers hepatologists information on CME courses, online practice guidelines, research grants, and policy issues. Access to their two online journals is for members only. (some features fee-based) http://www.aasld.org

American Association of Cardiovascular and Pulmonary Rehabilitation   Annual meeting details, a search engine for locating certified programs nationwide, and a link to information on this organization's publications are offered. Clinical guidelines, media kits, programs for consumers, and a searchable online directory of cardiopulmonary rehabilitation programs are, additionally, featured. http://www.aacvpr.org

American Association of Immunologists   The purpose of this site is to provide immunologists with information on job opportunities, research funding, and member access to the online version of the *Journal of Immunology.* In addition, articles on educating the public and a membership directory are offered. (some features fee-based) http://12.17.12.70/aai/default.asp

***Don't type in long URLs** –* add the site number to the eMedguides URL: www.eMedguides.com/**G-1234**.

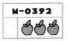

American Board of Internal Medicine (ABIM) Information for examination and certification in internal medicine is featured at the ABIM Web site. The site contains certification test dates, request for application forms, examination statistics, general test guidelines, and pass rates. In addition, the site provides an online directory of actively certified diplomats, information on ABIM certification policies and procedures, ABIM newsletters, and pages for certification in a variety of subspecialties. A list of links to medical societies and organizations affiliated with the ABIM is also provided.

(some features fee-based) http://www.abim.org/

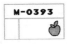

American Board of Obstetrics and Gynecology (ABOG) This site provides information on examination dates, official statements regarding certification, and guides to learning for obstetrician-gynecologists and subspecialists in maternal-fetal medicine, reproductive endocrinology/infertility, and gynecologic oncology.

http://www.abog.org

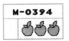

American Cancer Society The society provides this comprehensive site for information on all aspects of cancer, primarily directed toward the public. The home page includes links to information on a variety of cancer types, prevention, treatment options, therapies, research, statistics, and media resources. A state-by-state scroll menu connects visitors to local organizations and an online directory of medical resources. Each cancer description is quite thorough and is augmented by additional links to other resources on the same topic, such as specialized glossaries, imaging, drugs, and alternative therapies.

http://www.cancer.org

American Chronic Pain Society Facilitating patient support and professional and public awareness, this page discusses various aspects of chronic pain and offers information about pain management, answers to a variety of frequently asked questions, and a helpful reading list.

http://www.theacpa.org

American College of Allergy, Asthma, & Immunology (ACAAI) Information for patients, physicians, and other interested visitors is available at this research, advocacy, and educationally-oriented organization. Consumers will find fact sheets on the role of the allergist, information on a variety of allergic diseases, and a document related to immunotherapy. Online CME, publications on the role of the allergist in the treatment of various diseases, and news about allergy and asthma are offered.

http://allergy.mcg.edu

American College of Cardiology (ACC) A major professional society with over 24,000 members from around the world, the American College of Cardiology (ACC) provides rigorous criteria to improve the quality of care delivered by its members. The society actively participates in healthcare policy debate, and users may access information about its position on specific issues. A searchable database of ACC publications, programs, and products is provided,

along with links to clinical information, conferences, information on advocacy, industry relations, and patient education. Summaries from the ACC Scientific Session and downloadable medical guidelines are found. The site contains numerous links to heart and health information, medical information, and cardiovascular specialists, all accessible after a simple, free registration process.
(free registration) http://www.acc.org

American College of Chest Physicians This site serves as a comprehensive resource page for healthcare practitioners and researchers involved in various multidisciplinary aspects of chest medicine. Resources include CME courses, links to relevant publications including *CHEST-The Cardiopulmonary and Critical Care Journal,* advocacy activity details in public and government affairs, consensus statements, and clinical guidelines. Information about the Chest Foundation is also included.
http://www.chestnet.org

American College of Clinical Pharmacology Activities, member benefits, and journal pages are available at this organization site, dedicated to pharmacology education. Pharmacology educational links are compiled, including CME resources, a pharmacology tutorial, and drug interaction tutorial. Meetings, links, and news are provided, as well as a members-only forum.
(some features fee-based) http://www.accp1.org/index.html

American College of Clinical Pharmacy This professional and scientific society offers a site map, which guides visitors through the publicly accessible side of the ACCP Web site. News released during the past 12 months, meeting information, a calendar of upcoming meetings, and the organization's online bookstore are freely offered. Visitors are encouraged to download Adobe Acrobat documents, including ACCP commentaries, practice papers, research information, and position statements. Practice guidelines and opinions are also included, as is the table of contents of the member-only portion of the site.
(some features fee-based) http://www.accp.com/

American College of Emergency Physicians Dedicated to maintaining high standards of care for patients in emergency situations, the American College of Emergency Physicians offers information about educational conferences, publications, legislation, advocacy, and research at its Web site. Recent headlines, a book store, a calendar of events, and relevant links add value to the site.
(some features fee-based) http://www.acep.org

American College of Endocrinology Clinical endocrinologists interested in becoming fellows of the American College of Endocrinology may be interested in this site, dedicated to explaining the benefits of membership. The Web site offers an online application.
http://www.aace.com/college

American College of Gastroenterology Created by the American College of Gastroenterology (ACG), this site offers physicians information on research grants, clinical updates, and several publications. Members of ACG have access to practice guidelines as well as the online version of the *American Journal of Gastroenterology*. A comprehensive collection of patient fact sheets is also provided.

(some features fee-based) http://www.acg.gi.org

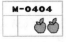

American College of Obstetricians and Gynecologists (ACOG)

Resources for physicians can be found at the ACOG home page under the technical help section. Once there, visitors can access a resident job bank, information on the National Fetal and Infant Mortality Review program, and advice on practice management. There are also educational materials on women's issues, policy updates, and a searchable database for ordering free patient education pamphlets. (some features fee-based) http://www.acog.org

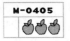

American College of Occupational and Environmental Medicine

Providing preventive services, education, research, and clinical care, the ACOEM organization and home page offer review of upcoming conferences, online position statements and guidelines, and access to abstracts of recent articles from *The Journal of Occupational and Environmental Medicine*. The reader will also find an assortment of additional publications of the organization as well as links to other occupational and environmental medicine resources. http://www.acoem.org/

American College of Physicians-American Society of Internal Medicine (ACP-ASIM)

Resources offered by the American College of Physicians-American Society of Internal Medicine (ACP-ASIM) site include clinical information, guideline reports, practice tips, discussion groups, and the *Annals of Internal Medicine*. The site also features CME information and discussion groups. (some features fee-based) http://www.acponline.org

American College of Preventive Medicine

Sponsored by the American College of Preventive Medicine (ACPM), this Web page offers information on CME workshops, policy issues, and ACPM publications. Additionally, clinical preventive service guidelines are available under the resource section of the site. http://www.acpm.org

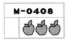

American College of Radiology

This Web site offers information on accreditation and continuing education programs, fellowship and resident information, and career services. Educational materials for physicians include CME information, resident education, and home study materials. In addition, there are sections on advocacy, radiology research, and related links.

(some features fee-based) http://www.acr.org/

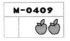

American College of Rheumatology (ACR)

Physicians will find treatment guidelines, an online catalog of abstracts, research grants, and classification criteria for rheumatic diseases at this site. Members can access online journals. A special section is dedicated to patient information with fact sheets on a variety of conditions. (some features fee-based) http://www.rheumatology.org

American College of Sports Medicine Information provided by the American College of Sports Medicine (ACSM) covers research grants and reports as well as CME programs and online self-testing. A variety of publications are offered such as the online version of ACSM's *Health and Fitness Journal*.
(some features fee-based) http://www.acsm.org

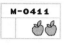

American College of Surgeons Maintained by the American College of Surgeons, this site provides the latest detailed news in surgical topics, CME information, a comprehensive online library, and a catalog for related publications. Patients can click on the public information link to find fact sheets on some of the most frequently performed procedures.
http://www.facs.org

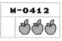

American Diabetes Association The American Diabetes Association (ADA), whose mission is to prevent and cure diabetes, features a section for healthcare professionals that contains clinical practice guidelines, other ADA professional publications, information on their research and grant program, and a variety of continuing education resources. Patients will find fact sheets on nutrition, exercise, and treatment as well as details regarding the organization's outreach programs. Additional resources at the site include an online diabetes book store, advocacy and legal information, and a comprehensive listing of related links.
http://www.diabetes.org/default.asp

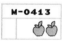

American Dietetic Association Information on nutrition is featured at the American Dietetic Association's Web page. Although primarily intended for consumers, healthcare professionals will find publications designated specifically for clinicians. Consumers are offered nutrition tips, fact sheets, coverage of policy issues, and an online marketplace.
http://www.eatright.org

American Gastroenterological Association Examining the field of gastroenterology, the American Gastroenterological Association offers this physician-oriented Web page with clinical information, practice management tools, practice guidelines, CME courses, and research grants. A section of the site is devoted especially to training program information and financial resources. Consumers will find many patient wellness brochures through the digestive health resource center link.
(some features fee-based) http://www.gastro.org/index.html

American Geriatrics Society (AGS) Dedicated to the well-being of older adults, the American Geriatrics Society Web page provides healthcare professionals with the latest news, continuing education information, electronic publications, public policy information, and an electronic job bank. Numerous publications are offered to consumers, and a list of related resources is provided.
(some features fee-based) http://www.americangeriatrics.org

American Heart Association (AHA) To increase awareness of heart disease, the American Heart Association offers this site. Healthcare professionals can choose from a special drop-down menu at the top of the page to jump to advocacy information, online publications, AHA journals, research grants, and statistics. Within the professional education section, practice guidelines and online CME programs are available. Patients can click on a variety of topics such as disease warning signs, family health, and risk awareness and read fact sheets on heart disease.
http://www.americanheart.org

American Hospital Association Intended for hospital administrators, the American Hospital Association site features information on their advocacy and research efforts. The site also contains descriptions of their programs such as their "Campaign for Coverage" and a resource library.
(some features fee-based) http://www.aha.org

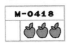

American Lung Association (ALA) The home page of the American Lung Association provides extensive coverage of asthma, tobacco control, air quality, and diseases from A-to-Z. Each Web division offers a brief overview of the topic accompanied by National Heart, Lung, and Blood Institute (NHLBI) guidelines, fact sheets, data and statistics, and therapeutic interventions. ALA events and programs, occupational lung health, and ALA research highlights are all accessible, as well as publication subsites containing online press releases, newsletters, and additional references that may be ordered from the site.
http://www.lungusa.org

American Medical Association (AMA) The American Medical Association Web site provides information about the organization, policy and advocacy, ethics, education, science, public health, quality, and accreditation. In addition, there are journals and medical news, consumer health information, and information for physicians. The AMA site is very extensive and warrants careful exploration. http://www.ama-assn.org

American Medical Informatics Association The use of information technology in healthcare is the focus of the American Medical Informatics Association (AMIA) site. The resource center section offers information on products, policy issues, and research grants. Visitors can view the online version of the AMIA journal and access related publications.
(some features fee-based) http://www.amia.org

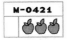

American Medical Student Association Medical students will find a wealth of information at the Web page of the American Medical Student Association, including career development resources, discussion groups for special interests such as bioethics and primary care, financial resources, and advocacy help. Additional sections are geared toward medical education, health policy, global health issues, and public health issues.
(some features fee-based) http://www.amsa.org

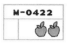 **American Medical Women's Association** Visitors to the American Medical Women's Association (AMWA) Web site will find patient brochures on a variety of women's health topics, advocacy information, and AMWA publications. Women medical students will find the student information and AMWA Foundation sections of use for financial resources. The *Journal of AMWA* is available online to subscribers only.

(some features fee-based) http://www.amwa-doc.org/index.html

 American Neurological Association (ANA) With a focus on academic neurology, this site features information for medical students, such as an enhanced clinical neuroscience program in medical school, student interest group, a match program, and a fellowship directory. The site also contains a comprehensive list of neurology resources.

(some features fee-based) http://www.aneuroa.org

 American Orthopaedic Society for Sports Medicine Professionals interested in orthopaedic surgery and sports medicine will find information on CME courses, research grants, and the online version of the *American Journal of Sports Medicine* at this Web page. Under the publications section, links for patient and professional educational materials are available.

(some features fee-based) http://www.sportsmed.org

 American Osteopathic Association Providing support to the osteopathic physician, this Web site offers CME information, full online reports of the AOA's health news updates, and the opportunity to view a multimedia Webcast of presentations made of a recent Women's Health Symposium. News, online publications, and information specifically for members are offered, including postdoctoral and research and grant opportunities. A variety of AOA brochures about osteopathic medicine are available to consumer audiences.

(some features fee-based) http://www.aoa-net.org/

 American Pain Society The American Pain Society (APS) is a multidisciplinary, scientific organization that offers information on publications, advocacy, career opportunities, and upcoming events. A pain facility database allows the user to search for facilities by classifications, and additional resources for both patients and professionals provide contact information for related organizations. The APS site provides an abstract search engine to their database of internal documentation on pain-related topics.

http://www.ampainsoc.org

 American Podiatric Medical Association For those interested in podiatry, the American Podiatric Medical Association site features the *Journal of the American Podiatric Medical Association,* information on clinical workshops providing CME accreditation, and links to related organizations. Information for consumers includes online fact sheets on a number of podiatric disorders and a searchable database of podiatrists in the United States.

(some features fee-based) http://www.apma.org/

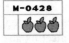
American Psychiatric Association (APA) The American Psychiatric Association is a national and international association of psychiatric physicians. Their site includes sections on policy, clinical practice guidelines, research grants, CME information, and publications.
http://www.psych.org

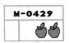
American Public Health Association At the forefront of disease control and prevention, the American Public Health Association provides a forum for exchange of information on national and international health practice, standards, and policy. Scientific program review, organization publications, and information on advocacy efforts are provided at the site, with relevant sections on programs and policies related to infectious disease control and a smoke-free society. http://www.apha.org

American Red Cross Dedicated to providing a range of health and safety services, the American Red Cross offers descriptions of its programs at this page. Disaster services, biomedical services, and health and safety commitments are discussed. News presentations and spotlight information are found, including school safety tips, the safety of the nation's blood supply, and the rapid responses initiated by the organization to national and international disasters. Visitors are able to locate their local Red Cross chapter by entering a postal code or browsing a complete nationwide listing.
http://www.redcross.org/

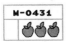
American Social Health Association This organization is dedicated to providing education and patient support for sexually transmitted diseases. Statistical data, sexual health glossaries, national and local hotlines, support groups, and prevention information is featured. Press releases, articles, and other publications are also online to provide current information on outlined topics. http://www.ashastd.org

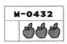
American Society for Gastrointestinal Endoscopy The professional society for gastroenterologists, surgeons, and other health professionals provides information about GI disease and the use of endoscopy. One can view an online database of clinical updates, policy and position statements, and patient care guidelines. Patient information comes in the form of educational documents that discuss upper endoscopy, flexible sigmoidoscopy, colonoscopy, and more. http://www.asge.org

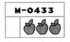
American Society of Clinical Oncology Supported by the American Society of Clinical Oncology (ASCO), this site features resources for professionals such as ASCO abstracts, CME information, practice guidelines, and publications. A section of the site is dedicated to patients and includes a directory of oncologists, patient guides, and news of the latest research. A list of related Internet resources is provided both for professionals and consumers. (some features fee-based) http://www.asco.org

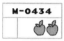

American Society of Hematology   Examining hematology, this site for clinicians and scientists contains links to the organization's journal entitled *Blood,* educational materials on a variety of conditions, and annual meeting abstracts. Research awards and grants are also described.
(some features fee-based) http://www.hematology.org

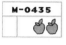

American Society of Hypertension   Physicians who specialize in hypertension will find educational materials, information on the organization's hypertension specialist program with qualifying exams, and a list of related resources. In addition, members can view the current and archived editions of the society's journal online.
(some features fee-based) http://www.ash-us.org

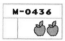

American Society of Nephrology   Resources offered by the American Society of Nephrology include full access to the online version of their journal, research grant information, postgraduate education information, kidney disease statistics, and a fee-based job placement service. A frequently asked questions section is available to patients.
(some features fee-based) http://www.asn-online.org

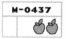

American Society of Plastic Surgeons   Hosted by the American Society of Plastic Surgeons, the Plastic Surgery Information Service site offers medical professionals access to national statistics, the online version of the *Journal of Plastic and Reconstructive Surgery,* and physician counseling guides on procedures. Readers will find helpful information on international volunteer work, a consumer-oriented set of FAQs, advocacy information, and a plastic surgeon locator service useful.
(some features fee-based) http://www.plasticsurgery.org

American Stroke Association   A division of the American Heart Association, the American Stroke Association provides healthcare professionals with CME information, scientific statements, statistics, and research funding information for strokes. A link within the "Professional" section takes visitors to a page containing a directory of current and ongoing therapeutic trials. The site also features an online risk assessment quiz for patients and several consumer education brochures.
(some features fee-based) http://www.strokeassociation.org

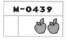

American Thoracic Society   As an association that seeks to establish standards for the prevention, treatment, and control of respiratory diseases, much of the content of the society's site is dedicated to educational programs, assemblies and conferences, publications, and clinical research. Additionally, the site provides related news updates, advocacy information, and details on membership. Contact information for local chapters of the society and an online store are offered.
(some features fee-based) http://www.thoracic.org

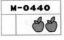

American Urological Association This site of the American Urological Associatiion details information about the organization, its publications, guidelines, and managed care issues. The education section offers a residency program database and facts about home study and other CME programs. A Web Forum limits access to members, and a section devoted to the public offers disorder and general urology information.
http://www.auanet.org

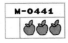

Arthritis Foundation Intended for patients, their families, and caregivers, the Arthritis Foundation Web page features fact sheets on many types of arthritis, advocacy information, and volunteer opportunities. The organization's online store offers a variety of publications to consumers and physicians, intended as patient education tools. Some Spanish-language materials are available. http://www.arthritis.org

Association of American Medical Colleges Created to provide information on medical education, the Association of American Medical Colleges site offers prospective medical students information on applying to medical schools, medical school directories, and related publications. Research publications and databases on medical education can be accessed by going to the "Jump to" box and selecting "Research." Medical school faculty and staff may find certain publications and the policy sections useful.
http://www.aamc.org

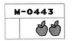

Association of Program Directors in Internal Medicine The Association of Program Directors in Internal Medicine promotes excellence in the training of internal medicine. Their site provides visitors with member-developed software, answers to FAQs, a job bank of faculty and resident positions, and a catalog of their lending library. Policy issues and a link to the electronic resident application service are also provided.
(some features fee-based) http://apdim.med.edu

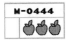

Canadian Medical Association This neighboring major medical association offers several useful features at its site, including full access to evidence-based clinical practice guidelines, practice management tools, a publications catalog, and a clinical discussion bulletin board. Medical database search tools, a problem-oriented drug formulary for primary care practitioners, and a compilation of health and medicine-related Internet links are provided.
(some features fee-based) http://www.cma.ca

Canadian Society of Internal Medicine This resource, available in English and French, provides visitors with access to the Canadian Society of Internal Medicine newsletter, a list of employment opportunities for internists, and links to related resources.
http://csim.medical.org

Endocrine Society The Web site for the Endocrine Society provides information about scientific meetings, ethics, special interest groups, awards and grants,

and related publications. Information for patients includes fact sheets about endocrinology and animal research, breast cancer, endometriosis, female infertility, and hormone rhythms.
http://www.endo-society.org

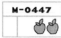

Epilepsy Foundation of America   Healthcare professionals will find information on research grants and fellowships at the Epilepsy Foundation of America (EFA) site. Patients can be directed to the site for fact sheets, advocacy information and opportunities, and to read the online version of the foundation's publication, *Epilepsy USA News*. Information on EFA-sponsored programs, such as a women-and-epilepsy initiative, are also provided.
http://www.efa.org

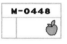

Gerontological Society of America   Visitors interested in the field of gerontology will have access to the organization's most recent newsletter, grant information, an online job bank, and publications of the Gerontological Society of America at this Web page. Link to related resources are available.
http://www.geron.org

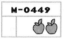

Institute of Medicine   The focus of the Institute of Medicine site is on health and science policy. Visitors can find online research reports as well as information pertaining to ongoing studies and programs. Emerging infectious diseases, sex differences in medicine, controversy over marijuana use in medicine, and the science base for tobacco harm reduction are a selection of recent topical coverage available online. Descriptions of program units in ongoing study and their goals can be viewed and include the Food and Nutrition Board, the National Cancer Policy Board, and the Board on Global Health.
http://www.iom.edu

Internal Medicine Interest Group (IMIG)   Maintained by medical students at Michigan State University, this site offers links to residency information and to other organizations covering a variety of medical subspecialties. For those interested in the specialty of internal medicine, this page serves as a gateway to further information about many medical fields.
http://www.echt.chm.msu.edu/~chmimig/

International Society of Internal Medicine   The International Society of Internal Medicine comprises more than 50 national societies of internal medicine. Their site provides an international directory of society members and information on upcoming International Congress of Internal Medicine meetings.
http://www.acponline.org/isim/

Leukemia and Lymphoma Society   The Society seeks to provide information, education, patient services, and community services, and fund research dealing with leukemia, lymphoma, Hodgkin's disease, and myeloma. The site describes educational materials, publications, and services offered. A research link provides workshop information and applications, a professional education calendar, and grant information.   http://l3.leukemia-lymphoma.org/hm_lls

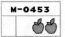

Lupus Foundation of America Commonly asked questions about lupus are addressed at a library of current information about the disease, and an event listing, a research resource link, and the opportunity to learn more about local programs and services are provided. Visitors will also find a comprehensive article, authored by Dr. Richard Lahita, which addresses the causes, symptoms, and management of the disease. The Lupus Foundation of America's Health Forum provides alternate Web sites for exchange of experiences and expertise.
http://www.lupus.org/

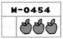

Muscular Dystrophy Association (MDA) A searchable database of MDA clinics nationwide, numerous publications for both consumer and professional audiences, and online publications of the MDA are available at its Web site. An "Ask the Experts" forum, coverage of the recent Ross Report, and an active clinical trials listing for MDA-covered diseases are provided. Additional research resources include listings of current research from the scientific literature, the latest in gene therapy information, and links to major research sites. A master list of neuromuscular diseases in the MDA program connects visitors to basic references, special materials, FAQs, clinical trials, and research updates and digest information for each specific disease.
http://www.mdausa.org/

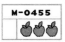

National Headache Foundation In addition to membership, visitors to this site will find online brochures on a variety of headache conditions, a listing of educational resources and materials available for purchase, headache support groups nationwide, and excerpts from the organizations award-winning publication, *Head Lines*. Online educational treatment modules, a future calendar of events, CME, topical monographs, and current clinical trial listing are offered.
http://www.headaches.org/

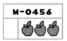

National Kidney Foundation This award-winning site is dedicated to providing both clinicians and consumers with information and educational resources regarding kidney disease. General public brochures and articles, a variety of clinical practice guidelines, and a variety of organization council support are available. Future meeting information is provided.
http://www.kidney.org/

National Multiple Sclerosis Society Visitors to this site will find a national directory of society chapter offices and articles presented for use by both physicians and other healthcare professionals. Resources for physicians include grant applications, clinical trial information, clinical publications, and status reports on scientific progress. A section on research and clinical studies provides a listing of recent bulletins and links to further details on new therapies. A presentation on gender-specific study initiatives may be downloaded from the site, and a schedule of educational Internet programming on various aspects of MS is provided.
http://www.nmss.org

National Osteoporosis Foundation Dedicated to osteoporosis, this site offers physicians information on CME programs, clinical guidelines, research grants, and reimbursement for bone density tests. Consumers will find fact sheets, prevention tips, support groups, and a directory of doctors. In addition, the online store has separate sections for the both the public and health professionals. http://www.nof.org

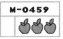

National Parkinson Foundation Physicians interested in Parkinson's disease will find research grant information, research reports, and a library of online publications at the National Parkinson Foundation (NPF) site. Information for patients includes links to support groups, online tests for various conditions, clinical study information, and NPF programs. Caregivers of Parkinson patients can click on a link to a separate site with resources and support especially for them.
http://www.parkinson.org

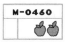

National Psoriasis Foundation Within the programs and events section of the National Psoriasis Foundation site, medical professionals can find workshops and a members-only newsletter. Resources for patients with psoriasis include fact sheets on the disease, treatment therapies, and the latest research findings. A comprehensive listing of related Internet links is provided.
http://www.psoriasis.org

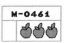

National Stroke Association Resources provided at the National Stroke Association home page include a Stroke Information Library that includes patient overviews of such topics as acute treatment research, effects of stroke, prevention and reducing risk, and recognizing symptoms. In addition, the site has survivor and caregiver resources, including a list of regional stroke centers, regional stroke support groups, and regional chapters by state. A glossary and links to related Web sites are also included. http://www.stroke.org/index.cfm

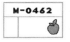

Society for Medical Decision Making Based out of George Washington University Medical Center, the Society for Medical Decision Making offers free education modules and members-only access to the *Medical Decision Making* journal, newsletter, and member directory. In addition, there is an electronic LISTSERV to facilitate an e-mail discussion group for members.
(some features fee-based) http://www.hfni.gsehd.gwu.edu/~smdm/

Society of General Internal Medicine Internists will find links to a residency directory, a fellowship directory, and a clerkship guide on the Society of General Internal Medicine site. Other resources include funding opportunities and professional development information, such as position openings, an interest group mail list, and a mentor program. In addition, publications, such as the *Journal of General Internal Medicine* (members only) and a newsletter are available. (some features fee-based) http://www.sgim.org

World Health Organization (WHO) Coverage of World Health Day, disease outbreaks, and other news just off the press is available at the WHO

online Mediacentre. A large variety of health topics is addressed by this international organization, including communicable/infectious diseases, vaccine preventable diseases, noncommunicable diseases, and environmental health and safety issues, aging, mental health, and tobacco-related disease. The WHO Headquarters Library may be searched, as well as the WHO Statistical Information System (WHOSIS). A variety of World Health Reports and other publications and periodicals issued by the organization are provided.
http://www.who.int/

7.2 GOVERNMENT ORGANIZATIONS

AGENCIES AND OFFICES

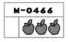

Administration on Aging (AOA) This division of the U.S. Department of Health and Human Services offers information intended for older Americans and for those concerned about them. Information on the nationwide network of state agencies intended to enrich the lives of older persons is available, such as day care programs, transportation, legal services, and counseling opportunities. In addition to complete details about these programs, a Practitioners Page is offered, which provides links and addresses selected issues in the field of aging. Both a comprehensive site index and quick index page make site navigation simple. http://www.aoa.dhhs.gov/

Agency for Healthcare Research and Quality (AHRQ) Several navigational tools are available at this Web site, including search and browse features for all of the agency's quality assessments, research findings, consumer health guides, and clinical information. Included in this collection of medical information are evidence-based practice reports, clinical practice guidelines sponsored by the agency and from the National Guidelines Clearinghouse, and Spanish-language documents. Also found are research findings across primary care, healthcare financing, and managed care, as well as several additional fields that are part of this agency's focus.
http://www.ahcpr.gov/

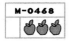

Agency for Toxic Substances and Disease Registry As an agency of the U.S. Department of Health and Human Services, this division strives to prevent exposure and adverse health effects of hazardous substances from a variety of pollution sources. Public health assessments, applied research, and educational goals of the organization are available for review at this site. Visitors can instantly access national alerts, health advisories, news, and ATSDR archives.
http://www.atsdr.cdc.gov/atsdrhome.html

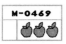

Centers for Disease Control and Prevention (CDC) The lead federal agency for the protection of the health of people in the United States offers up-to-date, credible information on an A-to-Z listing of health topics. The "In the

News" connection brings visitors to press summaries and releases and also sheds light on current health-related hoaxes and rumors. The National Center for Health Statistics, the online *Emerging Infectious Disease Journal, Morbitidy and Mortality Weekly Report,* and CDC Prevention Guidelines are all available at this agency of the U.S. Department of Health and Human Services.
http://www.cdc.gov/

Centers for Medicare & Medicaid Services Information about the Medicare, Medicaid, and State Children's Health Insurance Programs of the Health Care Financing Administration is available at this site, with both fee-for-service and managed - care plans reviewed. Regulatory activities of the division are discussed at the site, and information specifically geared toward providers and researchers is available.
http://www.hcfa.gov/

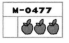

Department of Health and Human Services Housing the majority of federally-affiliated programs and agencies, the U.S. Department of Health and Human Services (HHS) offers access to its primary divisions from its site. A pull-down menu of commonly requested health information leads visitors to various starting points for research, accessing several, prominent HHS agencies and initiatives. Also featured are the news and public affairs page, which allows visitors to search for press releases and fact sheets, and a display of department headlines at the home page.
http://www.os.dhhs.gov/

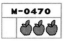

Food and Drug Administration (FDA) FDA news is the focus of this Health and Human Services site, including "Hot Topic" coverage, press releases, and safety alerts. A recent FDA product approval link and connections to newly approved drugs, medical devices, and biologicals are provided. Divisions within the FDA can be accessed from the site, including the Center for Food Safety and Applied Nutrition, the Center for Drug Evaluation and Research, the Center for Devices and Radiological Health, and the Center for Biologics Evaluation and Research. Information for health professionals about regulated products, adverse reactions, and clinical trials is available, as well as consumer-oriented health issue coverage.
http://www.fda.gov/

Health Resources and Services Administration Key program areas are highlighted at this government division, including HIV/AIDS services and primary healthcare resources for the medically underserved. In an effort to assure equitable and comprehensive healthcare to all, this organization also details its State-funded programs and health workforce training campaign.
http://www.hrsa.dhhs.gov/

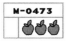

National Institutes of Health (NIH) One of the world's foremost medical research centers, the NIH offers access to a multitude of separate centers and institutes within its online domain. As part of the Public Health Service, its Web site boasts an A-to-Z topic health index, access to news and current events, and

the scientific resources link, which details intramural research, training, and laboratories of the Institute. ClinicalTrials.gov, MEDLINEplus, and the NIH Health Information Index are all valuable starting points for research.
http://www.nih.gov/

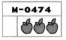 **Office of Disease Prevention and Health Promotion** Activities of this federal division include the Healthy People Initiative and healthfinder, an award-winning gateway to health information. This division of the Office of Public Health and Science also offers several online publications and a variety of Internet links supported by the division, including the National Health Information Center, a national health information referral service.
http://odphp.osophs.dhhs.gov/

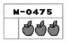 **Office of Public Health and Science** Program offices of this federal government division include the National Vaccine Program, the Office of HIV/AIDS Policy, the Office of the Surgeon General, and the Office on Women's Health. Any one of these and a number of other subdivisions can be accessed from the site, which also provides connections to a variety of supported agency, clearinghouse, and resource- center links.
http://www.surgeongeneral.gov/ophs/

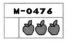 **Substance Abuse and Mental Health Services Administration** This federal agency is responsible for improving both the quality and availability of prevention and treatment programs to serve those affected by substance abuse and mental illness. The Center for Mental Health Services, the Center for Substance Abuse Prevention, and the Center for Substance Abuse Treatment can all be accessed from the site.
http://www.samhsa.gov/

7.3 FOUNDATIONS AND GRANT SUPPORT

Hundreds of major foundations offer financial support for research in medicine. Below are Web sites that provide access to foundation grants, grant organizations, areas of focus, eligibility, and other relevant data. In addition, several major sources of government research funding are provided, as well as Web sites for grants that are catalogued by specialized organizations and clearinghouses. Major associations and societies that appear in the "Associations" section frequently include information on research grants, and many offer annual awards for research and study.

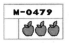 **Foundation Center** The Foundation Center provides direct, "hot links" to thousands of grant-making organizations, including foundations, corporations, and public charities, along with a search engine to enable the user to locate sources of funding in specific fields. In addition, the site provides listings of the largest private foundations, corporate grant makers, and community foundations. There is also information on funding trends, a newsletter, and grant-seeker orientation material. More than 900 grant-making organizations are accessible through this useful site. http://fdncenter.org

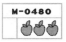

M-0480

National Institutes of Health (NIH): Funding Opportunities Funding opportunities for research, scholarship, and training are extensive within the federal government. At this site of the National Institutes of Health, a Grants Page exists with information about NIH grants and fellowship programs, information on Research Contracts containing information on Requests for Proposals (RFPs), Research Training Opportunities in biomedical areas, and an NIH guide for Grants and Contracts. The latter is the official document for announcing the availability of NIH funds for biomedical and behavioral research and research training policies. Links are provided to major divisions of the NIH that offer additional information on specialized grant opportunities.
http://grants.nih.gov/grants

M-0481

Polaris Grant Central For the grant seeker, this site provides resources that are derived from numerous organizations pertaining to grant identification and application. Books and publications on grant sources, descriptions of grant information providers, grant information clearinghouses, federal contracts, grant training materials, and resources on disk or CD-ROM are offered. Within the site, useful sections provide "Tips and Hints" on writing grant proposals, "Grant News" from various government agencies and other organizations, "Scholarships or Grants to Individuals," and information on grant workshops.
http://www.polarisgrantscentral.net

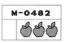

M-0482

Society of Research Administrators: GrantsWeb The Society of Research Administrators has created an extremely useful grant information site, with extensive links to government resources, general resources, private funding, and policy/regulation sites. The site section, devoted to U.S., Canadian, and other international resources, provides links to government agency funding sources, the Commerce Business Daily, the Catalog of Federal Domestic Assistance, scientific agencies, research councils, and resources in individual fields, such as health and education. Grant application procedures, regulations, and guidelines are provided throughout the site, and extensive legal information is provided through links to patent, intellectual property, and copyright offices. Associations providing funding and grant information are also listed, with direct links. http://www.srainternational.org/cws/sra/resource.htm

7.4 GRADUATE SCHOOL DEPARTMENTS

M-0483

Baylor College of Medicine: Department of Medicine The Department of Medicine at Baylor College of Medicine maintains a Web site with links to nearly 20 departmental sections. Although there is not a separate page for internal medicine, the general site provides an overview of the training programs, teaching conferences, and research centers. Current research focuses on thrombosis, atherosclerosis, gene therapy for cancer and AIDS, cellular mechanisms of aging, MRI and bone measurement technology, and lung inflammation. http://public.bcm.tmc.edu/medicine/

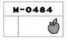

Case Western Reserve University: School of Medicine Departments Although Case Western Reserve University does not offer a separate Web site for its department of internal medicine, this page provides visitors with links to other sites within the School of Medicine.
http://mediswww.cwru.edu/academicdept.htm

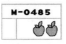

Columbia University College of Physicians and Surgeons: Division of General Medicine The Division of General Medicine at Columbia University College of Physicians and Surgeons features information about the clinical research and fellowship programs. Topics of research include cardiovascular or pulmonary diseases, diseases of aging, medical ethics, medical informatics, and telemedicine. http://cpmcnet.columbia.edu/dept/medicine/generalmed/

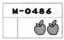

Duke University Medical Center: Division of General Internal Medicine This site provides an overview of the Division of General Internal Medicine. Research areas include ethics in medicine, quality of patient care, cancer prevention, and development of clinical guidelines for disease management. Visitors may visit two Web sites to obtain additional information on clinical practice and research activities.
http://dukegim.duke.edu/home.asp?divisionID=47

Emory University: Department of Medicine Emory University offers this site with descriptions of its Department of Medicine, including specific division information, patient care, research projects, and residency programs. Current research focuses on diabetes, geriatrics, cancer, infectious diseases, obstructive lung disease, epidemiology, and heart disorders.
http://www.emory.edu/MED/DEPT/

Harvard Medical School Family Health Guide: Department of Medicine This general site of Harvard Medical School presents information about the different academic and clinical departments, affiliated hospitals, and institutes. By clicking on "Research" then "Clinical Departments," visitors will access contact information for the Department of Medicine. At this time, there is not a separate site for the Department of Internal Medicine.
http://www.hms.harvard.edu/

Indiana University, Indianapolis: Division of General Internal Medicine and Geriatrics The Division of General Internal Medicine and Geriatrics provides limited information about its programs on its Web site, but the Department of Medicine serves as an adequate resource. By using the menu at the bottom of the page, visitors may access the department's research centers and active clinical trials, which include Alzheimer's disease, autism, cancer, diabetes, high blood pressure, arthritis, pediatric asthma, schizophrenia, and stroke. http://medicine.iupui.edu/genintme.html

Johns Hopkins University: Department of Medicine The Johns Hopkins University Department of Medicine focuses on research, teaching, and patient care. Although there is not an individual site for the Internal Medicine

Division, visitors may find general information about the department's research centers by selecting "overview" from this page.
http://www.med.jhu.edu/deptmed/

Mayo Medical School: Internal Medicine Program   This Web site highlights the general internal medicine fellowship and residency programs of the Mayo Clinic. The program description summarizes clinical, educational, and research training.
http://www.mayo.edu/mgsm/rgim.htm

New York Hospital - Cornell Medical Center: Division of General Internal Medicine   The Division of General Internal Medicine at Cornell Medical Center details its research and education programs. Research activities focus on improving the quality of patient care, assessing new technologies and intervention procedures, and developing new strategies to treat and prevent disease and disability.
http://www.nycornell.org/medicine/gim/index.html

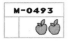

Northwestern University: Department of General Internal Medicine
The primary areas of focus of the Department of General Internal Medicine are cancer control, mental health, and cardiovascular epidemiology. Current and ongoing research projects include such topics as hypertension, mammography recommendations, diet as a risk factor for breast cancer, weight management, and domestic violence. The site also provides links to other divisions of the medical school site.
http://www.medicine.northwestern.edu/

St. Louis University: Division of General Internal Medicine   This Web page of St. Louis University provides links to divisions of the medical departments, such as the Division of General Internal Medicine. By clicking on this heading, visitors will find specific information about patient and clinical services. Research studies include hepatitis C, diabetes, chronic obstructive pulmonary disease, asthma, and hypertension.
http://internalmed.slu.edu/index.html

Stanford University: General Internal Medicine Division   Although Stanford University does not maintain a separate Web page for the General Internal Medicine Division, it does provide an outline of divisions within the Department of Medicine, including research centers and residency programs.
http://www-med.stanford.edu/school/depts.html

University of Alabama: Division of General Internal Medicine   The Division of General Internal Medicine at the University of Alabama, Birmingham, maintains a Web site with descriptions of its clinical activities, conferences, research interests, and fellowships. Some research projects focus on provider-patient communication, healthcare referral system, quality of patient care, and medical informatics.
http://info.dom.uab.edu/gim/index.htm

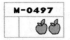 **M-0497**

University of California Los Angeles (UCLA): Division of General Internal Medicine   The Division of General Internal Medicine summarizes its patient care, residency program, continuing medical education, research activities, and fellowships at its Web site.
http://gim.med.ucla.edu/

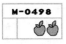 **M-0498**

University of California San Diego (UCSD): Division of General Internal Medicine/Geriatrics   The Division of General Internal Medicine/Geriatrics focuses on teaching, research, and clinical care. Its site offers information about fellowships, clinical trials, residency, and research programs. Research and clinical programs address such topics as Alzheimer's disease, cholesterol, dementia, asthma, diabetes, and hypertension.
http://medicine.ucsd.edu/dgim/

 M-0499

University of California San Francisco (UCSF): Division of General Internal Medicine   The Division of General Internal Medicine at the University of California, San Francisco, offers basic information about patient care, research and clinical activities, residency and fellowship programs, publications, and conferences. Current research interests include osteoporosis, thyroid disease, metabolism, cancer prevention, and HIV and sexually transmitted disease prevention. The division also offers an extensive listing of continuing medical education courses.
http://dgim.ucsf.edu/

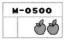 **M-0500**

University of Chicago: Department of General Internal Medicine
The University of Chicago Department of General Internal Medicine specializes in the care of patients with acute or chronic diseases and conditions. Physicians provide services in gynecology, allergy testing, nutrition counseling, and hypertension screening.
http://www.uchospitals.edu/areas/medicine.html#GIM

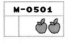 **M-0501**

University of Colorado Health Sciences Center: Division of General Internal Medicine   The Web site of the Division of General Internal Medicine provides information about the division's programs and projects directed toward patients, physicians, and medical students. It also offers schedules of medical conferences and seminars.
http://www.uchsc.edu/uh/gim/index.html

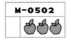 **M-0502**

University of Iowa: Department of Internal Medicine   The Department of Internal Medicine at the University of Iowa details the services of its individual divisions, including allergy, pharmacology, endocrinology, gastroenterology, hematology, oncology, nephrology, and rheumatology. Faculty contacts, grand rounds schedules, continuing education courses, residency and fellowship programs, and internal medicine news are all available online.
http://www.int-med.uiowa.edu/

 M-0503

University of Michigan, Ann Arbor: Department of Internal Medicine   The Department of Internal Medicine Web site serves as a comprehensive resource for information about the department. Topics include a patient glossary of clinical services and health terms, a physician and clinic directory, funding and grant support details, and information on research programs in such areas as cardiology, gastroenterology, geriatric medicine, hematology and oncology, infectious diseases, medical genetics, nephrology, nuclear medicine, and rheumatology. http://www.med.umich.edu/intmed/

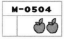

University of North Carolina at Chapel Hill: Department of Internal Medicine The Department of Internal Medicine Web site provides details about the specific centers and divisions of the department. The site also offers links to other academic units and programs and highlights research projects and residency training programs.
http://www.med.unc.edu/depts_medicine.htm

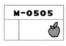

University of Pennsylvania Health System: Division of General Internal Medicine This site of the University of Pennsylvania Division of General Internal Medicine is in the process of being created. In the future, it will provide information about clinical care, education, research, and directory of the health system. http://www.med.upenn.edu/dgim/

University of Pittsburgh: Division of General Internal Medicine The Division of General Internal Medicine maintains a Web site that provides an annual report about the division; a directory of services, facilities, and research centers; a listing of clinical and teaching activities; and recent press releases. Focus areas include women's health, AIDS, medical ethics, and biomedical informatics. http://www.dept-med.pitt.edu/genmed.html

University of Texas Southwestern Medical Center, Dallas: Department of Internal Medicine The Department of Internal Medicine Web site offers information about the department's many divisions, the residency program, the lecture schedule, and internal medicine clinics.
http://www3.utsouthwestern.edu/internalmed/

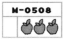

University of Virginia: Department of Internal Medicine The University of Virginia Department of Internal Medicine offers a wealth of information on its Web site. Of interest are the clinical divisions, residency program, schedule of seminars and conferences, and inpatient/outpatient clinics and consultations. Selected research activities focus on asthma, hypertension, heart, lung, pituitary and thyroid disorders, influenza, cancer genetics, sexually transmitted diseases, and lung disease.
http://www.med.virginia.edu/medicine/clinical/internal/

University of Washington: Division of General Internal Medicine The Web site of the Division of General Internal Medicine at the University of Washington describes the clinics and research centers of the division. It summarizes the various research projects, including Alzheimer's disease, breast cancer, chronic fatigue syndrome, diabetes, dementia, and women's health.
http://depts.washington.edu/gim/

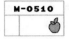

University of Wisconsin, Madison: General Internal Medicine Section This page of the University of Wisconsin, Madison, Department of Medicine provides information about the department's more than 15 clinical sections, including internal medicine.
http://www.medicine.wisc.edu/sections/

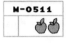

Vanderbilt University: Division of General Internal Medicine The Division of General Internal Medicine at Vanderbilt University provides research, clinical, and educational programs. Special attention is given to the field of geriatrics, and a section of geriatric medicine and a center on aging are developing within the division. Faculty research topics include diabetes, hypertension, geriatric nutrition, biomedical informatics, and alcohol and drug addiction. http://medicine.mc.vanderbilt.edu/divisions/im/index.cfm

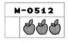

Washington University in St. Louis: Department of Internal Medicine Washington University in St. Louis presents this site for the Department of Internal Medicine. Visitors may access information about numerous divisions and sections within the department, conference schedules, faculty research topics, online journals and publications, and professional societies.
http://internalmed.wustl.edu/

Yale University: Department of Internal Medicine The Department of Internal Medicine provides information about its clinical sections, research interests, residency programs, and physician referral directory. Of specific interest is research in AIDS, cancer, sleep disorders, diabetes, dialysis, and women's health. Visitors may access additional information on these research topics.
http://info.med.yale.edu/intmed/

7.5 INTERNAL MEDICINE DEPARTMENTS

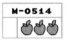

Academic Internal Medicine Departments Online Organized by state, this site offers more than 100 links to academic internal medicine departments with Web pages. Some of the sites do not contain a section for the department of internal medicine but do have general information on the school and/or other subspecialties. http://www.im.org/departme.htm

National Institutes of Health (NIH): Ranking of Internal Medicine Departments This site offers a list of more than 100 departments of internal medicine, ranked according to NIH funding. Many of the departments have hyperlinks to their Web pages.
http://www.residentphysician.com/Medicine_rankings.htm

7.6 HOSPITALS

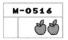

American Hospital Association: Metropolitan and Regional Hospital Associations A listing of metropolitan and regional hospital associations is

provided on this Web page by the American Hospital Association. There are more than 30 associations listed, most with hyperlinks to their Web sites. http://www.aha.org/resource/links.asp#9

American Hospital Association: Healthcare Organizations A directory of more than 100 healthcare organizations is featured on this Web page. The organizations include the Acute Long Term Hospital Association, America's Blood Centers, and the Council of Teaching Hospitals and Health Systems. http://www.aha.org/resource/links.asp#10

American Hospital Association: Links More than 40 sites are listed in this directory of American Hospital Association links. The links lead to AHA-sponsored Web pages, as well as to related societies and nonprofit organizations. http://www.aha.org/resource/links.asp#1

American Hospital Association: State Hospital Associations Links to state hospital associations are provided on this Web page, including Puerto Rico. A few states without a Web page offer contact information instead. http://www.aha.org/resource/links.asp#2

Cable News Network Online: The 100 Top Hospitals Drawn from a survey by Solucient, this site offers a list, organized by state, of the top 100 hospitals. http://www.cnn.com/2000/HEALTH/12/12/top.100.hospitals.list/

U.S. News & World Report: Best Hospitals by Specialty The *U.S. News & World Report* hospital rankings are featured on this Web page. Visitors can search for top hospitals by specialty or geographic region. Numerous articles related to the best hospitals are also found. http://www.usnews.com/usnews/nycu/health/hosptl/tophosp.htm

U.S. News & World Report: Top Hospitals A listing of the top 15 hospitals in the United States, according to *U.S. News & World Report,* is provided on this Web page. http://www.usnews.com/usnews/nycu/health/hosptl/honroll.htm

CLINICAL PRACTICE

8.1 GENERAL RESOURCES

M-0523

American College of Physicians-American Society of Internal Medicine Online: Web Sites for Internists Professionals may browse this site by category and access clinical practice guidelines, CME resources, full-text journal collections, and other general practice information resources. Offering a wide selection of clinical practice tools, this site of the American College of Physicians and the American Society of Internal Medicine boasts condition-specific information, medical news, and sites relevant to evidence-based practice, computers in medicine, and other decision support tools.
http://www.acponline.org/computer/ccp/bookmark/

M-0524

Canadian Medical Association: Clinical Resources Providing easy access to clinical information, evidence-based research, and resources in primary care, this site offers visitors links to the CMA Infobase of practice guidelines, direct connection to the OSLER medical databases search engine, a problem-oriented formulary entitled *Drugs of Choice,* and the WebMedLinks compilation of medicine-related Internet connections. Clinical question and answer discussion groups are also provided.
http://www.cma.ca/clinical/index.htm

M-0525

University of Alabama: Clinical Resources The Clinical Digital Libraries Project of the University of Alabama provides collections of general clinical resources, diagnostic clinical resources by symptom, the Lister Hill Library Databases, and a listing of practice management resources in diagnostic procedures. Clinical resources by topic are accessible at the site and include a variety of online textbook chapters, pathology databases, clinical guidelines, trials, and news. Drug reference, patient/family, and preventive medicine links are offered at this one-stop reference and teaching resource for physicians and other interested visitors. Although some features are fee-based, a wide selection of free material is available.
(some features fee-based) http://www.slis.ua.edu/cdlp/uab/uasom/

8.2 CLINICAL CALCULATORS AND ONLINE DECISION-MAKING

M-0526

Clinical Decision-Making Calculators Physicians can utilize clinical decision-making calculators for decision analyses, disease/test relations, expo-

sure/disease relations, and treatment/outcome relations. Sponsored by the University of Oklahoma Health Sciences Center, useful clinic calculators offered include the body-mass- index, the family-practice-incidence rate, and the number-needed-to-treat calculator. Statistical analysis tools are also provided, addressing odds and probabilities and confidence intervals.
http://www.fammed.ouhsc.edu/robhamm/cdmcalc.htm

MedCalc 3000   The frequently updated Medcalc 3000 can be utilized at this site, combining various equations, clinical criteria scores, and decision trees used in healthcare. In addition, subscribers are provided with a quick converter to the unit values and a math calculator. Alphabetical lists of the medical equations and clinical criteria topics are presented, with links to the actual calculators. http://calc.med.edu

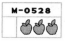

Medic8.com: Medical Tools, Calculators, and Scores   Medic8.com provides visitors to its Web site with numerous medical calculator connections to measure body function, dosing, and other vital data, such as blood oxygen content and body mass. Scores such as coronary disease probability, the geriatric depression scale, and the Glasgow coma scale are generated from input data. Over 60 connections offer individual scoring methods, algorithms, and assessments across a variety of medical specialties.
http://www.medic8.com/MedicalTools.htm

Online Clinical Calculators   More than 25 clinical calculators are featured on this personal Web page. Calculators include an acid-base calculator, steroid converter, Baysean analysis, body mass index, growth charts, and pregnancy dates. http://www.medcalc.com/

8.3 CLINICAL PRACTICE GUIDELINES

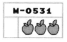

Agency for Healthcare Research and Quality (AHRQ): Clinical Practice Guidelines   Guidelines are presented in various categories of healthcare, including acute pain management, depression in primary care, heart failure, post-stroke rehabilitation, and cardiac rehabilitation. Physicians can also access several quick reference guides, including the management of cataract, cancer pain, sickle cell disease, and urinary incontinence.
http://text.nlm.nih.gov/ftrs/pick?collect=ahcpr&dbName=0&cc=1&t=929043260

American College of Physicians-American Society of Internal Medicine Online: Guidelines/Condition-Specific Information   At this Web-Sites-for-Internists page, professionals will find a wide selection of disease-specific guidelines. Accompanied by annotated entries that list guideline source and content, visitors are offered both disease-oriented information and practical guides to diagnosis and management. Preventive care, hypertension and hyperlipidemia, HIV, diabetes mellitus, cancer, and asthma are represented.
http://www.acponline.org/cgi-bin/im-bookmarks.pl?
d=s&c1=Guidelines/Condition-specific%20Information

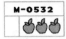

Canadian Medical Association: Clinical Practice Guidelines Produced or endorsed in Canada, this collection of guidelines can be browsed by entering keywords or phrases. Basic and advanced search interfaces are available for access to more than 1500 evidence-based clinical practice guidelines.
http://www.cma.ca/cpgs/

Medscape: Multispecialty Practice Guidelines Encompassing published guidelines from a variety of sources within several medical specialties, this site is an indispensable tool for healthcare practitioners. By clicking on one of 25 medical concentrations, visitors are taken to lists of available subjects that lead to further listings of acceptable practice documents. Guidelines are drawn from authoritative, specialty-specific organizations, education programs, consensus conferences, and governmental divisions. (some features fee-based)
http://www.medscape.com/Home/Topics/
multispecialty/directories/dir-MULT.PracticeGuide.html

Medscout: Medical Specialty Guidelines Medscout offers access to a variety of practice guidelines across many medical specialties at this large online collection. The American Academy of Family Physicians, the American Association of Clinical Endocrinologists, the American Heart Association, the American Diabetes Association, and several additional specialty organizations are represented at this address. By accessing any individual recommendation or consensus statement link, visitors are taken to individual organization collections. http://www.medscout.com/guidelines/medical_specialty/

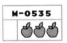

National Guideline Clearinghouse (NGC) Visitors can search the National Guide Clearinghouse (NGC), a principal U.S. government database, by typing keywords in the search box or browsing the NGC by disorder, treatment, or organization sponsor. Clinical practice guidelines can be compared, and the NGC provides guideline syntheses for guidelines regarding various conditions. This comprehensive database, offering structured abstracts, links to full-texts, and an electronic forum for information exchange, is produced by the Agency for Healthcare Research and Quality in partnership with the American Medical Association and the American Association of Health Plans.
http://www.guideline.gov/index.asp

University of California San Francisco (UCSF): Primary Care Clinical Practice Guidelines This searchable site offers primary care clinical practice guidelines in over 20 specialty categories. By entering keywords or clicking on infectious disease, mental disorders, cardiovascular system, skin, pregnancy, or any other listing, visitors are taken to large collections of online guidelines, sponsored by a variety of reputable professional organizations, government divisions, and academic institutions.
http://medicine.ucsf.edu/resources/guidelines/

8.4 DRUG INFORMATION SOURCES

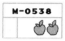

Drug InfoNet: Pharmaceutical Manufacturer Information   Links, addresses, e-mail contacts, and telephone numbers are provided for numerous ethical drug manufacturers, such as Allergan, Inc., Biocraft Laboratories, Bristol-Myers Squibb, the Immunex Corporation, and the Wyeth-Ayerst Laboratories, as well as for over-the-counter/consumer drug manufacturers.
http://www.druginfonet.com/maninfo.htm

DrugKnowledge Databases   Visitors can access drug information through DrugKnowledge databases by brand name, generic name, manufacturer, indication, contraindication, side effect, or drug category through the integrated index at this site. The DrugKnowledge database includes the DrugDex System, the Poisindex System, Martindale, *Physicians' Desk Reference,* Index Nominum, and Complementary and Alternative Medicine databases.
http://www.micromedex.com/products/pd-drugk.htm

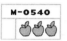

MEDLINEplus Health Information: Drug Information   This guide, provided by the National Library of Medicine, offers alphabetized information on more than 9,000 prescription and over-the-counter medications, provided by the United States Pharmacopeia. The database may be browsed by the first letter of the generic or brand name of the drug, with contents of individual drug sites including its category, description, indications, precautions, and side effects.   http://www.nlm.nih.gov/medlineplus/druginformation.html

MICROMEDEX: DRUGDEX System   DRUGDEX offers subscribers an information service for unbiased drug information that includes an overview of each drug, dosing information, pharmacokinetics, cautions, and clinical applications. The independently reviewed data is gathered from the medical literature for FDA-approved and investigational drugs, along with over-the-counter products and non-U.S. preparations.
(fee-based) http://www.micromedex.com/products/pd-drugdxsys.htm

PDR.net   Information for consumers, physicians, pharmacists, and other healthcare professionals is available at this single location. PDR Online and PDR Multi-drug Interactions are available, as well as new drug information, pricing, and related medical news from Reuters sources. Registration for free access to PDR.net is available.
http://www.pdr.net/

8.5 EVIDENCE-BASED MEDICINE

Agency for Healthcare Research and Quality (AHRQ): Evidence-based Practice   Evidence-based reports from the Agency for Healthcare Research and Quality (AHRQ) and a listing of evidence-based practice centers nationwide are found at this AHRQ site. Summaries of available evidence reports

regarding a broad range of diseases can be accessed and include findings, decision analyses, future research considerations, and links to full evidence reports. http://www.ahcpr.gov/clinic/epcix.htm

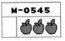

Boston University: Evidence-Based Medicine Evidence-based medicine resources from the Alumni Medical Library of Boston University provide access to instructional slide shows, tutorials, medical glossaries, library, and information resources, including textbooks and primary literature sources and tips for searching MEDLINEplus. In addition, links are presented to information on journals, including *Evidence-Based Health Policy and Management* and *Best Evidence,* as well as links to related Internet sites, such as the American College of Physicians, the Agency for Healthcare Research and Quality, CenterWatch, and the National Library of Medicine's Health Services/Technology Assessment Text. http://med-libwww.bu.edu/library/ebm.html

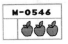

HealthLinks: Evidence-Based Practice and Guidelines As its name implies, this HealthLinks site offers an assortment of tools and full-text publications of authoritative evidence-based practice. Guides to finding the best available studies and guidelines; definitions, glossaries, and calculators in evidence-based practice; reviews related to understanding evidence-based papers; and links to scientific centers of evidence-based research are provided. http://healthlinks.washington.edu/clinical/guidelines.html

New York Online Access to Health (NOAH): Evidence-Based Medicine (EBM) Those seeking information on evidence-based practice will find a variety of useful links at this site. EBM is defined for both consumers and physicians at a variety of articles on the subject, and numerous discussions of laboratory and outcomes research, clinical trials, and levels of evidence are accessible. Documents addressing research methods, statistical terms in EBM, and special considerations with regard to medical decision-making, understanding news stories, and using systematic reviews are examined at this educational collection of links. http://www.noah-health.org/english/ebhc/ebhc.html

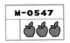

University of Sheffield: Core Library for Evidence-Based Practice A virtual library of full text documents can be accessed from this compilation of sites, including articles on literature-searching and evidence- interpretation, review of research, and specifics on how best to utilize a variety of study types. Basic statistics for clinicians, systematic reviews, guidelines on interpreting various papers, and meta-analysis approaches are addressed. Additional sections of the library examine controlled trials and practical applications of research and primary care. http://www.shef.ac.uk/~scharr/ir/core.html

8.6 INFORMATICS

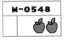

Agency for Healthcare Research and Quality (AHRQ): Healthcare Informatics Healthcare informatics, including public health data sources,

standard activities for federal agencies, medical informatics and health services research data, and clinical vocabulary links are available at this site from the Agency for Healthcare Research and Quality. Links to information on research findings, funding opportunities, consumer health, clinical details, and medical news are also featured.
http://www.ahcpr.gov/data/infoix.htm

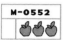

American College of Physicians-American Society of Internal Medicine (ACP-ASIM): Computers in Medicine ACP-ASIM online offers valuable resources for professionals in clinical practice, including newsgroup access, a Telemedicine Resource Center, and a link to the American Medical Informatics Association. "Web Sites for Internists" is a compilation of sites reviewed by the ACP-ASIM, which may prove to be useful resources in Continuing Medical Education, medical news, and medical specialty supersites. Information on electronic products and several articles provide authoritative medical informatics reference for practicing professionals.
http://www.acponline.org/computer/cim.htm

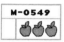

American Medical Informatics Association The home page of the American Medical Informatics Association presents information on press releases, news and developments, research and grants, and the Association's missions, goals, and objectives. Access to AMIA publications, such as the *Journal of the American Medical Informatics Association,* and Guidelines for the Use of Electronic Mail with Patients are provided. Details about the various AMIA working and special interest groups are presented, along with information about the organization's academic and training programs. Additional informatics resources on the Web can be accessed from the site.
http://www.amia.org

Duke University Medical Center: Clinical Informatics Links to worldwide medical informatics Web sites are provided at this site, hosted by the Division of Clinical Informatics at the Duke University Medical Center. Over fifty organizations, associations, institutes, and divisions are presented, including the American Health Information Management Association, the Medical Records Institute, the Yale Center for Medical Informatics, and the American Medical Informatics Association. Program details, research, and event links are provided. http://dmi-www.mc.duke.edu/

International Medical Informatics Association: Medical Informatics The International Medical Informatics Association (IMIA) offers a downloadable flyer describing the association, as well as access to the recommendations of the IMIA on education in health and medical informatics. Electronic editions of IMIA newsletters are presented, as well as links to IMIA working groups, member societies located worldwide, and institutional members.
http://www.imia.org

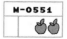

Medscout: Medical Informatics Medical informatics is presented at this site from Medscout, with approximately one-hundred links to sites that include

the American Medical Informatics Association, various medical informatics newsletters and journals, and medical informatics on the Internet. Medical informatics resources for various health topics, such as death, diseases, ethics, education, aging, and telemedicine can also be accessed through this site.
http://www.medscout.com/informatics/index.htm

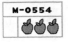

National Library of Medicine (NLM) Health information sources, including MEDLINEplus, ClinicalTrials.gov, DIRLINE, and the NLM Gateway are made available at this site from the United States National Library of Medicine. Links to information about research programs in the areas of computational molecular biology, medical informatics, digital computing and communications, digital library research, extramural funding opportunities, interactive multimedia technology, and medical informatics training are provided. In addition, visitors to this site can access announcements, press releases, information on what's new at the National Center for Biotechnology and exhibitions and public programs of the NLM.
http://www.nlm.nih.gov/

8.7 LAW AND MEDICINE

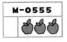

American Medical Association (AMA): Legal Issues for Physicians
Addressing legal concerns of healthcare practitioners, providers can access information in the areas of business and management, patient-physician relationships, and compliance. Various medical case summaries are provided, as well as a Compliance Interactive Tutorial System, and information on the litigation center, which serves as a legal advocate for the medical profession.
http://www.ama-assn.org/ama/pub/category/4541.html

American Society of Law, Medicine, and Ethics Information about two peer-reviewed journals, access to research projects on pain and undertreatment, a news section containing information on recent developments in the field, and details on free Web membership are offered at this multidisciplinary domain. Upcoming conference details, real audio presentations addressing the impact of new technologies on medicine and public policy, current news, publications, and related links are provided.
(some features fee-based) http://www.aslme.org/

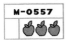

MedNets: Medical Law Links to greater than 30 medical law resources, including the American Bar Association Health Law Section, AMA Statements on Advanced Directives, Expert Witness Net, the Health Care Liability Alliance, Medical Care Law, the U.S. States Abortion Laws, and the Law and Legislative Center, are provided at this site. Additional information on medical malpractice carriers, medical law databases, health law journals, and related medical ethics issue coverage are available.
http://www.mednets.com/medlaw.htm

8.8 MANAGED CARE

American Medical Association (AMA): Other Managed Care Issues
A definition of this continuously evolving trend in healthcare delivery is found at this page, in addition to a connection to the AMA's Principles of Managed Care in Adobe Acrobat format. Geared toward physician readers, chapters on managed care contracts, utilization management, and disease management are provided, offering key components of the AMA's efforts to address ethical and policy issues of the system.
http://www.ama-assn.org/ama/pub/category/3371.html

Medscape: Managed Care Helping to keep physicians and other health-care professionals abreast of the most current medical, economic, and legal issues surrounding managed care delivery, this site's assortment of connections is an indispensable reference for practitioners and others interested in managed care developments. Regularly updated managed care news, current conference coverage, and articles on new developments and implementation of programs are found at this Medscape specialty center.
(free registration) http://www.medscape.com/Home/Topics/managedcare/managedcare.html

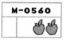

National Committee for Quality Assurance Reporting on the state of the nation's managed care plans, this non-profit organization evaluates health-care and provides its visitors with information to help decide on health plan selection. Online publications and products, the annual "State of Managed Care Quality Report," and the committee's "Health Plan Report Card" on accredited plans are all easily and freely accessible.
http://www.ncqa.org/

Northern Light: Special Edition Managed Care Providing a wide selection of managed care resources, this site of Northern Light offers access to consumer issues and information, prescription drug discussions, information geared toward healthcare professionals, and links to individual managed care plan Web sites. Attention to industry standards and developments, current articles, Web sites, and updates in healthcare legislation are offered. Important links include health insurance reform proposals of the American Medical Association and the American College of Physicians-American Society of Internal Medicine page on effective medical practice and managed care delivery.
http://special.northernlight.com/managedcare/index.html#hmo

8.9 MEDICAL CREDENTIALS AND LICENSURE

Federation of State Medical Boards The Federation of State Medical Boards (FSMB) online provides visitors with policy documents, details on post-licensure assessment, the credentials verification service, state medical board information, and subscription information for FSMB publications, such as the

Journal of Medical Licensure and Discipline. The FSMB Library is accessible to members of the organization.

(some features fee-based) http://www.fsmb.org

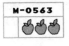

National Board of Medical Examiners After entering this Web site, visitors gain access to information on the United States Medical Licensing Examination, including services provided to medical schools and healthcare professionals. Post-licensure assessment and pages on research and development supported by the board are available.

http://www.nbme.org/

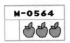

United States Medical Licensing Examination News regarding scoring, answers to FAQs about the exam, and samples of test questions and test formats are presented at this site, sponsored by the Federation of State Medical Boards of the United States and the National Board of Medical Examiners. Testing accommodations, practice session information, and important related links are all provided, including connections to the Education Commission for Foreign Medical Graduates and the Association of American Medical Colleges.

http://www.usmle.org/

8.10 MEDICAL ETHICS

American Medical Association (AMA): Ethics Standards The AMA provides links to its Council on Ethical and Judicial Affairs, Ethics Resouce Center, and Institute for Ethics at the AMA, along with faculty biographies, and selected publications and presentations. Particular topics covered are end-of-life care and guidelines to accepting gifts from industry. Ethics resources are provided in the areas of professionalism, outreach activities, research, and federation activities. http://www.ama-assn.org/ama/pub/category/2416.html

American Medical Association (AMA): Principles of Medical Ethics Principles adopted by the American Medical Association (AMA) as the essentials of honorable behavior for the physician are listed at this ethics standards page. Seven points addressing physicians' dealings with both patients and colleagues are presented. Links to fundamental elements of the physician-patient relationship and printable ethics reports of the Council on Ethical and Judicial Affairs adopted by the AMA are available.

http://www.ama-assn.org/ama/pub/category/2512.html

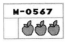

Medscout: Medical Ethics Over one-hundred medical ethics resources are presented at this site from Medscout, including connections to the American Society of Bioethics and Humanities, the Center for Ethics and Professionalism, Values and Biotechnology, Disease Intervention, the Center for Clinical Ethics and Humanities in Health Care, and the National Human Genome Research Institute. http://www.medscout.com/ethics

8.11 PRACTICE MANAGEMENT

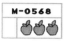

American College of Physicians-American Society of Internal Medicine (ACP-ASIM): Practice Operation and Ownership Provided by the American College of Physicians and the American Society of Internal Medicine, this site offers several articles on the managed care environment, effective office operations, selection of practice management systems, and employment and ownership considerations. To take advantage of this collection, membership in the ASP-ASIM is required. However, overviews of the material are available to all.

http://www.acponline.org/cca/practice.htm

Galaxy: Information and Practice Management Services and technology links for medical practice management are offered at this Web listing, including FamilyPractice.com, Health Card Technologies, Inc., the Healthcare Marketplace, MedComm International, PharmComm, Inc., and the Summex Corporation Home Page. Communication systems, medical records management, and multimedia tools for diagnosis are offered at this Internet selection of pages.

http://www.galaxy.com/galaxy/Business-and-Commerce/General-Products-and-Services/Health-and-Medicine/Information-and-Practice-Management.html

Medical Group Management Association Practice solutions, practice tools, and access to the Virtual Exhibit Hall with resources by category are featured at this site from the Medical Group Management Association. A leading organization for professional practice management, this group offers access to information on educational events, government affairs, networking details, interactive tools, survey reports, and MGMA publications.

http://www.mgma.com

MedMarket.com MedMarket.com, a medical industry Web site, provides healthcare professionals with information and resources for coding and compliance products, computer systems, financial services, insurance, medical billing, office organizing systems, travel and meetings, consulting, continuing education, equipment repair, and training.

http://www.medmarket.com/index.cfm?id=pract_mgmt

Medscape: The Journal of Medical Practice Management Abstracts and full-text articles are available to registered users at this online journal site of Medscape. Available content includes current feature articles and archived issues that address software systems, managed care, economic trends in healthcare delivery, and billing and coding topics.

(free registration) http://managedcare.medscape.com/JMPM/public/JMPM-journal.html

Practice Development Insights Updated daily, this practice resource site provides connections to online forums, facilitating professional communication in the field. Insights on budgeting time and clinical resources, details on practice

development on the World Wide Web, and ideas for generating referrals are supplied. Hiring practices and additional topics in marketing are addressed. http://www.wpicomm.com/pdi/

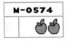 **PrimeMedical.Net**   Information on practice management is provided through a list of links at this site that connect to a variety of administrative service organizations for the business support of a medical practice. Coding and billing resources, medical reference sites, a physician educational resource corner, medical organization links, and online medical journal listings are provided. http://www.primemedical.net/practicemangement.htm

8.12 TELEMEDICINE

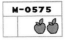 **American Telemedicine Association**   This nonprofit organization, a leader in advocating telemedicine technologies, serves as a clearinghouse for telemedical information and services and promotes research and education in the field. Members of the organization have access to the online version of the *TeleMedicine Journal,* newsletter archives, and access to member product and service discounts. A listing of upcoming events is posted at the site. (some features fee-based) http://www.atmeda.org/

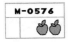 **Galaxy: Telemedicine**   Telemedicine resource listings and links are provided at this site from Galaxy, a medical portal. Featured pages include online centers for telemedicine and telemedicine law, the Association of Telehealth Service Providers, and multimedia workstation information. http://www.galaxy.com/cgi-bin/dirlist?node=53155

 Telemedicine Information Exchange   Created and maintained by the Telemedicine Research Center with support from the National Institutes of Health, this page offers access to frequently asked questions about telemedicine, articles providing basic information for newcomers to telemedicine, and a searchable Telemedicine Programs Database of programs nationwide and abroad. Special coverage of home health and telemedicine, citations from current telemedicine journals, and links to related online resources are included. http://tie.telemed.org/

 Telemedicine Today   This online magazine provides visitors with connections to articles that cover a broad range of telemedicine subspecialties. Telehome healthcare, telecardiology, general telemedicine, and emergency telemedicine are all included in the listing of abstract and article collections. A state-by-state legal guide, an online telemedicine forum, and tables of contents and some articles to back issues of the newsletter are provided. http://www.telemedtoday.com/

9

PRESENTING CONDITIONS

9.1 ABDOMINAL PAIN

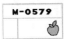

Abdominal Pain Gastoenterology Consultants offer this review of abdominal pain as a frequent symptom with various causes. Questions that might be asked of the patient by the physician are presented, as well as a brief discussion of the nature of the pain, which, once noted, is useful in delineating various etiologies. http://www.gastro.com/abdpain.htm

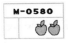

Flowcharts on Familydoctor.org: Abdominal Pain, Chronic From the American Academy of Family Physicians *Family Health and Medical Guide,* this familydoctor.org page offers a self-care algorithm for evaluation of dull, ongoing pain in the abdomen. The flowchart allows each visitor to reach a fast conclusion regarding the most appropriate way to proceed, which may warrant over-the-counter remedies, dietary interventions, or immediate physician consultation. http://familydoctor.org/flowcharts/528.html

9.2 ACID BASE DISORDERS, GENERAL

eMedicine: Metabolic Acidosis eMedicine's instant access textbook offers a complete review of the differential diagnosis of metabolic acidosis, as well as a method for determining the underlying cause with laboratory testing. Authored by Karen L. Stavile, a physician at the State University of New York Health Science Center, the page provides clinical strategies for treatment that include emergency care and alkalinizing agents.
http://www.eMedicine.com/cgi-
bin/foxweb.exe/showsection@d:/em/ga?book=emerg&topicid=312

Postgraduate Medicine: Acid-Base Disorders Originally published in the March 2000 issue of *Postgraduate Medicine,* this full-text article takes a stepwise approach to acid-base disorders. The article offers a table of common clinical states and associated acid-base disorders, along with a discussion regarding diagnostic tests and assessing the accuracy of data. Compensation formulas for simple acid-base disorders are covered, and several illustrative case studies are examined. A bibliography is provided.
http://www.postgradmed.com/issues/2000/03_00/fall.htm

9.3 ALKALOSIS

Alkalosis Precipitating causes, differential diagnosis, and treatment for both metabolic and respiratory alkalosis are outlined at this site of the Pepid database. Variable treatment, according to underlying cause and distinction between chloride-responsive and chloride-resistant metabolic varieties, are presented.
http://www.pepid.com/pepidce/meh/meh140.htm

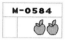

Temple University: Metabolic Alkalosis The primary processes associated with metabolic alkalosis and the related respiratory and renal compensatory mechanisms are described at this Web outline. Conditions in which metabolic alkalosis may occur, differentiation between saline sensitive and saline resistant metabolic alkalosis, and diagnostic criteria are discussed.
http://blue.temple.edu/~pathphys/renal/metabolic_alkalosis.html

9.4 ANEMIA

Blood Cells and Anemia: Pathophysiologic Consequences Authored by a diplomate of the American Board of Pathology, this page is the second of a five-part series on blood cells and anemia. Information on the physiological compensations for decreased blood mass in nutritional anemias, anemias of chronic disease, hemolytic varieties, and hemoglobinopathies and thalassemias is discussed. Clinical signs and symptoms and classifications are presented.
http://www.neosoft.com/~uthman/anemia/anemia.html

MEDLINEplus Health Information: Anemia An assortment of site links related to anemia is accessible from this site of the National Library of Medicine, with overviews, anatomy and physiology, and specific aspects of the symptom discussed. Pages on treatment and information specific to individual disorders and different populations are accessible.
http://www.nlm.nih.gov/medlineplus/anemia.html

9.5 APNEA

Agency for Health Care Policy and Research: Systematic Review of the Literature Regarding the Diagnosis of Sleep Apnea MetaWorks investigators present a summary review of the current literature on sleep apnea, with key questions guiding the review, research methodology, and findings from various studies relayed. Future research directions and a connection to the full report of the former Agency for Health Care Policy and Research are offered.
http://www.ahcpr.gov/clinic/apnea.htm

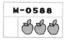

American Sleep Apnea Association This organizational site contains information for healthcare professionals and publications for patients regarding sleep apnea evaluation and treatment. Pages on personal experiences are accessible, and an online or mail order information packet may be obtained free of charge. http://www.sleepapnea.org/

9.6 ASCITES

Virtual Hospital: Ascites From University of Iowa Health Care, information at this page provides an examination of diagnostic and therapeutic paracentesis and other important interventions for reduction of serous fluid in the abdomen. http://www.vh.org/Providers/ClinRef/FPHandbook/Chapter04/14-4.html

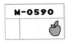

Virtual Hospital: Introduction to Clinical Radiology: Ascites Virtual Hospital's introduction to clinical radiology offers information on the clinical presentation of ascites accompanied by an X-ray film of a patient with massive ascites. http://www.vh.org/Providers/Lectures/icmrad/abdominal/parts/Ascites.html

9.7 BLEEDING, ABNORMAL MENSTRUAL

Abnormal/Irregular Menstrual Bleeding A discussion of normal menstrual bleeding is discussed and accompanied by a table comparing some common causes of irregular or abnormal bleeding. Nine conditions are listed, with the causes, symptoms, diagnosis, and treatment options reviewed, courtesy of the Web site, "A World for Women."
http://www.mjbovo.com/AbnlBleed.htm

Women's Diagnostic Cyber: Abnormal Menstrual Bleeding Authored by Frederick R. Jelovsek, M.D., this series answers common inquiries regarding changes in menstrual flow and various aspects of abnormal bleeding. From the menu at the right side of the page, visitors can find related article access, a document discussing differential diagnosis, and a list of related publications.
http://www.wdxcyber.com/mbleed.htm

9.8 BLEEDING, GASTROINTESTINAL

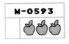

Merck Manual of Diagnosis and Therapy: Gastrointestinal Bleeding Hematemesis, hematochezia, and melena are introduced, with symptoms and signs, a discussion of diagnosis based on exam and diagnostic testing, and assessment and restoration of blood loss reviewed. An emphasis on the prevention of complications, as well as accessible tables and chapters outlining causes of GI bleeding, shock, and peptic ulcer treatment are provided.
http://www.merck.com/pubs/mmanual/section3/chapter22/22a.htm

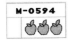

National Institute of Diabetes and Digestive and Kidney Diseases (NIDDK): Bleeding in the Digestive Tract An information sheet offered by the National Digestive Diseases Information Clearinghouse offers a discussion of causes, recognition, diagnosis, and treatment of bleeding in the digestive

tract, with a table outlining causes based on various gastrointestinal tract locations. http://www.niddk.nih.gov/health/digest/pubs/bleeding/bleeding.htm

9.9 BLEEDING, GENERAL

International Federation of Red Cross and Red Crescent Societies: Bleeding   Management of uncontrolled bleeding, external bleeding, and internal bleeding is addressed at this page, with review of symptoms and signs and immediate actions to take.
http://members.tripod.com/RCSSAS/bleeding.html

Virtual Hospital: Bleeding Disorders   The focus of the site is on determining the type and causes of specific bleeding disorders. Presentation of bleeding conditions, physical exam, and differential diagnosis of abnormal bleeding are outlined at this peer-reviewed site of the University of Iowa.
http://www.vh.org/Providers/ClinRef/FPHandbook/Chapter05/01-5.html

9.10 CHEST PAIN

Chest Pain Simulator Computer Program Manual: The Approach to Chest Pain   Ten specific causes of chest pain are identified at this site of the *Chest Pain Simulator Computer Program Manual*. General information regarding symptoms and the physical examination in angina, myocardial infarction, pneumonia, pericarditis, mitral prolapse, and other conditions are examined. Approaches to the clinical management of chest pain are introduced.
http://www.madsci.com/manu/indxches.htm

Flowcharts on Familydoctor.org: Chest Pain, Acute   The American Academy of Family Physicians offers visitors to this page a chest pain flowchart for identifying symptoms and causes, as well as the proper self-care or emergency action to take. A series of questions leads viewers to an appropriate conclusion based on subjective answers regarding symptoms.
http://www.familydoctor.org/flowcharts/523.html

9.11 CLAUDICATION

American Family Physician: A Primary Care Approach to the Patient with Claudication   Authored by physicians of the Cleveland Clinic in Florida, this publication site of the American Academy of Family Physicians provides information on the proper evaluation and examination of patients presenting with intermittent claudication. Tables and figures outline differential diagnosis, stages of peripheral arterial occlusive disease, and pulse volume recording. An information handout on the subject intended for patient distribution may be accessed from the page. http://www.aafp.org/afp/20000215/1027.html

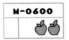

Heart Canada: Intermittent Claudication As a service of Heart Canada, a description of intermittent claudication, as well as a discussion of causes, other symptoms of arterial insufficiency, assessment, and both conservative and surgical interventions are reviewed at this LifeMD.com site.
http://www.heartcanada.com/claudication.php

9.12 CONFUSION

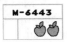

Elder Advocates: Helping to Prevent Symptoms of Confusion in the Elderly Delirium brought on by depression, nutritional imbalances, infection, and other problems specific to the elderly is addressed at this page. A list of medications frequently known to cause confusion in elderly patients is presented at the site, which emphasizes the importance of identification of the causes of confusion. http://www.eldercareadvocates.com/pages/art14.htm

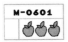

National Institutes of Health (NIH): Priority Expert Panel on Long-Term Care for Older Adults: Confusion Discussion of confusion in the aging population is addressed at this site of the National Institutes of Health. Five sources of confusion are identified, including compromised brain support, sensoriperceptual problems, and the true dementias. Review of studies relating to acute and chronic confusional states and the state of science regarding delirium, sundown syndrome, irreversible dementias, Alzheimer's disease and related states, treatment in the institutional setting, and research needs are addressed.
http://www.nih.gov/ninr/research/vol3/Confusion.html

9.13 CONSTIPATION

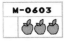

MEDLINEplus Health Information: Constipation A wide range of information on constipation can be accessed at this site. Links provide information on the condition, diagnostic procedures, nutrition tips, and self-care. Documents on lower-GI tract radiology, organization connections, and subsections dedicated to children and seniors are found.
http://www.nlm.nih.gov/medlineplus/constipation.html

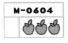

National Digestive Diseases Information Clearinghouse: Constipation In addition to an "Easy-to-Read" site on the topic, visitors will find details on causes, diagnostic tests, and treatment for constipation. Points to remember, dietary considerations, and related conditions and diseases are discussed. http://www.niddk.nih.gov/health/digest/pubs/const/const.htm

9.14 CONVULSIONS/SEIZURES

Health at Home: Seizures A chapter of *Health at Home,* offered as a service of the American Institute for Preventive Medicine, reviews causes and symptoms of seizures, as well as self-care tips and first aid for seizure victims.
http://www.mcare.org/healthtips/homecare/SEIZURES.HTM

National Center for Emergency Medicine Informatics: Seizures Emergency medicine resources from the National Center for Emergency Medicine Informatics include this guideline on seizures, which discusses the patient presentation, immediate measures to take, and a discussion of grand mal seizures. Diagnostic studies to be obtained are reviewed.
http://www.ncemi.org/cse/cse0104.htm

9.15 COUGH

PathoPlusPage: Tutorial on Cough The physiology of cough as an important defense mechanism is discussed at this site, with information on effective versus ineffective cough, protussive and antitussive therapies, and conditions in which cough is a symptom. Additional authoritative resources may be accessed from the site, including the full text of the American College of Chest Physicians (ACCP) Consensus Statement on cough presented by Medscape.
http://www.pathoplus.com/cough.htm

Patient-Oriented Evidence That Matters: Diagnosis of Chronic Cough Information geared toward the primary care clinician reviews the differential diagnosis of chronic cough. The most common causes of chronic cough among patients referred for evaluation and the symptoms associated with specific diagnoses are presented.
http://www.infopoems.com/POEMs/JC099602.htm

9.16 CYANOSIS

Merck Manual of Diagnosis and Therapy: Cyanosis *Merck Manual of Diagnosis and Therapy* differentiates peripheral and central cyanosis at this site, which discusses the primary problems that may result in reduced blood Hg. Links to related topics, such as dyspnea, chest pain, and cough, are found.
http://www.merck.com/pubs/mmanual/section6/chapter63/63h.htm

University of Arkansas for Medical Sciences: Cyanosis Authored by Gary D. Wright of the University of Arkansas for Medical Sciences, this article suggests a variety of factors that may contribute to the subjective presence of cyanosis. Clinical features of central and peripheral cyanosis, differential diagnosis, and emergency standards of care are presented.
http://www.statdoc.com/Emerald/pubs/Wright_pubs/cyanosis.htm

9.17 DEHYDRATION

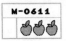

eMedicine: Dehydration Dehydration in the pediatric population is presented at this eMedicine article, authored by Ann G. England, M.D. The pathophysiology of dehydration; isonatremic, hyponatremic, and hypernatremic volume depletion; potassium considerations; and acid and base problems are reviewed. Clinical presentation, causes, a host of convenient links to diagnostic differentials, and MEDLINE reference connections are provided.
http://www.emedicine.com/emerg/topic372.htm

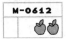

Information On Dehydration The definition, causes, and symptoms of dehydration, specifically in those with eating disorders, are presented at this fact sheet from Support, Concern, and Resources for Eating Disorders. Dangers of dehydration, dehydration prevention, and treatment sections are offered for consumer reference.
http://www.eating-disorder.org/dehydration.html

9.18 DELIRIUM

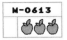

Internet Mental Health: Delirium Internet Mental Health's complete American and European diagnostic criteria and features of delirium are available for viewing, as well as current research in the area, online booklets and related articles, and a PDF quick reference guide for physicians from the American Psychiatric Association.
http://www.mentalhealth.com/dis/p20-or01.html

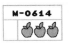

Merck Manual Home Edition: Delirium and Dementia Differences between delirium and dementia are recognized at this online Merck publication. Common causes of both, symptoms, diagnosis, treatment, and side-by-side comparisons are made at the page.
http://www.merck.com/pubs/mmanual_home/sec6/76.htm

9.19 DIZZINESS/VERTIGO

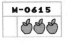

MEDLINEplus Health Information: Dizziness and Vertigo Links to overviews, clinical trials, images and diagrams, and specific conditions related to dizziness and vertigo may be accessed at this National Institutes of Health presentation. A directory of organizations with a focus on health issues relating to hearing, balance, voice, speech, and language is provided as a service of the National Institutes on Deafness and Other Communications Disorders.
http://www.nlm.nih.gov/medlineplus/dizzinessandvertigo.html

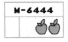

Northwestern University: Dizziness in the Elderly Five causes of dizziness in the geriatric population are considered in this article, including otologic, central, medical, psychogenic, and unlocalized etiologies. Thorough

definitions of each and a summary of the diverse causes and the diagnostic process are included. Tables at the site profile vestibular suppressants, as well as drugs that may cause ataxia.
http://www.galter.nwu.edu/geriatrics/chapters/dizziness.cfm

9.20 DYSMENORRHEA

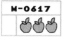

American Family Physician: Primary Dysmenorrhea The American Academy of Family Physicians offers a full-text article on primary dysmenorrhea, including its epidemiology, a figure outlining menstrual fluid prostaglandin levels, and a table which lists circumstances indicative of secondary dysmenorrhea. Clinical presentation, diagnosis, possible causes, and complete treatment information are presented. http://www.aafp.org/afp/990800ap/489.html

eMedicine: Dysmenorrhea Authored by Alan D. Clark, M.D., a member of the American College of Emergency Physicians, this article provides comprehensive educational material on the pathophysiology, clinical presentation, and diagnostic differentials for dysmenorrhea. Laboratory and imaging studies are listed, and information on treatment with nonsteroidal anti-inflammatory agents, further outpatient care, and patient education is provided.
http://www.emedicine.com/emerg/topic156.htm

9.21 DYSPEPSIA

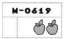

Mayo Clinic: Non-ulcer Dyspepsia Non-ulcer dyspepsia is the focus of the MayoClinic Health Oasis article, which discusses persons affected, typical symptoms, causes, and controllable factors, such as stress and fatigue. Behavioral therapy details and links to additional, related articles are provided.
http://www.mayohealth.org/home?id=HQ01120

Virtual Hospital: Dyspepsia and Peptic Ulcer Disease The *University of Iowa Family Practice Handbook* presents a peer-reviewed document on dyspepsia and peptic ulcer disease, which outlines duodenal ulcer, the role of acid control measures, complications and other considerations, gastric ulcers, and NSAID-induced gastroduodenal ulcers. Authored by Peter P. Toth, M.D., Ph.D, this chapter offers comprehensive, yet concise information on predisposing factors in peptic ulcer disease.
http://www.vh.org/Providers/ClinRef/FPHandbook/Chapter04/08-4.html

9.22 DYSPHAGIA

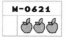

Dysphagia Resource Center Links are compiled at this page to an assortment of case studies, articles, and information related to the causes and diseases associated with dysphagia. Conference announcements, related Internet sites, research information and funding, journals and other publications, and connections offering online tutorials are provided at this large Internet collection. http://www.dysphagia.com/

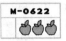

MEDLINEplus Health Information: Dysphagia   The National Library of Medicine's MEDLINEplus Health Information contains several connections to information on dysphagia, as provided by the National Institutes of Health, the American Gastroenterological Association, and additional private organizations. Fact sheets and other accessible publications address specific conditions and aspects of dysphagia, as well as diagnosis and current clinical trials. http://www.nlm.nih.gov/medlineplus/dysphagia.html

9.23 DYSPNEA

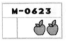

Alliance for Lung Cancer: Dyspnea   Providing advocacy, support, and educational material, this organization offers a fact sheet on symptom management, providing tips for quick relief of dyspnea. Sections of the text contain information on controlled breathing, relaxation, and supplemental oxygen and medications. http://www.alcase.org/education/bestcare/dyspnea.html

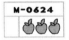

American Family Physician: Diagnostic Evaluation of Dyspnea Authors from Kaiser Permanente Medical Center discuss the pathophysiology, differential diagnosis, history and physical examination, and other assessment details at this full text article. This American Academy of Family Physicians site includes information on arterial blood gas analysis and pulmonary function testing, and is supplemented by tables regarding clues to causative conditions and spirometric parameters in diagnosis.
http://www.aafp.org/afp/980215ap/morgan.html

9.24 DYSTONIAS

National Institute of Neurological Disorders and Stroke (NINDS): The Dystonias   A description of the dystonias and information on early symptoms, disease classifications, and known brain abnormalities are reviewed at the National Institute of Neurological Disorders and Stroke Web site. An outline of surgery, medications, and other treatments, and ongoing NINDS research studies and goals are presented.
http://www.ninds.nih.gov/health_and_medical/pubs/dystonias.htm

Society for Neuroscience: Dystonias   The Society for Neuroscience offers this "Brain Briefing," addressing individuals affected by the involuntary muscle contractions associated with dystonias. Current research demonstrating genetic factors and alterations in dopamine are discussed, and discoveries surrounding diagnosis, treatments, and further complexities of the illness are reviewed.
http://www.sfn.org/briefings/dystonias.html

9.25 EDEMA

M-0627

MEDLINEplus Medical Encyclopedia: Swelling The National Library of Medicine offers MEDLINEplus Medical Encyclopedia for consumers, including a review of edema and overall swelling. Visitors will find an enlargeable image of pitting edema of the leg, an overview of the condition, and a connection to treatment information.
http://www.nlm.nih.gov/medlineplus/ency/article/003103.htm

M-0628

ThriveOnline: Swelling ThriveOnline's Medical Library offers this page on swelling, with related links provided to information on angioedema and several other specific types of swelling. Edema, generalized swelling or massive edema, links to information on common causes, and five enlargeable thumbnail images are offered to visitors.
http://thriveonline.oxygen.com/medical/library/article/003103.html

9.26 FATIGUE, EXCESSIVE

M-6445

Lycos Health with WebMD: Fatigue Created by adam.com, this page offers access to information on several diseases that may have fatigue as a main symptom. Considerations in differentiating between fatigue and drowsiness, possible causes, and medical questions documenting fatigue are included. Diagnostic tests that may be performed in the diagnostic workup are listed, with links available to further information on assessment and management.
http://webmd.lycos.com/content/asset/adam_symptoms_lethargy

M-0630

National Cancer Institute (NCI): Fatigue This CancerWeb site introduces the challenges of fatigue as they pertain to cancer. Definitions of acute and chronic fatigue, instruments used in the measurement of fatigue, and mechanisms that contribute to fatigue are examined. Complete assessment and interventions are reviewed.
http://www.graylab.ac.uk/cancernet/304461.html

9.27 FEVER/HYPERTHERMIA

M-0631

Matrix: Fever and Rash Viral and non-viral diseases manifested by various rashes and fever; other diseases manifested by fever and vesicles; and conditions presenting with red macules/papules or wheals and fever are outlined and listed at this page of the University of California at Davis.
http://matrix.ucdavis.edu/tumors/fever.html

M-0632

MEDLINEplus Medical Encyclopedia: Fever An overview of fever, otherwise known as hyperthermia or pyrexia, is found at this page. A definition of normal body temperature and considerations regarding temperature variations, and links to information on febrile seizures, heat stroke, and related con-

ditions are found, as well as connections to common causes of fever, such as infection and dehydration.
http://www.nlm.nih.gov/medlineplus/ency/article/003090.htm

9.28 HEARTBURN

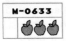

Hospital Practice: A Practical Approach to Heartburn Including a complete case presentation, as well as diagnostic and management algorithms, this Hospital Practice site offers an informative discussion of the treatment of gastroesophageal reflux disease (GERD). Adjustments in treatments and therapeutic result discussions, review of lifestyle modifications, medications, step-up and step-down approaches, and surgical interventions are reviewed, as well as the controversy surrounding *H. Pylori* infection and GERD.
http://www.hosppract.com/issues/1999/11/dmmcas.htm

St. Luke's Fact Sheets: Heartburn and Other Esophageal Problems This fact sheet, presented as a service of St. Luke's Episcopal Health System, discusses causes of heartburn or reflux, self-care tips for prevention, and further treatment measures for those who do not respond to medications and lifestyle modification measures.
http://www.sleh.com/FactSheets/fact-d06-esoph.html

9.29 HEMATEMESIS

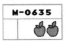

MSN Health: Vomiting Blood Consumer viewers will find information, powered by adam.com, on common causes, considerations, and what to expect regarding the physical exam in documenting hematemesis. Links to diagnostic tests, interventions, and a host of conditions associated with the regurgitation of blood from the stomach are found.
http://content.health.msn.com/content/asset/adam_symptoms_hematemesis

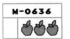

University of Alabama: Hematemesis Clinical Resources The *Merck Manual* chapter on gastrointestinal bleeding, clinical guidelines from the National Guidelines Clearinghouse, news resources, and miscellaneous hematemesis clinical resource links are compiled at this site of the Clinical Digital Libraries Project.
http://www.slis.ua.edu/cdlp/WebDLCore/
clinical/gastroenterology/symptoms/hematemesis.htm

9.30 HEMATOCHEZIA

American Journal of Gastroenterology: The Outpatient Evaluation of Hematochezia A useful discussion of hematochezia and appropriate di-

agnostic assessment is found at this online article, which emphasizes the use of flexible sigmoidoscopy in diagnosing significant colonic lesions.
http://www-east.elsevier.com/ajg/issues/9302/ajg90fla.htm

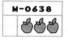

Gastroenterology Therapy Online: Acute Lower Intestinal Bleeding
The passage of bloody stool, with various descriptions and designations of lower intestinal tract bleeding, are reviewed at this article, which addresses the incidence, clinical presentation and course, and bedside diagnosis associated with color and diagnostic and physical examinations. Diagnostic procedures, criteria for diagnosis of site or level, and references are provided at this article, authored by physicians of the Washington University School of Medicine.
http://www.gastrotherapy.com/literature/articles/l2034h10.asp

9.31 HEMATURIA

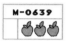

Digital Urology Journal: Hematuria Microscopic and gross hematuria are the subjects of this *Digital Urology Journal* page. The necessity of a thorough evaluation is emphasized, including intravenous pyelogram (IVP) and cystoscopy. Common, less serious reasons for hematuria and more serious conditions are outlined, and a summary of proper treatment is provided.
http://www.duj.com/hematuria.html

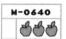

Urology Channel: Hematuria A comprehensive article denotes types of hematuria, associated symptoms, causes, classification of, and diagnostic information at site of the Urology Channel. Purposes of examination and diagnostic testing in differential diagnosis, as well as hematuria-associated symptoms suggestive of the cause of bleeding are reviewed.
http://www.urologychannel.com/Hematuria/index.shtml

9.32 HEMOPTYSIS

Pulmonology Channel: Hemoptysis The most common and least serious causes of hemoptysis are reviewed, along with distinctions between hemoptysis and hematemesis as an integral part of the diagnosis. Classifications of hemoptysis are reviewed, and connections to similar pages on causes, symptoms, diagnosis, and treatment follow the discussion. Many additional pages on related conditions and therapies are found throughout the Pulmonology Channel site.
http://www.pulmonologychannel.com/hemoptysis/

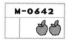

Virtual Hospital: Hemoptysis This peer-reviewed CME module offers a case presentation of hemoptysis, a discussion of the evaluation and diagnosis, and treatment related to specific etiology. Media for diagnosis can be enlarged and viewed at the site.
http://www.vh.org/Providers/TeachingFiles/
PulmonaryCoreCurric/Hemoptysis/Hemoptysis.html

9.33 HYPERPIGMENTATION/HYPOPIGMENTATION

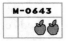

Merck Manual of Diagnosis and Therapy: Hypopigmentation   The three main types of hypopigmentation, including vitiligo, albinism, and postinflammatory hypopigmentation, are reviewed in terms of their incidence, characterizations, and treatments for cosmetic disfigurement. This Merck chapter offers a connection to its related page on hyperpigmentation management.
http://www.merck.com/pubs/mmanual/section10/chapter123/123a.htm

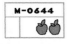

Skin Delivery: Skin Problems: Hyperpigmentation   The Skin Delivery domain offers visitors a chance to review external and internal causes of hyperpigmentation, with additional sections on treatment and information on some encouraging new breakthroughs.
http://www.rci.rutgers.edu/~zatz/Skinprobs/Hyperpig.html

9.34 HYPERVENTILATION

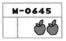

Health at Home: Hyperventilation   Provided as a service of the American Institute for Preventive Medicine, this page offers viewers information on the causes of hyperventilation, measures for prevention, and self-care tips in a concise, user-friendly format.
http://www.mcare.org/healthtips/homecare/HYPERVEN.HTM

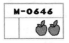

National Center for Emergency Medicine Informatics: Hyperventilation   The National Center for Emergency Medicine Informatics provides visitors with a description of the clinical presentation of hyperventilation, along with measures to take to reduce ventilatory rate and volume. A discussion of the acute metabolic acidosis of hyperventilation is found.
http://www.ncemi.org/cse/cse0102.htm

9.35 HYPOTENSION

American Family Physician: Evaluation and Treatment of Orthostatic Hypotension   The diagnosis of orthostatic hypotension, classification and clinical features, and tables outlining the nonneurogenic and neurogenic causes are presented at this full text article. Initial steps in evaluation, in addition to diagnostic tests and treatment measures are provided as a service of the American Academy of Family Physicians.   http://www.aafp.org/afp/971001ap/engstrm.html

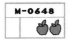

MEDLINEplus Health Information: Low Blood Pressure   A variety of information on low blood pressure can be accessed from this collection of sites, courtesy of the National Library of Medicine. Specific conditions and aspects of low blood pressure, clinical trials in hypotension, and a connection to information on the tilt-table test are found.
http://www.nlm.nih.gov/medlineplus/lowbloodpressure.html

9.36 JAUNDICE

Evaluation of the Jaundice Patient in Clinical Practice   A variety of information and definitions related to jaundice and conditions causing jaundice are presented at this page, authored by Harold Jeghers, M.D. Clinical detection of jaundice, differential of the yellow skin color, prehepatic jaundice, and medical history and examination for patients with jaundice are examined. The author also presents a list of selected references applicable to bilirubin metabolism, differential diagnosis, neonatal jaundice, cholestatic jaundice, jaundice in cirrhosis and alcoholism, and jaundice in pregnancy.
http://www.jeghers.com/annts/jaundice.htm

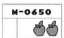

Rush-Presbyterian-St. Luke's Medical Center: Jaundice   Causes of excess bilirubin in the body, other symptoms that may occur with jaundice, and details on diagnosis of liver disease, bilirubin metabolism disorders, and hemolytic diseases are found. Links to additional information from Rush-Presbyterian-St. Luke's and World Book, Inc., are offered, including hepatitis, bilirubin, and cholelithiasis.
http://www.rush.edu/worldbook/articles/010000a/010000001.html

9.37 JOINT PAIN/ARTHRALGIAS

MEDLINEplus Medical Encyclopedia: Joint Pain   Adam.com's encyclopedic articles include this review of joint pain, which offers information on common causes and links to additional details on the symptoms and treatment for arthritis, bursitis, osteoarthritis, and a host of diseases that may be related to arthralgias.   http://www.nlm.nih.gov/medlineplus/ency/article/003261.htm

New Zealand Family Physician Focus: Assessment of the Patient with Joint Pain   This review focuses on musculoskeletal emergencies, monoarticular and polyarticular joint pain, back pain, and non-specific arthralgia/myalgia. Key musculoskeletal red flags, a discussion of articular versus periarticular disease, attention to inflammatory versus mechanical conditions, and notable considerations in the diagnosis of polyarticular joint pain are outlined. Essential points regarding examination and clinical findings are concisely summarized.   http://www.rnzcgp.org.nz/nzfp/ISSUES/June00/FOCUS_CHAPMAN.htm

9.38 LYMPHADENOPATHY/SWOLLEN GLANDS

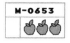

American Family Physician: Lymphadenopathy: Differential Diagnosis and Evaluation   The American Academy of Family Physicians' online articles include this review of the causes of lymphadenopathy, epidemiology, and diagnostic approaches. An algorithm for evaluation, lymph node groupings, and initial management are discussed at this authoritative, one-stop reference.
http://www.aafp.org/afp/981015ap/ferrer.html

Don't type in long URLs – add the site number to the eMedguides URL: www.eMedguides.com/**G-1234**.

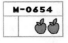

MEDLINEplus Medical Encyclopedia: Glands, Swollen: Overview
Visitors to this site will find general information on the function of the lymphatic system and a listing of common infectious, immune or autoimmune, malignancy-related, and other causes of swollen lymph glands. Hyperlinks within the text provide specific information on selected conditions, and an additional connection to diagnostic information is found.
http://www.nlm.nih.gov/medlineplus/ency/article/003097.htm

9.39 MEMORY LOSS

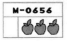

MEDLINEplus Health Information: Memory The latest news in memory impairment, clinical trials of memory disorders, current research in the field, and articles addressing specific conditions and aspects of memory loss are provided at this National Library of Medicine collection.
http://www.nlm.nih.gov/medlineplus/memory.html

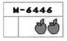

Rutgers University: Memory Disorders Project The Memory Disorders Project at Rutgers University is a group of researchers involved in promoting the understanding of memory impairing disorders and the development of accurate assessment tools. Navigation of the site brings users to answers to FAQs about memory impairment, recommended book and Web site listings, and the free *Memory and the Brain* newsletter, which provides articles about memory impairment as a result of aging, disease, or injury.
http://www.gluck.edu/memory/

9.40 MOOD ALTERATION

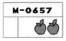

Geocities: Mood Disorders Contents of this page include symptoms and criteria for mood episodes and mood disorders, such as major depression, bipolar disorders, dysthymic and cyclothymic disorders, and mood disorders due to a general medical condition or induced by substance abuse.
http://www.geocities.com/morrison94/mood.htm

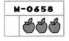

Merck Manual of Diagnosis and Therapy: Mood Disorders, General
The epidemiology, etiology of primary and secondary mood disorders, and diagnostic information are contained at this online Merck reference. The document offers links throughout to more in-depth information on the symptomatic pictures of depression, dysthymic disorder, bipolar depression, and cylothymic disorders, as well a link to information on mood disorders in children.
http://www.merck.com/pubs/mmanual/section15/chapter189/189a.htm

9.41 MOUTH SORES

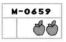

MEDLINEplus Medical Encyclopedia: Mouth Sores An overview of information and treatment details of mouth ulcers, nodules, and hemorrhagic lesions can be found on this site, which offers information on the many origins of mouth lesions and common causes.
http://www.nlm.nih.gov/medlineplus/ency/article/003059.htm

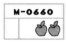

Oral Medicine Forum: Mouth sores A definition, considerations with regard to diseases that start with oral lesions, common causes, and home care suggestions are offered, as a service of Dr. Song's Oral Medicine Forum.
http://user.chollian.net/~yunheon/msore.html

9.42 MUSCLE SPASMS/CRAMPS

Physician and Sports Medicine: Skeletal Muscle Cramps During Exercise In this issue of the *The Physician and Sports Medicine* users are introduced to exercise-associated muscle cramping. The causes of cramping are discussed, and important risk factors are considered. A review of acquired syndromes, congenital abnormalities, and other acquired disorders associated with muscle cramping is found, with traditional theories of etiology presented. Management information, prevention details, and references are included.
http://www.physsportsmed.com/issues/1999/11_99/schwellnus.htm

WebMDHealth: Muscle Spasms (Cramps) WebMDHealth's Internet encyclopedic reference is powered by adam.com and offers this concise yet complete overview on the common causes of muscle spasms and muscular twitching. Diagnostic tests that may be performed are listed with respective hyperlinks to further details.
http://my.webmd.com/content/asset/adam_symptoms_spasms,_muscle

9.43 MUSCLE WEAKNESS

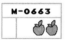

MEDLINEplus Medical Encyclopedia: Weakness Adam.com and the National Library of Medicine bring viewers background information on muscle weakness that addresses the importance of the symptom and its common causes. Visitors will find connections to metabolic, neurologic, primary muscular, toxic, and other diseases known to be associated with measurable weakness by accessing the topic in the site index.
http://www.nlm.nih.gov/medlineplus/ency/article/003174.htm

Merck Manual Home Edition: Causes of Muscle Weakness The *Home Edition* provides a table outlining the major causes of muscular weakness, with the underlying problem, related example, and important consequences re-

viewed. Muscle weakness in cases of brain or spinal cord damage, diseases of the neuromuscular junction, and psychological causes are addressed.
http://www.merck.com/pubs/mmanual_home/boxes/65b1.htm

9.44 NAUSEA AND VOMITING

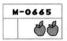

Familydoctor.org: Self-Care Flowcharts: Nausea and Vomiting As one of several self-care flowcharts provided by the American Academy of Family Physicians, this page offers an overview of the myriad of illnesses related to nausea and vomiting. The emphasis of the site is on distinguishing between mild sickness and serious illness requiring immediate medical care.
http://familydoctor.org/flowcharts/529.html

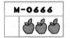

MEDLINEplus Health Information: Nausea and Vomiting As a service of the National Library of Medicine, this MEDLINEplus site offers a collection of connections to information on nausea and vomiting, with a general overview provided by the American Academy of Otolaryngology-Head and Neck Surgery, Inc. Clinical trial details, diagnosis and symptoms fact sheets, and a page on nutrition tips for managing symptoms are found. Facts on nausea and vomiting in children are provided at an assortment of selected sites.
http://www.nlm.nih.gov/medlineplus/nauseaandvomiting.html

9.45 NEURALGIAS

drkoop.com: Neuralgias Provided by adam.com, this site describes the causes and risks of various neuralgias, including tic douloureux, neuralgias resulting from blood vessel or tumor pressure, and nerve disorders. Prevention; symptoms; signs and tests; and treatment, aimed at pain control, are presented.
http://umm.drkoop.com/conditions/ency/article/001407.htm

University of Iowa Health Care: Neuralgias A single fact sheet at this site examines several disorders associated with nerve-related pain. Possible causes, drug to relieve pain, and surgical treatment options are explored.
http://www.uihealthcare.com/topics/neurologicalhealth/neur3535.html

9.46 NOCTURIA

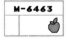

Harvard Health Letter: Nocturia This health topic from the *Harvard Health Letter* considers the significance of nocturia, with various etiologies outlined. Night time urination as a symptom of sleep problems, normal patterns of urination, and nocturia associated with prostate problems are considered.
http://www.webpoint.com/tms/harvard/special/dis_urinary/urinary1.htm

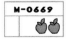

MEDLINEplus Medical Encyclopedia: Urination, Excessive at Night
The frequent need to urinate at night is defined at this encyclopedic reference of

the National Library of Medicine. Links to additional information on common causes, such as diabetes mellitus and benign prostatic hyperplasia are accessible after locating the main topic from the site index.

http://www.nlm.nih.gov/medlineplus/ency/article/003141.htm

9.47 OVERACTIVE BLADDER

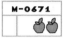

American Medical Women's Association: Overactive Bladder   An article reprinted from the American Foundation for Urological Disease presents information on the effect of overactive bladders on people's lives, urgency symptoms, and myths and facts about the condition. Control and treatment measures, and statistics on treatment and in the elderly are outlined.

http://www.amwa-doc.org/Education/OBI8.htm

UROlog: Overactive Bladder   Based on information provided by Pharmacia and Upjohn, this series of sites addresses the anatomy of the lower urinary tract, neuronal control, receptors, the mechanisms of continence, overactive bladder and types of incontinence, and management of the condition.

http://www.urolog.nl/artsen/features/bladder.asp

9.48 PAIN SYNDROMES

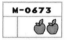

Johns Hopkins Medicine: Chronic Pain Syndromes in Women   Johns Hopkins Medical Institutions provides an overview of chronic pain syndromes in women, including chronic pelvic pain, interstitial cystitis, chronic urogenital syndromes, and vulvodynia described in terms of medical presentation, etiology, and disorder characteristics.

http://www.neuro.jhmi.edu/PelvicPain/home.html

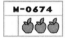

Merck Manual of Diagnosis and Therapy: Pain   Classifications of pain, pain evaluation, and pharmacologic treatment are addressed at this site, which also includes links to pain that may be psychophysiologically-related. Examples given of psychogenic pain syndromes and links to information on other pain disorders are provided. Pain clinical management, cognitive approaches to therapy, and non-drug treatments are examined.

http://www.merck.com/pubs/mmanual/section14/chapter167/167a.htm

9.49 PARESTHESIAS

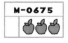

American Family Physician: Parasthesias: A Practical Diagnostic Approach   A problem-oriented diagnostic presentation of the American Academy of Family Physicians offers clinicians information on the pathophysiology and etiology of paresthesias, as well as tables detailing selected causes of paresthesias and peripheral neuropathy. Diagnosis of common nerve root le-

sions and nerve entrapment syndromes are outlined, and an overview of the patient history documentation process and examination is discussed. Figures at the site illustrate nerve distributions.
http://www.aafp.org/afp/971200ap/mcknight.html

 Building Better Health: Numbness and Tingling   A consumer-oriented description of numbness and tingling and an interesting discussion of causes of paresthesias are found, along with information on several symptoms that may accompany paresthesias. Diagnosis, treatment, prevention details, and definitions of key terms within the text are provided.
http://www.buildingbetterhealth.com/article/gale/100083774

9.50 PELVIC PAIN

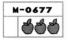 **International Pelvic Pain Society**   This Society Web site offers an overview of pelvic pain, with definitions, differences between acute and chronic conditions, sources of pain, and general guidelines for gynecologic extrauterine, urologic, gastrointestinal, musculoskeletal, and neurological diagnoses. Patient examination approaches, a related online newsletter, a calendar of events, and a printable patient booklet in PDF format on *Understanding the Principles of Chronic Pelvic Pain* are presented.
http://www.pelvicpain.org/clinical_problem.asp

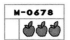 **Merck Manual of Diagnosis and Therapy: Pelvic Pain**   Information on categorizing pelvic pain and establishing an accurate diagnosis are provided at this online Merck reference. Aspects of the physical examination and special laboratory and diagnostic procedures are reviewed, in addition to treatment directions and considerations with regard to differential diagnosis.
http://www.merck.com/pubs/mmanual/section18/chapter237/237a.htm

9.51 PHOTOPHOBIA

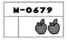 **MEDLINEplus Medical Encyclopedia: Vision, Light Sensitive**   Common causes of sensitivity to sunlight, otherwise known as photophobia, can be accessed from this site topic, with connections available to further information on specific conditions. Self-care measures and tools used in diagnosis are reviewed.   http://www.nlm.nih.gov/medlineplus/ency/article/003041.htm

 Photophobia   Located within the Texas School for Blind and Visually Impaired Web site, this page offers visitors a look at a description of photophobia; its treatment, aimed at correcting the underlying cause; and implications with respect to mydriatics and other drugs that dilate the pupils.
http://www.tsbvi.edu/Education/anomalies/photophobia.htm

9.52 PHOTOSENSITIVITY

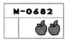

InteliHealth: Photosensitivity   Symptoms, prevention, and treatment related to photosensitivity are discussed at this online information sheet, provided as a service of InteliHealth of Harvard Medical Schools.
http://www.intelihealth.com/IH/ihtIH/WSIHW000/331/10710.html

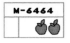

New Zealand DermNet: Photosensitivity   Patient information on photosensitivity is found at this site, maintained by the New Zealand Dermatological Society. A variety of reasons why photosensitivity may occur, confirmation with photosensitizing materials and testing, and basic sun protection techniques are introduced. A number of related pages can be accessed, examining polymorphic light eruptions, discoid lupus, patch tests, and photo testing methods.   http://www.dermnet.org.nz/index.html

9.53 POLYDIPSIA

HealthAnswers.com: Excessive Thirst   Authored by Adam Brochert, M.D., this article from an online medical encyclopedia reviews the signs and causes of polydipsia, as well as diagnosis of specific conditions associated with the symptom. Treatment, directed at the cause, is summarized.
http://www.healthanswers.com/library/MedEnc/enc/3240.asp

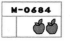

HealthCentral: Thirst, Excessive   Sections of this fact sheet include considerations, common causes, and home care for compulsive thirst. Links to further information on profuse sweating, diabetes mellitus and insipidus, drug-induced thirst, and other causes of polydipsia are found.
http://www.healthcentral.com/mhc/top/003085.cfm

9.54 POLYURIA

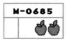

Doctor Resources Symptom Sorters: Polyuria   The causes of polyuria are outlined at a table at this site, including common, less common, and rare conditions. Possible investigations and several red flags in diagnosis are presented, such as weight loss and cough in a smoker or polydipsia with blood and protein on urinalysis.
http://www.docres.co.uk/s_sorters/s61.html

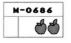

MEDLINEplus Medical Encyclopedia: Urination, Excessive Volume
Enlargeable illustrations at this particular site topic review the anatomy of the male and female urinary tract. Common causes of excessive urination are listed, and links to further information on specific conditions are provided, including diabetes insipidus and diabetes mellitus, renal failure, and sickle cell anemia.
http://www.nlm.nih.gov/medlineplus/ency/article/003146.htm

9.55 PROTEINURIA

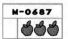 **American Family Physician: Proteinuria in Adults: A Diagnostic Approach**   Authored by professors of the University of Wisconsin-Madison Medical School, this article of the American Academy of Family Physicians provides a problem-oriented diagnosis module. A table outlining common causes of proteinuria, classification details, and detection and quantification of proteinuria are presented. Selected causes by type and the complete diagnostic evaluation are discussed, including a flowchart algorithm, diagnostic criteria, and selected tools of investigation.
http://www.aafp.org/afp/20000915/1333.html

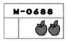 **National Institute of Diabetes and Digestive and Kidney Diseases (NIDDK): Proteinuria**   The National Kidney and Urologic Diseases Information Clearinghouse offers this National Institutes of Health publication on the signs of proteinuria and kidney failure, tests for proteinuria, treatment, and recent research of the division. A summary of "Points to Remember" completes this informative fact sheet.
http://www.niddk.nih.gov/health/kidney/pubs/proteinuria/proteinuria.htm

9.56 PRURITIS

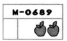 **MEDLINEplus Medical Encyclopedia: Itching**   An overview of itching or pruritus is available on this site, sponsored by the National Institutes of Health and adam.com. Causes of localized or generalized itching and links to more in-depth information on common causes are provided. A figure of the dermal layers and home care measures are presented.
http://www.nlm.nih.gov/medlineplus/ency/article/003217.htm

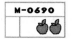 **Virtual Hospital: Dermatology: Pruritus**   A dermatology chapter of the *University of Iowa Family Practice Handbook* offers an overview, etiology, diagnostic details, and treatment information for pruritus originating from cutaneous, systemic, and psychogenic causes.
http://www.vh.org/Providers/ClinRef/FPHandbook/Chapter13/01-13.html

9.57 RASH

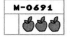 **Flowcharts on Familydoctor.org: Skin Rashes and Other Changes**   The American Academy of Family Physicians at familydoctor.org provides this user-friendly algorithm for determining possible diagnosis and self-care measures for skin rashes and changes. More than forty "yes" or "no" questions lead patients to succinct information on many conditions, as well as advice on when to consult a physician.
http://www.familydoctor.org/flowcharts/545.html

University of Alabama: Rash: Clinical Resources The Clinical Digital Libraries Project of the University of Alabama provides collections of online professional resources, including this page of hyperlinks to assessment, diagnosis, and management documents on skin lesions and rashes. Many references are free of charge. However, some connections may require a user subscription.
(some features fee-based)
http://www.slis.ua.edu/cdlp/uab/clinical/dermatology/vascularreactivity/rash.htm

9.58 SHOULDER PAIN

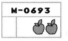

Family Practice Notebook.com: Shoulder Pain This Family Medicine Resource offers an outline of the musculoskeletal causes of shoulder pain, in addition to referred pain and etiologies, thoracic causes, and miscellaneous diseases related to shoulder discomfort. Links to additional details on etiologies and treatment for rotator cuff tears, degenerative joint disease, and a host of other conditions are provided.
http://www.fpnotebook.com/ORT237.htm

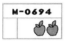

Martha Jefferson Hospital: Shoulder Pain and Problems A review of basic shoulder anatomy is found, and several paragraphs on different types of shoulder problems and injuries are offered, such as impingement syndrome, adhesive capsulitis, and rotator cuff tear. The causes of shoulder problems and examples of diagnostic procedures are summarized.
http://www.mjh.org/modules/ortho/shoulder.htm

9.59 STRIDOR

American Family Physician: Diagnosis of Stridor in Children Authors from the University of Calgary and the Asian Medical Centre in Calgary describe larnyngomalacia, croup, other conditions associated with stridor, and classifications of stridor in children. The etiology and clinical manifestations of the harsh, vibratory sound; a table outlining causes; and historical information in the evaluation of stridor are presented. Physical examination findings, diagnostic tools, and an algorithm for evaluation are all available to interested clinicians. http://www.aafp.org/afp/991115ap/2289.html

Family Practice Notebook.com: Stridor An outline of congenital conditions, inflammatory disorders, neoplasms, and neurogenic causes of stridor are presented at this pediatric reference of the Family Practice Notebook. Visitors are able to easily connect to etiologies, signs, symptoms, and diagnostic information for specific conditions.
http://www.fpnotebook.com/PED108.htm

9.60 SWEATING, EXCESSIVE (HYPERHIDROSIS)

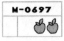

Excessivesweating.org: What Is Hyperhidrosis? Hyperhidrosis, otherwise known as excessive sweating, is discussed at this article, which reviews symptoms, specific conditions associated with hyperhidrosis, and links to a glossary of information on diseases and terminology.
http://www.excessivesweating.org/what.html

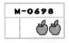

Hyperhidrosis An overview, classification and causes, symptoms and manifestations, and treatments for hyperhidrosis are presented at this online brochure, authored by Ivo Tarfusser, M.D. A link to comprehensive information on endoscopic thoracic sympathectomy is offered.
http://www.parsec.it/summit/hyper1e.htm

9.61 SYNCOPE

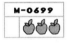

Merck Manual of Diagnosis and Therapy: Syncope (Fainting)
Etiology and pathophysiology, bradyarrhythmias causing syncope or fainting, supraventricular tachyarrhythmias, symptoms, laboratory findings, diagnosis, and treatment are all included at this searchable Merck publication.
http://www.merck.com/pubs/mmanual/section16/chapter200/200b.htm

National Institute of Neurological Disorders and Stroke (NINDS): Syncope Information Page Treatment, prognosis, and current research being conducted by the National Institute of Neurological Disorders and Stroke on syncope and fainting are presented at this Web resource.
http://www.ninds.nih.gov/health_and_medical/disorders/syncope_doc.htm

9.62 TINNITUS

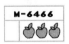

American Tinnitus Association The American Tinnitus Association offers a variety of resources for information on tinnitus at this Web address. A listing of FAQs covers several likely causes of the disorder and connects users to tinnitus treatment options. Support and self-help sections, programs of the organization, and connections to other tinnitus resources are available.
http://www.ata.org/

Tinnitus FAQ This companion FAQ to the ALT.SUPPORT.TINNITUS newsgroup is provided as a service for better understanding tinnitus. A compilation of site links and information on research and treatment centers, tinnitus diagnosis and treatment possibilities, living with tinnitus with masking techniques, and details on related symptoms and conditions are offered. The "What's New" topic offers quick summary updates.
http://www.bixby.org/faq/tinnitus.html

9.63 URINARY FREQUENCY

 eMedicine: Urinary Frequency, Urgency, or Burning eMedicine's Consumer Treatment Guidelines stand out in their ability to offer patients and other interested individuals useful overviews of the signs and symptoms, potential treatments, precautions, and medications often associated with worrisome symptoms. This review provides drug profiles for urinary frequency and urgency treatment, as well as advice on when to contact a physician.
http://www.emedicine.com/general/topic168.htm

 MEDLINEplus Medical Encyclopedia: Urinary Frequency/Urgency Included in the encyclopedic reference of the National Library of Medicine is this adam.com review of urinary frequency and urgency. Common causes are listed, and links to detailed information on urinary tract infections, pregnancy, and additional conditions related to changes in frequency of urination are accessible. http://www.nlm.nih.gov/medlineplus/ency/article/003140.htm

9.64 URINARY INCONTINENCE

 eMedicine: Incontinence Authored by Pilar Guerrero, M.D., of Mount Sinai Medical Center, this eMedicine page offers a discussion of factors responsible for incontinence, demographic information, clinical considerations and presentation, assessments, and diagnostic differential site links. Laboratory work-up, imaging studies, and a guideline for management make the site a comprehensive reference for practicing professionals.
http://www.emedicine.com/emerg/topic791.htm

 Merck Manual of Diagnosis and Therapy: Incontinence General information on the involuntary leakage of urine, as well as review pages specific to transient and established incontinence are offered and provide causes, specific conditions, and diagnosis. Laboratory findings, detrusor overactivity treatment, outlet incompetence deficiency treatment, and considerations in obstruction are addressed. http://www.merck.com/pubs/mmanual/section17/chapter215/215a.htm

9.65 URINARY RETENTION

 National Center for Emergency Medicine Informatics: Urinary Retention The National Center for Emergency Medicine Informatics (NCEMI) offers a summary of the presentation of urinary retention, information on clinical intervention, and a discussion addressing causes, such as anticholinergics or urethral strictures.
http://www.ncemi.org/cse/cse0709.htm

 Wellington School of Medicine: Urinary Retention Viewers are led through a series of slides on the causes, clinical assessment and investigations,

and management of urinary retention at a this site of the Wellington School of Medicine, authored by Dr. John Nacey. Broad categorizations of urinary retention illustrate key points of the text.
http://medmic02.wnmeds.ac.nz/groups/rmo/urinary_retention/retention_toc.html

9.66 WEIGHT LOSS, UNINTENTIONAL

MEDLINEplus Medical Encyclopedia: Weight Loss-Unintentional
Causes of unintentional weight loss are reviewed, and links to further information on symptoms and management of these conditions are offered, as a service of the National Library of Medicine and adam.com.
http://www.nlm.nih.gov/medlineplus/ency/article/003107.htm

Virtual Hospital: Watch Weight Loss in Older People   This site of the University of Iowa Hospitals and Clinics summarizes the main categories of causes of unintentional weight loss. Directions in diagnosis are introduced, including mouth examination, depression assessment, and laboratory testing.
http://www.vh.org/Patients/IHB/IntMed/ABA30/1999/9-23-99Elderweightloss.html

9.67 WHEEZING

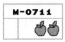

Asthma and Wheezing   Approved by the American Academy of Family Physicians Foundation, this article of Protocare Corporation demonstrates the chain of events associated with reactive airway or asthma, signs and symptoms, a table outlining trigger factors for wheezing, and treatment options.
http://www.quickcare.org/resp/cough.html

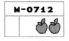

MEDLINEplus Medical Encyclopedia: Wheezing   Details regarding this abnormal breathing sound, links to information on additional abnormal breath sounds, the clinical importance of wheezing, and a variety of links to details on common causes are available from this National Library of Medicine site.
http://www.nlm.nih.gov/medlineplus/ency/article/003070.htm

10

COMMON DIAGNOSTIC
TESTS AND PROCEDURES

10.1 ALLERGY AND IMMUNOLOGY DIAGNOSTICS

IMMUNOLOGIC TESTS

Basic Immunologic Laboratory Tests The Medical College of Georgia provides a list of links at this page, which offers information on assessments and screening tests based on a case example. Pathogenesis, molecular immunology, various clinical disease features, and associated laboratory diagnostics are featured. http://www.ufrgs.br/favet/imunovet/immuno/casehist/basic.htm

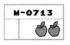

CliniWeb International: Immunologic Tests PubMed search links are available from this site, which lists a variety of immunologic test techniques. By clicking on a selected test, visitors are able to access complete listings of PubMed entries or review abstracts for the chosen procedure. http://medir.ohsu.edu/cliniweb/E1/E1.450.495.html

NASAL SMEAR

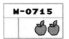

Lexi-Comp's Clinical Reference Library: Eosinophil Count, Nasal Specimen collection details and a synopsis on use and methodology are presented at this site of the Laboratory Corporation of America and Lexi-Comp, Inc. The significance of eosinophil increases and the test's use in the diagnosis of allergy and other conditions are stated. http://www.labcorp.com/datasets/labcorp/html/chapter/mono/he002000.htm

WebMDHealth: Nasal Smear for Eosinophils Based on the *Yale University School of Medicine Patient's Guide to Medical Tests,* this information includes where and how the test is performed, test purpose, preparations, procedure, and a review of diagnostic advantages and disadvantages. http://my.webmd.com/content/asset/yale_lab_
tests_test_name_nasal_smear_for_eosinophils.html

RADIOALLERGOSORBENT TEST (RAST)

Lexi-Comp's Clinical Reference Library: Quantitative Radioallergosorbent Test The Laboratory Corporation of America and Lexi-Comp provide this review of scoring classifications, test indications, and limitations of clinical laboratory findings associated with quantitative radioallergosorbent testing. Additional information on test methodology is outlined at the site, and links to specific allergen profiles are available.
http://www.labcorp.com/datasets/labcorp/html/chapter/mono/al002600.htm

Testuniverse.com: Radioallergosorbent Test Providing general information on the allergen profile, also known as the IgE allergen specific test, this page describes test indications, the procedure, and diagnostic variations. Details concerning test interpretation, advantages, factors affecting results, and disadvantages are presented.
http://www.testuniverse.com/yale/YALE-153.html

SKIN TESTS: PUNCTURE, INTRADERMAL

WebMDHealth: Skin Tests A table at the site outlines basic information about allergy skin testing. A concise discussion of test purpose, procedures, and expectations is presented, along with a summary of interpretation, advantages over other testing methods, and disadvantages.
http://my.webmd.com/content/asset/yale_lab_tests_test_name_skin_tests.html

10.2 CARDIOLOGY DIAGNOSTICS

CARDIAC CATHETERIZATION AND ANGIOGRAPHY

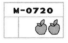

Internet Medical Education, Inc.: Cardiac Catheterization Sections of this cardiac catheterization tutorial include information on left heart and coronary angiography, right heart catheterization, left and right heart catheterization, and cardiac biopsy. Test requirements, procedures, and risks involved are addressed. http://www.med-edu.com/patient/cad/cardiac-cath.html

Virtual Hospital: Cardiac Catheterization Procedure University of Iowa Health Care presents a review of catheter insertion, blood sampling, dye injection, and other components of catheterization procedures. An enlargeable diagram illustrates the catheter pathway, and several additional images of the technique are provided.
http://www.vh.org/Patients/IHB/IntMed/Cardio/Cath/Procedure.html

COMPUTED TOMOGRAPHY

ACC/AHA Expert Consensus Document on Electron-Beam Computed Tomography for the Diagnosis and Prognosis of Coronary Artery Disease   For those interested in this highly sensitive technique, information is offered on its use in the screening of asymptomatic high-risk individuals and for the diagnosis of coronary artery disease. Its greatest potentials, discussion of the technology, and recommendations based on review of the literature are provided.   http://www.acc.org/clinical/consensus/electron/dirIndex.htm

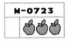

Yale University: Cardiothoracic Imaging: Computed Axial Tomography   Explanation of this digitally-based imaging technique, an animated image illustrating the ability to achieve numerous pictures based on transformation of density and position information, an audio lecture explaining the equipment, and notes on computed tomography techniques are offered at this multimedia presentation.   http://info.med.yale.edu/intmed/cardio/imaging/techniques/ct_imaging/

ECHOCARDIOGRAPHY

ACC/AHA Guidelines for the Clinical Application of Echocardiography   This Scientific Statement of the American College of Cardiology and the American Heart Association summarizes recommendations in the clinical applications of Doppler echocardiography, color Doppler, stress Doppler, and transesophageal echocardiography techniques. A systematic review of the literature includes guidelines for echocardiography in specific diseases and in diagnostic evaluations.   http://www.americanheart.org/Scientific/statements/1997/039703xec.html

Heart Site.com: Echocardiogram   Discussion of ultrasound technology is found at this Heart Site page, with information on M-mode and 2-D echocardiography, electrocardiography during echocardiography, and Doppler techniques for assessment of blood flow. Diagnostic capabilities of echocardiography are fully described, and a controllable ultrasound inset presents moving images of the procedure.   http://www.heartsite.com/html/echocardiogram.html

ELECTROCARDIOGRAPHY

American College of Cardiology (ACC): Guidelines for Electrocardiology   A clinical publication of the American College of Cardiology and the American Heart Association provides practitioners with a statement of indications for electrocardiography in different patient populations, including those with known disease, those suspected of cardiovascular illness, and those with no apparent dysfunction.
http://www.acc.org/clinical/guidelines/electro/

University of Alabama: Electrocardiography Clinical Resources (ECG) The *Merck Manual,* the ECG Library of the Heart Information Network, and many additional resource links on diagnosis and evaluation with electrocardiography are accessible from this page of the Clinical Digital Libraries Project. Clinical guidelines and diagnostic handbook pages are included in this document collection.
http://www.slis.ua.edu/cdlp/WebDLCore/clinical/
cardiology/procedures/electrocardiography.htm

ELECTROPHYSIOLOGY STUDIES

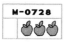

ACC/AHA Guidelines for Clinical Intracardiac Electrophysiological and Catheter Ablation Procedures Developed in collaboration with the North American Society of Pacing and Electrophysiology, this downloadable guideline discusses the role of electrophysiological study in the evaluation of a variety of cardiac arrhythmias in guiding drug therapy, and for the purposes of catheter ablation. A chapter on pediatric differences is also offered at this publication of the American Heart Association and the American College of Cardiology. http://www.acc.org/clinical/guidelines/ablation/dirIndex.htm

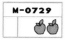

Virtual Hospital: Electrophysiology Studies: A Guide for Patients Internally peer-reviewed, this guide discusses anatomy and physiology of the normal heart, arrhythmias and their classifications, and the purpose of electrophysiological studies. Preparations, intravenous catheter insertion and positioning, and other educational review of postprocedural care are found.
http://www.vh.org/Patients/IHB/IntMed/Cardio/HeartFailure/EP.html

EXERCISE STRESS TESTS

American Family Physician: Ordering and Understanding the Exercise Stress Test This page of the American Academy of Family Physicians offers clinicians a practical therapeutic approach to implementation of the cardiac stress test in practice. Pretest evaluations, relative and absolute contraindications, findings, and formats for reporting results are reviewed. A connection to guidelines of the American College of Cardiology and the American Heart Association is available.
http://www.aafp.org/afp/990115ap/401.html

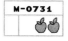

American Heart Association (AHA): Exercise Stress Test A description of the exercise stress test is provided at this site. Connections to related publications on exercise, stress and heart disease, and heart damage detection are offered. AHA Scientific Statements and clinical guidelines for professionals are also available.
http://www.americanheart.org/Heart_and_Stroke_A_Z_Guide/exercises.html

Holter Monitoring (Ambulatory Electrocardiography)

ACC/AHA Guidelines for Ambulatory Electrocardiography   Guidelines developed in collaboration with the North American Society of Pacing and Electrophysiology include this downloadable review of current and emerging technologies, heart rate variability, and symptom assessment in ambulatory electrocardiography. Additional sections on evaluation of pacemaker function, monitoring of myocardial ischemia, and pediatric considerations are provided. http://www.acc.org/clinical/guidelines/ae/dirIndex.htm

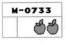

Holter Monitoring   A general description of Holter monitoring, clinical indications, technique, and interpretation via modern computer analysis systems are discussed at this site of the University of Medicine and Dentistry of New Jersey. http://www.umdnj.edu/rspthweb/crt/holter.htm

Intravascular Ultrasound

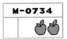

Annals of Thoracic Surgery: Intravascular Imaging and Physiologic Lesion Assessment   Discussion of alternatives to coronary angiogram is found at this article, including intravascular ultrasound, invasive physiologic assessment, and myocardial fractional flow reserve measurement. This *Annals of Thoracic Surgery* supplement provides details on clinical studies and diagnostic accuracy of emerging techniques. http://www.ctsnet.org/journal/ats/68/1547?item=main

Intravascular Ultrasound   A viewable intravascular ultrasound guided coronary stent implantation is available at this site with a download of the RealPlayer software. Discussion of this emerging technique, its importance in cardiology research, as well as hyperlinks to related terminology and procedures are offered, courtesy of the Florida Cardiovascular Institute. http://www.fcvi.org/ivus.htm

Magnetic Resonance Imaging

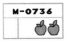

WebMDHealth: Heart MRI   Powered by adam.com, this page offers visitors an overview of cardiac magnetic resonance imaging, including reasons for test performance, procedures involved, and patient preparation. In addition to special considerations concerning accuracy, facts on abnormal results and risk information are provided. http://my.webmd.com/content/asset/adam_test_heart_mri

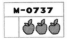

Yale University: Cardiothoracic Imaging: Magnetic Resonance Imaging   Images of MRI equipment and a technical discussion of the strong magnetic field necessary to create images of vasculature and blood velocity characteristics are found. Coronal, axial, and sagittal MRI images, as well as

links to case studies employing MRI technology, are provided at this multimedia presentation of Yale University.
http://info.med.yale.edu/intmed/cardio/imaging/techniques/mri_diagram/

POSITRON EMISSION TOMOGRAPHY

First Virtual Congress of Cardiology: Positron Emission Tomography (PET) This online presentation provides a summary of the current and emerging roles of PET in clinical cardiology. The sensitivity and specificity of PET for detection and localization of coronary artery disease (CAD), its use as an accurate preoperative predictor of functional recovery, and discussion of careful patient selection are addressed.
http://pcvc.sminter.com.ar/cvirtual/cvirteng/cienteng/mneng/mnm3004i/idicarli/dicarli.htm

University of Iowa Health Care: Positron Emission Tomography (PET) Patient information, procedures and protocols for positron emission tomography, and downloadable PDF files of cardiac protocols are provided. A case study of myocardial viability and additional PET Internet links are offered, courtesy of major research and teaching institutions.
http://pet.radiology.uiowa.edu/

TILT TABLE TEST

ACC Expert Consensus Document on Tilt Table Testing for Assessing Syncope Intended to inform practitioners concerning an evolving area of clinical practice, this publication offers a review of the diagnostic capabilities of tilt table testing in patients presenting with syncopal symptoms. Rationale for and history of its use, a description of current protocols, recommendations and indications, and economic impact are examined.
http://www.acc.org/clinical/consensus/tilt.htm

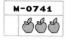

Heart Site.com: Tilt Test Answers to questions about neurally mediated syncope and tilt table test procedures are answered at this illustrated fact sheet of the Heart Site. Safety considerations and information provided by the test are addressed in easy-to-understand terms.
http://www.heartsite.com/html/tilt_test.html

TRANSESOPHAGEAL ECHOCARDIOGRAM

aHealthyMe!: Transesophageal Echocardiography A definition of this diagnostic tool accompanies additional information on transesophageal echocardiography in detecting abnormal tissue growth and abnormalities in pattern flow or in cases where conventional echocardiography results may not be obtained. A test description, aftercare, and normal and abnormal result information are presented. http://www.ahealthyme.com/article/gale/100084805

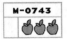

Heart Site.com: Transesophageal Echocardiogram   The manner in which the transesophageal echocardiogram differs from a standard echocardiogram test is discussed, with reference to select cases that may require this modified procedure. Explanations of procedure performance are accompanied by illustrations, and preparations, safety considerations, and information obtainable are addressed.
http://www.heartsite.com/html/tee.html

10.3 DERMATOLOGY DIAGNOSTICS

GENERAL RESOURCES

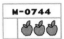

American Family Physician: Recognizing Neoplastic Skin Lesions: A Photo Guide   In addition to its patient information counterpart, this site offers a diagnostic collection of images of primary malignancies of the skin. Common forms and distinctions in appearance are discussed.
http://www.aafp.org/afp/980915ap/rose.html

DermIS: Dermatology Online Atlas   The menu at this page offers visitors diagnostic information and images sorted and batched by body part and locale. Special features include a guided tour and an interactive quiz mode for dermatologic diagnosis. http://www.dermis.net/doia/mainmenu.asp?zugr=d&lang=e

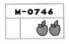

University of Rochester Medical Center: Dermatology Laboratory Tests   General information on diagnostic laboratory tests is available at this Department of Dermatology Web site. Intended to provide overviews of collection and interpretation procedures, the site offers notes for each test on clinical interpretation and its role in diagnosis.
http://wwwminer.lib.rochester.edu/Miner/dermdb/DLTtests/DermaDiagTest.html

SKIN BIOPSY, GENERAL

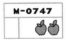

Skin Biopsy   Providing hyperlinks to information on related terms throughout the text, this resource on skin biopsies offers viewers details on biopsy types, microscopic examination, and distinctions of appearance among various lesions. Enlargeable images of biopsy procedures are displayed.
http://www.skincancerinfo.com/sectionb/biopsy.html

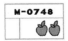

ThirdAge: Skin Lesion Biopsy   Methods of obtaining skin samples, test preparations, and access to pages on risks and results are presented at this page of the adam.com encyclopedic database.
http://thirdage.adam.com/ency/article/003840.htm

10.4 ENDOCRINOLOGY AND METABOLISM DIAGNOSTICS

ADRENAL CORTEX FUNCTION TESTS

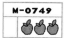

Postgraduate Medicine: Assessment of Adrenal Glucocorticoid Function Options for assessment of hypoadrenalism and hyperadrenalism are presented at this current review of test outcome interpretation and diagnosis. Screening tests, scanning techniques, and the best methods for pursuing an accurate diagnosis are evaluated at this online journal symposium.
http://www.postgradmed.com/issues/1998/07_98/hasinski.htm

University of Alabama: Adrenal Gland Evaluation Clinical Resources Links to MD Consult reference publications, pathology resources, and clinical guidelines in adrenal function assessment are presented at this collection of the Clinical Digital Libraries Project. Although many resources are available free of charge, MD Consult documents require a user library subscription.
(some features fee-based)
http://www.slis.ua.edu/cdlp/uab/clinical/endocrinology/procedures/adrenal.htm

BLOOD GLUCOSE SELF-MONITORING

American Diabetes Association: Self-Monitoring of Blood Glucose This *Diabetes Care* supplement contains a review of the American Diabetes Association Consensus Conference on dealing with issues surrounding self-monitoring. A discussion of the epidemiology of self-monitoring, potential indications, and review of the current technology and system limitations are provided. http://www.diabetes.org/diabetescare/Supplement/s62.htm

Juvenile Diabetes Research Foundation International: Monitoring Your Blood Sugar Directed toward the general public, this fact sheet explains the importance of diabetes self-monitoring and offers information on the use of commercially available systems for monitoring blood sugar. Procedures for using blood glucose meters, testing urine for ketones, and data on essential blood glucose reference ranges are presented, for obtaining optimal blood sugar control. Further information on the hemoglobin A1c (HBA1c) test in cases of frequent hypoglycemia is available.
http://www.jdf.org/living_w_diabetes/pages/monitor.php

BONE DENSITOMETRY

Bone Mineral Density (BMD) Testing: Incorporating BMD into Your Practice Consideration of a baseline BMD measurement, bone mass measurements and technologies, and answers to frequently asked questions, provided

by healthcare professionals, are found at the site. Information on interpreting reports, tables, and device selection are addressed.
http://www.bonemeasurement.com//hcp/bmd_testing/incorporate_practice.html

University of Washington: Bone Density Techniques for evaluating bone density are summarized at this tutorial, which introduces dual energy X-ray absorptiometry (DEXA), ultrasound, and quantitative computed tomography methods. T- and Z-score standard deviations are discussed, and several graphs at the page illustrate the prevalence of osteopenia and osteoporois. A discussion of ideal anatomic locations of measurement is found.
http://courses.washington.edu/bonephys/opbmd.html#tech

FASTING PLASMA GLUCOSE

Lexi-Comp's Clinical Reference Library: Glucose, Serum In addition to describing collection procedures, this site of the Laboratory Corporation of America includes summaries of causes for sample rejection, reference interval, and test indications and limitations. Causes of high or low serum or plasma concentrations are outlined, and the association of hypoglycemia with several organic causes is examined.
http://www.labcorp.com/datasets/labcorp/html/chapter/mono/pr004500.htm

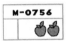

Testuniverse.com: Fasting Plasma Glucose Facts for consumers regarding the fasting blood sugar test are presented at this page, which describes the purpose of the test and offers a description of procedures and general information about normal and abnormal values. A list of medications and other factors that may affect test results is provided.
http://www.testuniverse.com/mdx/MDX-3163.html

GLUCOSE TOLERANCE TEST

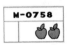

drkoop.com: Glucose Tolerance Test Powered by drkoop.com, this page offers consumer information on how the test is performed for a variety of patient populations. Preparation for the test, risks, normal values, and interpretation of abnormal results are outlined. Links to additional information on disorders that may be related to abnormal results can be accessed.
http://umm.drkoop.com/conditions/ency/article/003466.htm

Endocrine Dynamic Function Tests: Glucose Tolerance Test The glucose tolerance test for investigation of suspected acromegaly is discussed at this laboratory Web page. Information on precautions, the procedure, and guidelines to interpretation are offered.
http://www.poolehos.org/pathgp/edft/a_acrome.htm

GROWTH HORMONE STIMULATION TEST

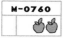

Lycos Health with WebMD: Growth Hormone Stimulation Test
Information on the growth hormone stimulation test, otherwise known as the arginine test, is presented at this site of the adam.com encyclopedic database. Test preparation, associated risks, and value interpretation are presented.
http://webmd.lycos.com/content/asset/adam_test_arginine_test

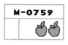

Vanderbilt Medical Center: Growth Hormone Challenge Indications for, procedures related to, and an interpretative summary for the arginine infusion test are presented at this site of Vanderbilt University Medical Center. Information on additional tests of pituitary function may be accessed from the site. http://www.mc.vanderbilt.edu/pituitarycenter/html/test.html

HORMONE LEVELS

Endocrinology Databases Authored by Armando G. Amador, this page leads visitors to a variety of databases specifying reference values for hormones. Pituitary, steroid, thyroid, insulin-like growth factors, and other hormones are included. Each database contains further links to a variety of serum and urine reference range tables.
http://www.il-st-acad-sci.org//data2.html

Laboratory Assessments Provided by Great Smokies Diagnostic Laboratory, this page offers information on laboratory assessments, categorized according to system, such as immunology, endocrinology, and metabolic assessments; condition; and test focus. Test descriptions and utility for each profile are detailed. Connecting to the FAQ link for each diagnostic category offers further information on test procedures and special test instructions.
http://www.gsdl.com/assessments/

INSULIN TOLERANCE TEST

Canterbury Health: Insulin Tolerance Test A consumer information brochure at the site describes the aims of the test and the normal hormonal response. Procedures for insulin administration, test safety and risks, and a summary of what to expect are included.
http://www.chl.govt.nz/chlabs/endo/insutole.htm

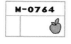

Technical Bulletin: Insulin Tolerance Test Provided by Meridian Valley Laboratory, this page reviews various aspects of the insulin tolerance test, including its clinical significance and benefits. Details are provided in a concise table format.
http://www.meridianvalleylab.com/2gitt/2gitt.html

METABOLIC TESTING, GENERAL

Case Western Reserve University: General Test Information A collection of general information on screenings for inherited disorders of energy metabolism is presented at this site, which includes overviews of enzyme assays and tests for metabolites in body fluids.
http://www.cwru.edu/med/CIDEM/assaygen.htm

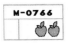
Royal Children's Hospital Division of Laboratory Services: Metabolic Disorders and Tests for Their Investigation A listing of metabolic disorders and tests for their investigation are found at this site, with links to the appropriate tests found within each disorder paragraph. Purposes of specific metabolic tests accessed and sample collection information are provided.
http://www.rch.unimelb.edu.au/biochem/metcond.htm

OVARIAN FUNCTION TESTS

Clinical Value of Hormonal Tests of Menopausal Status The diagnosis of both premature menopause and menopause are considered at this guideline, provided by the Broomfield Hospital in the United Kingdom. Summary recommendations respecting the use of hormone measurements are presented.
http://www.broombio.demon.co.uk/guidelines/hrt.htm

Infertility Diagnosis Investigation of the female endocrine system is the focus of this site, provided by Advanced Reproductive Care, Inc. Determination of the cause of infertility via basal body temperature charting, urinary leutinizing hormone detection, follicle-stimulating hormone and estradiol, imaging, cervical factor investigations, and male factor causes is addressed.
http://www.arcfertility.com/diagnosis.html

PITUITARY-ADRENAL FUNCTION TESTS

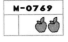
Investigation of Pituitary Function: Pituitary-Adrenal Function Definitions of several tests of pituitary-adrenal function are found at this test directory page. Connections to information on the principles, preparations, procedures, reference ranges, and interpretations of the dexamethasone suppression test, cortisol and ACTH assays, and the ACTH stimulation tests are provided. http://members.aol.com/Richstott/Pitfunc.htm

Postgraduate Medicine: Assessment of Adrenal Glucocorticoid Function Tests appropriate for screening of adrenal gland function are discussed at this article, which outlines dexamethasone suppression testing and cortisol measurement. Adrenal insufficiency, hypercortisolism, and causes of Cushing's syndrome are summarized.
http://www.postgradmed.com/issues/1998/07_98/hasinski.htm

TESTOSTERONE LEVEL

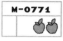

Bioavailable and Free Testosterone This laboratory page thoroughly discusses the significance of unbound and bound testosterone levels, as well as testing methodology and the test's clinical significance. Disorders that demonstrate increases or decreases in values are listed, along with test highlights and common reference ranges.
http://www.aruplab.com/testbltn/biofreetest.html

Lycos Health with WebMD: Testosterone A fact sheet at this page introduces reasons why testosterone testing may be indicated, normal values, and several possible meanings of abnormal results. Links to additional information on related diseases and conditions under which the test may be performed are provided, courtesy of adam.com.
http://webmd.lycos.com/content/asset/adam_test_testosterone

THYROID FUNCTION TESTS

Thyroid Disease Manager: Evaluation of Thyroid Function in Health and Disease From *The Thyroid and its Diseases,* this site contains a chapter on the evaluation of thyroid function in health and disease. The chapter provides a table listing all tests of thyroid function. Clinical descriptions are given for the tests, and result interpretation tables are found.
http://www.thyroidmanager.org/Chapter6/6-text.htm

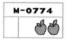

University of Missouri: Thyroid Function Tests Created to provide basic information on thyroid function tests, this page contains descriptions of thyroid hormone, pituitary measurements, related tests, factors that may affect values, and specific conditions associated with abnormality.
http://www.hsc.missouri.edu/~daveg/thyroid/thy_test.html

10.5 GASTROENTEROLOGY/HEPATOLOGY DIAGNOSTICS

ABDOMINAL CT

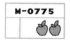

Harvard Medical School Family Health Guide: Abdominal CT Scan At this online brochure, the *Harvard Medical School Family Health Guide* offers connections to general information on computed tomography of the abdomen, with explanations of test preparations, performance, and risks for general consumer reference.
http://www.health.harvard.edu/fhg/diagnostics/abdominalCT/abdominalCT.shtml

MEDLINEplus Medical Encyclopedia: Abdominal CT General information about the abdominal CT scan, otherwise known as the retroperitoneum

CT, can be accessed from this site, courtesy of the National Library of Medicine. Several enlargeable images of abdominal CT scans and exploration, description of test performance, preparations for patients, and indications for its use are presented. Links to information on conditions under which the test may be performed and disorders that may be diagnosed are found.
http://www.nlm.nih.gov/medlineplus/ency/article/003789.htm

ABDOMINAL ULTRASOUND

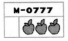 **eMedicine: Ultrasound, Abdominal**   This article describes the background of ultrasound as a clinical tool, patient history warranting abdominal ultrasound examination, and medical and legal pitfalls in diagnosis. Full-size and interactive images are included.
http://www.emedicine.com/emerg/topic621.htm

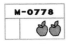 **Starting Abdominal Ultrasound**   From South Bank University, this site illustrates ultrasound investigation, with basic techniques and diagnostic processes examined. Practical hints for abdominal ultrasound procedures and links to case studies of gallstones, pleural metastasis, appendicitis, chronic pancreatitis, and iatrogenic ovarian cystosis are offered. The Medical Ultrasound Imaging WWW Directory at ultrasoundinsider.com contains a list of organizational links and other Web sites related to ultrasound imaging.
http://www.sbu.ac.uk/~dirt/museum/usnd-intro.html

COLONOSCOPY

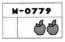 **American Gastroenterological Association: What is Colonoscopy?** A presentation of the colonoscopy procedure is offered for consumers at this site of the American Gastroenterological Association. The document discusses preparations for the procedure, procedure expectations, possible complications, and illustrations of the technique.
http://www.gastro.org/public/colonoscopy.html

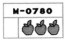 **University of Alabama: Colonoscopy Clinical Resources**   Clinical chapters on diagnostic and therapeutic gastrointestinal procedures are accessible from this collection, provided as a service of the Clinical Digital Libraries Project. Free clinical guidelines from the *American Society for Gastrointestinal Endoscopy Procedure Manual*, colonoscopy clinical guidelines, and pathology resources are collected at one location. (some features fee-based)
http://www.slis.ua.edu/cdlp/uab/clinical/gastroenterology/procedures/colonoscopy.htm

Esophageal Tests/Barium Studies

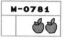

Harvard Medical School Family Health Guide: Barium Swallow
General information on the upper GI series is provided at this page, which connects visitors to answers to frequently asked questions about the test. Information on test preparations, what happens during the procedure, and associated risks are offered.
http://www.health.harvard.edu/fhg/diagnostics/upperGI/upperGIWhat.shtml

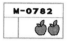

Mylifepath.com: Esophageal Function Tests The purposes of esophageal testing are summarized at this address, with definitions of manometry, esophageal pH testing, and barium fluoroscopy. Preparations, postcare, and examples of abnormal results and their meaning are presented.
http://www.mylifepath.com/article/gale/100272976

Fecal Occult Blood Test (Hemoccult)

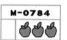

Annals of Internal Medicine: Suggested Technique for Fecal Occult Blood Testing and Interpretation in Colorectal Cancer Screening
Screening technique guidelines for fecal occult blood testing are presented by the American College of Physicians and the American Society of Internal Medicine at this online publication. Emphasis is on the interpretation of positive and negative results and subsequent work-up of those testing positive. Part II of the guideline, which further explores test performance and interpretation, may be freely accessed from the site.
http://www.acponline.org/journals/annals/15may97/ppcolo1.htm

Harvard Medical School Family Health Guide: Fecal Occult Blood Test Offering consumers online diagnostic test information, this page of the *Harvard Medical School Family Health Guide* describes the screening capabilities of fecal occult blood testing. Medicines that may interfere with test results and other considerations in sample collection are introduced.
http://www.health.harvard.edu/fhg/diagnostics/fecal/fecal.shtml

Flexible Sigmoidoscopy

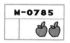

National Institute of Diabetes and Digestive and Kidney Diseases (NIDDK): Sigmoidoscopy The National Digestive Diseases Information Clearinghouse offers this consumer-oriented fact sheet on the sigmoidoscopy procedure. Expectations and preparation are summarized, and links to related gastrointestinal procedure publications are provided.
http://www.niddk.nih.gov/health/digest/pubs/diagtest/sigmo.htm

Postgraduate Medicine: Flexible Sigmoidoscopy Indications for sigmoidoscopy, goals of the procedure, and techniques employed in test performance are reviewed at this *Postgraduate Medicine* article. Clinicians will find valuable information on this important tool in primary care practice, emphasizing indications, contraindications, and essential maneuvers and rules of examination. http://www.postgradmed.com/issues/1999/06_99/davis.htm

GASTROSCOPY (UPPER ENDOSCOPY)

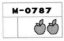

American Gastroenterological Association: What is Upper GI Endoscopy? Information, provided for consumer reference as a service of this professional organization, is grouped into procedure components, preparations, expectations, and possible complications. Simple illustrations of the upper endoscopic procedure are displayed.
http://www.gastro.org/public/uppergi.html

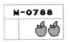

National Institute of Diabetes and Digestive and Kidney Diseases (NIDDK): Upper Endoscopy Provided by the National Digestive Diseases Information Clearinghouse of the National Institutes of Health, this fact sheet describes the upper endoscopy procedure. Reasons for performing the test and preparations are included, and fact sheets on related diagnostic tests can be accessed. http://www.niddk.nih.gov/health/digest/pubs/diagtest/uppend.htm

HYDROGEN BREATH TEST

Cleveland Clinic: What You Need to Know about the Hydrogen Breath Test General information on lactose intolerance and details about what happens during the hydrogen breath test are provided at this site. Visitors to the site will find guidelines to follow before, during, and after the procedure.
http://www.clevelandclinic.org/health/health-info/docs/0800/0845.HTM?index=5216

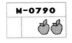

MedicineNet.com: Hydrogen Breath Test Answers to frequently asked questions about the hydrogen breath test are provided at this online fact sheet. Reasons for performing the test, how the results are interpreted, and other important details on limitations of the procedure are found.
http://www.focusondigestion.com/script/main/Art.asp?li=DIG&ArticleKey=8041

LIVER FUNCTION TESTS

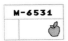

American Liver Foundation: Liver Function Tests A discussion of routine blood tests that assess true liver function, as well as liver or biliary tract disease, is found at this page, supplied by the American Liver Foundation. General categories of liver enzymes and several interpretations of enzyme elevations, increased bilirubin formation, and problems associated with abnormal serum albumin and prothrombin time are presented.
http://www.gastro.com/liverpg/lfts.htm

Postgraduate Medicine: Abnormal Findings on Liver Function Tests
Postgraduate Medicine provides a review of liver function test interpretations at this full-length article. Visitors to the page can learn about liver function test result abnormalities, patterns, and limitations in disease diagnosis. Tables at the site outline nonhepatic causes of abnormal results, reference ranges, and diagnostic approaches.
http://www.postgradmed.com/issues/2000/02_00/gopal.htm

STOOL CULTURE AND TESTING

drkoop.com: Fecal Culture
An overview of fecal culture tests discusses collection procedures, as well as testing purpose and result information. Microscopic culture images are found at this adam.com encyclopedic reference. Links to information on additional stool tests, such as the stool ova and parasites exam and fecal smear, are provided.
http://umm.drkoop.com/conditions/ency/article/003758.htm

Laboratory Guidelines for Ordering Stool Tests
Causes of infectious diarrhea and common enteric bacterial infectious agents are discussed at this PDF-format guide to ordering and interpreting laboratory tests. Recommendations for stool testing for bacterial cultures and ova and parasites are made, with definitions, information on pathogenic enteric protozoa, and viral infection lists presented. Links to additional information on sample collection, testing, and investigation are provided, as a service of the Alberta Medical Association and its Clinical Practice Guidelines Program.
http://www.albertadoctors.org/resources/cpg/cpg-infectious-diarrhea-guideline.pdf

10.6 INFECTIOUS DISEASE DIAGNOSTICS

GENERAL RESOURCES

Lycos Health with WebMD: Diagnosing an Infectious Disease
Of interest to both consumers and professionals, this site concisely outlines some of the most common infectious diseases, their symptoms, and appropriate diagnostic tests. The table serves as a useful quick reference for viral, bacterial, chlamydial, rickettsial, fungal, and parasitic infections and includes diagnostic details on everything from AIDS to toxoplasmosis.
http://webmd.lycos.com/content/asset/yale_
ab_tests_how_your_doctor_diagnoses_an_infectious_disease.html

ANTIGEN AND ANTIBODY TESTS

 Kirksville College of Osteopathic Medicine: Clinical Assays for Antigen-Antibody Interactions Serological assays for antigen-antibody reactions are reviewed at this page, which outlines agglutination reactions, precipitation reactions, and solid phase immunoassays. Immunofluorescence, assays for complement, and monoclonal antibodies are discussed at these illustrated lecture notes.
http://www.kcom.edu/faculty/chamberlain/Website/MSTUART/lect4.htm

 University of Melbourne: Antigen-Antibody Assays An interactive exercise, presented as a service of the University of Melbourne, tutors visitors on in-vitro antigen-antibody reactions used in laboratory assays. Animations demonstrate elementary principles involved, and visitors may access particular sections at any time by clicking on topics at the right or within text sections. Serology and immunoassay overviews give visitors background information, and performance sections for flow cytometry and enzyme immunoassays provide visitors with interactive practice presentations.
http://teach.microbiol.unimelb.edu.au/micro/interLab/sectionB/default.html

CHEST X-RAY AND OTHER IMAGING TESTS

 Bombay Hospital Journal: Imaging Infection and Inflammation Three questions clinicians must answer when dealing with febrile patients are reviewed at this page, which summarizes the basics of infective versus noninfective inflammation. Nuclear medicine techniques useful to the approach are reviewed. http://www.bhj.org/journal/1998_4003_july/sp_332.htm

 Virtual Hospital: American Thoracic Society Continuing Medical Education Testing Modules An internally peer-reviewed site, this Virtual Hospital page provides three test module groups for continuing medical education opportunities. Visitors will find histories and presentations, related radiographic images, and clinical discussions offered. Differential diagnosis information is found for each case, with tuberculosis, other infectious etiologies, malignant etiologies, and non-infectious possibilities explored, as well a synopsis of pathologic diagnosis.
http://www.vh.org/Providers/Simulations/ATS/ATS.html

CULTURES: BLOOD, CEREBROSPINAL (CSF), JOINT FLUID, URINE

 Body Fluid Culture Components of testing for culture and identification of pathogens from cerebrospinal, synovial, and peritoneal fluid are reviewed at this page, provided by the Laboratory Corporation of America. Visitors can also ac-

cess the laboratory's anaerobic culture page or a microbiology appendix, which contain culture recommendations, rationale, and specific procedure reviews.
http://www.labcorp.com/datasets/labcorp/html/chapter/mono/mb002700.htm

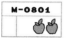 **Laboratory Processing of Samples in the Diagnosis of Infection** This site of the University of Leeds presents summary information on the use of samples from patients in the investigation of urinary tract, respiratory, and gastrointestinal tract infections, as well as in cases of sexually transmitted diseases and meningitis. Blood cultures and miscellaneous investigations, such as wound swabs, are addressed.
http://www.leeds.ac.uk/mbiology/ug/med/labdo.html

GRAM STAIN

 Infectious Disease Laboratory Notebook: Staining Index Links to Gram stain images of clinically important bacteria are provided at this image database, which includes page links on Gram positives and negatives, as well as flowcharts containing multimedia information on the acid-fast stain and additional office procedures. By accessing the main page of this Geocities site, visitors will find additional pages on Gram stain instructions and what physicians need to know about the process.
http://www.geocities.com/CapeCanaveral/3504/stain.htm

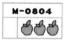 **Loyola University Medical Center: Gram Stain** Review of this common office procedure, including its usefulness in the presumptive diagnosis of several bacterial or pyogenic infections and for determining specimen adequacy, is presented as a service of Loyola University Medical Center. Reasons for examination, principles and procedures of technique, interpretation of smears, and an assortment of Gram stained images of medically important bacteria are provided. http://www.lumen.luc.edu/lumen/DeptWebs/microbio/med/gram/gram-stn.htm

MICROSCOPIC EVALUATION/SMEARS

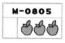 **Microbiology Lab Manual** Lessons in microbiology include an introduction to microscopic examination processes and chapters on aseptic technique and handling, enumeration of microorganisms, and specific staining procedures. Individual chapters on yeasts, molds, bacteriophages, enterobacteriaceae and pseudomonas, and streptococci are also offered at this complete course manual.
http://www.cat.cc.md.us/courses/bio141/labmanua/

 WWW Virtual Library: Microscopy By accessing the medically-oriented sites of the WWW Virtual Library, visitors will gain entrance to a variety of Internet pages on clinical microbiology and the use of electron microscopy in infectious disease diagnosis. The Histotech's Home Page, Microbiology and Virology of the MedWeb site, Microscopic Morphology, and Virus Ultrastructure

are just a few of the microscopy pages available. Visitors will find hundreds of images, discussions, and case reviews available from this collection.
http://www.ou.edu/research/electron/www-vl/

SPUTUM CULTURE

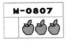

Diagnostic Procedures Handbook: Sputum Culture   The sputum culture's place in pneumonia diagnosis, collection procedures, reference range, and testing limitations are reviewed. The importance of the Gram stain is discussed, and test methodology, tables outlining bacteria, fungi, viruses, parasites, and additional species recovered from sputa are presented. Links to closely related information on additional culture types and specific organisms are accessible, courtesy of Lexi-Comp's Clinical Reference Library.
http://informatics.drake.edu/lth/html/chapter/mono/mb005900.htm

Testuniverse.com: Sputum Culture   A general outline of test purpose, preparation, and performance is found at this page, which is intended for consumer audiences or professional review. A summary of test result values and drugs and other factors that may affect results is presented.
http://www.testuniverse.com/mdx/MDX-3230

STOOL EXAMINATION

Laboratory Guidelines for Ordering Stool Tests for Investigation of Suspected Infectious Diarrhea   Causes of infectious diarrhea and common enteric bacterial infectious agents are discussed at this PDF-format guide to ordering and interpreting laboratory tests. Recommendations for stool testing for bacterial cultures and ova and parasites are offered, with definitions, information on pathogenic enteric protozoa, and viral infection lists presented. Links to additional information on sample collection, testing, and investigation are provided, as a service of the Alberta Medical Association and its Clinical Practice Guidelines Program.
http://www.albertadoctors.org/resources/cpg/cpg-infectious-diarrhea-guideline.pdf

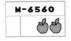

Stool Culture   Provided by the Laboratory Corporation of American, this site discusses components of stool isolation and identification for a variety of organisms. Collection methods, storage, and testing indications are reviewed, with limitations of testing stated. Additional information on diagnosis and a table summarizing specific syndromes, features, and characteristic etiologies are provided. Related links to information on cultures that have specific requirements for growth are available.
http://www.labcorp.com/datasets/labcorp/html/chapter/mono/mb012800.htm

TUBERCULIN SKIN TEST

M-6561

Centers for Disease Control and Prevention (CDC): Mantoux Tuberculin Skin Test Test administration, measurement of induration, and review of positive reactions are found at this site of the Division of TB Elimination. Images of appropriate needle insertion and millimeters of induration accompany the text.
http://www.nurse.net/clinical/tb/index.html

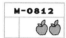
M-0812

Columbia University: Tuberculin Skin Test This fact sheet provided by Columbia University Medical Informatics offers answers to questions regarding the tuberculin skin test, including meanings of negative and positive results. Other issues addressed include possible side effects, Mantoux administration, caring for the test spot, and steps to be taken in light of positive results.
http://www.dmi.columbia.edu/resources/tbcpp/skintest.html

10.7 NEPHROLOGY/UROLOGY DIAGNOSTICS

CYSTOSCOPY

M-0813

MEDLINEplus Medical Encyclopedia: Cystoscopy Provided by the National Library of Medicine, this site describes how cystoscopy is performed and states details about test preparations, why the test is performed, and normal values. Links to information on conditions that may be diagnosed with abnormal results are offered.
http://www.nlm.nih.gov/medlineplus/ency/article/003903.htm

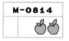
M-0814

Yale University School of Medicine Patient's Guide to Medical Tests: Cystourethroscopy Viewers may listen to or read the text of this audio presentation concerning diagnosis with cystoscopy. A brief review offers details on diagnostic uses, treatments that may be performed during the procedure, and patient preparation.
http://www.yourhealth.com/ahl/2155.html

INTRAVENOUS PYELOGRAM (IVP)

M-0815

Radiological Society of North America: Intravenous Pyelogram An online brochure summarizes common uses of the intravenous pyelogram, as well as equipment used, patient experience, and result interpretation. Risks versus benefits are examined, in addition to limitations of IVP studies.
http://www.radiologyinfo.org/content/ivp_radiology.htm

M-0816

ThriveOnline: Intravenous Pyelogram Also known as the excretory pyelogram, this test is described at the site, with reference made to conditions

indicated by abnormal results. Links to further information on these conditions are provided, as well as connections to over 25 additional conditions that may warrant performance of the test.
http://health.netscape.thriveonline.oxygen.com/medical/library/article/003782res.html

PROSTATE SPECIFIC ANTIGEN (PSA)

OncoLink: ProstateSpecific Antigen   A discussion of the positive predictive value of PSA and a variety of recent PSA-related concepts for diagnosis and management are reviewed at this OncoLink article. The need for improved methods of detection and further research directed at defining PSA function is addressed. http://oncolink.upenn.edu/disease/prostate/screening/Ablin.html

Review on Prostate Specific Antigen   This presentation reviews the role of PSA as one of the most well-known and useful tumor markers available. A history of testing; PSA's role in the screening, diagnosis, staging, and, monitoring of prostate cancer; its use in the diagnosis of benign prostatic hyperplasia (BPH); and discussion of PSA velocity are provided. Screening considerations and criteria, discussion of what PSA numbers indicate, and a summary of past trials and their implications are offered.
http://www.rph.wa.gov.au/labs/biochem/psa.html

RADIONUCLIDE KIDNEY SCAN

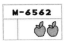

Applied Radiology Online: Renal Scintigraphy   Primarily for professionals, Applied Radiology Online provides this overview about recent developments in renal scintigraphy. The article highlights research relating to specific renal medical procedures.
http://www.appliedradiology.com/articles/article.asp?Id=405

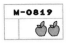

MEDLINEplus Medical Encyclopedia: Renal Scan   Sponsored by the National Library of Medicine, this page defines the kidney scan and provides information on how the test is performed, preparations, risks, and reasons it is ordered. Normal values, costs, and the meaning of abnormal results are included, with links offered to disorders associated with abnormal results.
http://www.nlm.nih.gov/medlineplus/ency/article/003790.htm

SPERM COUNT/SEMEN ANALYSIS

Fertility Institutes: Sperm Evaluation   Definitions of abnormalities in sperm count analysis are available at this site of the Fertility Institutes, which also includes a complete discussion of sperm motility studies and a new assay that may make analysis of sperm function more accurate. From this general in-

formation page, visitors can access more detailed information on advanced sperm testing procedures.
http://www.fertility-docs.com/sperm_eval.phtml

Semen Analysis and Male Infertility Information provided by both the World Health Organization and the British Andrology Society includes sample collection, procedure performance details, and normal results of semen analysis tests and measurements. Additional links offer greater details on individual components of the test, including sperm count, viscosity, liquefaction, morphology, motility, and anti-sperm antibodies. Problems arising from a badly taken sample are reviewed.
http://pages.unisonfree.net/norman.irene/

TRANSRECTAL ULTRASOUND AND BIOPSY

Technical and Clinical Aspects of Transrectal Ultrasound of the Prostate At this page of the Department of Urology, Nijmegen, the Netherlands, visitors have access to a complete publication addressing the clinical and technical aspects of transrectal ultrasound of the prostate. Ultrasound equipment, prostate anatomy, ultrasound and therapy, image processing, and the future of ultrasonographic technology chapters are presented, with treatment principles and illustrations included.
http://uroworld.azn.nl/uicbme/images/

Transrectal Ultrasound and Biopsy of the Prostate Offered as a service of Marin Urology, this presentation of the transrectal ultrasound gives consumers and clinicians an overview of diagnostic ultrasonography technology, with prostate imaging provided. A diagram and description of procedures for the prostate biopsy procedure are presented, along with images and information on biopsy findings.
http://www.marinurology.com/articles/cap/learning/trusp.htm

ULTRASONOGRAPHY: PELVIS, URINARY BLADDER, KIDNEYS

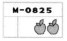

Radiological Society of North America: Ultrasound, Pelvis Common uses of pelvic ultrasonography are reviewed at this site's links. Preparations, equipment used, and frequently asked questions about the procedure are addressed. A review of benefits versus risks, as well as limitations of the procedure is presented. http://www.radiologyresource.org/content/ultrasound-pelvis.htm

Renal Ultrasound An online slide presentation offers details on renal anatomy and physiology, as well as indications for the renal ultrasound and ultrasound images of the extra renal pelvis and pelvic kidney. Congenital anomalies and several renal pathologies are presented, with outlines and related pathological images presented.
http://onlinelearning.tc.cc.va.us/faculty/tcjonef/renaleval/renal1/

URINALYSIS

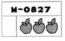

Internet Pathology Laboratory: Urinalysis Macroscopic urine inspection, urine dipstick chemical analysis, and microscopic examination are discussed at this page of the WebPath tutorial. Proper collection methods, common and uncommon crystals, epithelial cells, blood cells, and proper examination methods are explored at this comprehensive, illustrated site.
http://www-medlib.med.utah.edu/WebPath/TUTORIAL/URINE/URINE.html

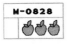

Virtual Hospital: Urinalysis Sponsored by University of Iowa Health Care, this page offers an introduction to specimen collection and gross urine examination, as well as chapters on urine chemical analysis and the microscopic evaluation. Images accompany this educational text, and a multi-part CME test for urinalysis is offered.
http://www.vh.org/Providers/CME/CLIA/UrineAnalysis/UrineAnalysis.html

URINE CULTURE

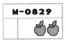

Family Practice Notebook.com: Urine Culture Part of the "Pathology and Laboratory Medicine" chapter, this site contains details on collection, specimen handling, and outlines of urine culture interpretation. By clicking on additional topics found throughout this family medicine resource, visitors can gain further information on urinary tract infections and specimen collection.
http://fpnotebook.com/URO37.htm

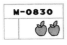

Lycos Health with WebMD: Urine Culture (Clean Catch) Offered as a consumer resource, this page describes reasons for performing the clean catch and complete procedure instructions. Normal and abnormal values are considered, with links available to several conditions associated with abnormal results.
http://webmd.lycos.com/content/asset/adam_test_clean_catch_urine_specimen

10.8 NEUROLOGY DIAGNOSTICS

ARTERIOGRAM (ANGIOGRAM)

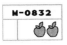

drkoop.com: Cerebral Angiography Angiography of the head is discussed at this encyclopedic reference of drkoop and the adam.com database. A description of testing procedures, preparations, and links to risks and test result information are provided. Visitors will also find several accessible images.
http://umm.drkoop.com/conditions/ency/article/003799.htm

Internet Stroke Center: Cerebral Angiography This online guide to imaging techniques offers a general discussion of this invasive test; information on the controversial role of conventional angiography in the management of stroke; and the advantages of magnetic resonance angiography over less advanced techniques. Both a frontal and lateral view of a carotid angiogram are displayed. http://www.strokecenter.org/pat/diagnosis/angio.htm

CEREBROSPINAL FLUID ANALYSIS AND LUMBAR PUNCTURE

eMedicine: Lumbar Puncture (Cerebrospinal Fluid Examination)
This eMedicine page outlines the therapeutic advantages of lumbar puncture for the diagnostic examination of cerebrospinal fluid. Lumbar puncture techniques and processes are examined, and multiple cases are presented.
http://www.eMedicine.com/NEURO/topic557.htm

WebMDHealth: Lumbar Puncture
Written in an easy-to-understand way, this site offers information on the lumbar puncture test. The purpose of the test is explained, along with how it works, preparation for the test, and the procedure itself. Post-test care, advantages and disadvantages of the test, and interpretation of the results are discussed.
http://my.webmd.com/content/asset/yale_lab_tests_test_name_lumbar_puncture_lp.html

COMPUTED TOMOGRAPHY (CT)

Radiological Society of North America: Computed Tomography of the Head
This physician-reviewed material describes various aspects of computed tomography scanning of the head, including common indications, equipment, procedure performance, and result interpretation. Benefits versus risks are addressed.
http://www.radiologyinfo.org/content/ct_of_the_head.htm

Testuniverse.com: Computed Tomography of the Spine
Excerpted from the *Complete Guide to Medical Tests,* this site offers general information, purpose and description of the test, and other details on equipment used. Test values and what abnormal results may indicate are also listed at this reference page. http://www.testuniverse.com/mdx/MDX-2934.html

ELECTRODIAGNOSTIC TESTS
(ELECTROMYOGRAPHY (EMG)/NERVE CONDUCTION STUDY)

American Academy of Physical Medicine and Rehabilitation: CME Online EMG Cases
With cases dating back to 1998, this online program provides opportunity for study of electrodiagnosis, with direct links to EMG presentations. For each connection, presenting symptoms, physical examination, electrophysiologic data, diagnostic impression, and commentary are provided. http://www.aapmr.org/cme/emg.htm

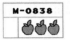 **TeleEMG.com: EMG and Nerve Conduction Homepage** Featuring nerve and muscular disease testing, this site offers physician and patient discussion groups, anatomical illustrations, and clinical discussion of EMG and nerve conduction testing. Links to an electronic EMG manual, nerve conduction set-ups, needle exam atlas, and answers to FAQs are offered, providing an educational experience for both professional and consumer audiences.
http://www.teleemg.com/

ELECTROENCEPHALOGRAM (EEG)

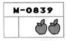 **EEG Course and Glossary** Authored by Sydney Louis, M.D., this discussion provides instruction on EEG interpretation, including wave forms, their frequency, and morphology. Discussions of various techniques and normal variants are offered.
http://www.brown.edu/Departments/Clinical_Neurosciences/louis/eegcrs.html

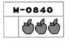 **eMedicine: EEG Seizure Monitoring** Presented by the Medical College of Georgia, this eMedicine article provides information on the diagnostic utility of EEG, advantages and disadvantages, cases and diagnosis, and technical considerations in EEG techniques. Graphic recordings of EEG monitoring are displayed, including temporal lobe and generalized epileptic seizures.
http://www.eMedicine.com/neuro/topic103.htm

EVOKED POTENTIALS

 Virginia Mason: Visual Evoked Potentials A description of visual evoked potentials, patient preparation details, and information on attachment and electrode removal are presented at this online information sheet.
http://www.vmmc.com/dbNeurophysiology/sec1824.htm

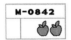 **Wake Forest University Baptist: Evoked Potential Laboratory** Three types of evoked potential tests are discussed at this hospital center Web site: brainstem auditory evoked potential, visual evoked potential, and somatosensory evoked potential. Testing indications are reviewed.
http://www.bgsm.edu/neurology/department/diagneuro/ep.html

MAGNETIC RESONANCE IMAGING (MRI)

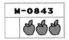 **MRI Tutorial** Presented by Doctors Groover, Christie, and Merritt, this site offers both a "PlainTalk" and "MedSpeak" version to accommodate all reading levels. A complete presentation on magnetic resonance imaging is offered, including pages on necessary equipment, image creation, image orientation, and safety considerations. By accessing brain MRI information, visitors are taken to

further consumer-oriented or clinical details on MRI imaging in brain tumors, metastases, stroke, multiple sclerosis, and cranial nerve tumor.
http://www.idsonline.com/gcm/mrtutpt.htm

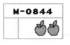

Neuroguide.com: Use of Functional Magnetic Resonance Imaging to Investigate Brain Function Neuroguide's Neuroscience on the Internet offers this page, authored by Thomas R. Gregg of the University of Medicine and Dentistry of New Jersey. Visualization of changes in chemical composition in the brain is discussed, including magnetic resonance of atomic nuclei, spin-echo magnetic resonance imaging, other MRI techniques, and functional MRI. The article is fully referenced.
http://www.neuroguide.com/gregg.html

MYELOGRAM

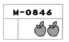

Canadian Association of Radiologists: Standards and Guidelines for Myelography A detailed definition of myelographic procedures, physician qualifications, and the radiographic facility for myelography are addressed at this comprehensive guideline. Indications for myelography, contraindications, and choice of contrast material are considered. Additional information on patient care and the myelogram examination are found, with a special section provided on diagnostic caveats.
http://www.car.ca/standards/myelography.htm

SpineUniverse: Myelogram (Myelography) A fact sheet at this site introduces visitors to the various components of myelography. Procedures, important considerations regarding medical conditions and current medications used, patient preparation, and common risks are addressed.
http://www.spineuniverse.com/conditions/072400spin_myelogram.html

NEUROLOGIC EXAMINATION

Merck Manual of Diagnosis and Therapy: Neurologic Examination Examining multiple components of the neurological evaluation, this Merck sponsored site offers visitors complete details on the mental status examination, cranial nerve testing, motor system examination, and assessment of muscle strength. Additional discussion on examination of coordination, stance, and gait; sensory testing; reflex testing; and the cerebrovascular examination are included. Hyperlinks throughout the text allows access to related portions of the online *Merck Manual*.
http://www.merck.com/pubs/mmanual/section14/chapter165/165c.htm

University of Florida: Neurologic Examination Equipment needed and general considerations of the neurological exam are presented at this complete tutorial, courtesy of the University of Florida College of Medicine. Nearly 10 categories of examination are presented, including mental status, coordination

and gait, and sensory evaluations. Visitors are presented with cranial nerve observations, a mini mental status link, oculomotor tests, grading of muscle strength, tendon reflex grading scale, and several additional tools and assessment techniques.
http://www.medinfo.ufl.edu/year1/bcs/clist/neuro.html

POSITRON EMISSION TOMOGRAPHY (PET)

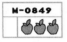

Positron Emission Tomography: The Power of Molecular Imaging
This 12-page color brochure discusses and illustrates the clinical uses and applications of positron emission tomography. PET's applications in brain diseases, such as Parkinson's disease, Alzheimer's, and seizure disorders, are addressed. Adobe Acrobat Reader, available free at this site, is required for downloading this document. http://149.142.143.86/html_docs/PET/

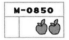

University of Iowa Health Care: Positron Emission Tomography (PET) The University of Iowa PET Imaging Center presents patient information, PET procedures and protocols for practitioners, and case studies for further review. Links to several PET institutes and research centers are provided.
http://pet.radiology.uiowa.edu/

10.9 ONCOLOGY DIAGNOSTICS

BONE MARROW BIOPSY

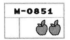

CBS HealthWatch by Medscape: Bone Marrow Aspiration Basic information on bone marrow aspiration and biopsy is provided at this site, excerpted from the *Patient's Guide to Medical Tests* by faculty at the Yale University School of Medicine. A review and illustration of the test procedure are found, in addition to factors affecting results and various test interpretations.
http://cbs.medscape.com/cx/viewarticle/170061

MDAdvice.com: Bone Marrow Aspiration and Biopsy Test preparation, description of the test itself, and indications of abnormal results are outlined at this online fact sheet on bone marrow aspiration and biopsy.
http://www.mdadvice.com/library/test/medtest109.html

BONE SCAN

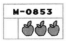

Postgraduate Medicine: When to Use Bone Scintigraphy Authored by Aaron Hendler, M.D., and Marlon Hershkop, M.D., this article examines important applications of bone scintigraphy and its particular value in assess-

ment of metastatic and other diseases. Findings indicating malignant versus benign tumors and guidelines for optimal use in various cancers are provided.
http://www.postgradmed.com/issues/1998/11_98/hendler.htm

SpineUniverse: Bone Scan Uses of the bone scan and components of the procedure are summarized at this article of SpineUniverse. Images and important considerations regarding allergies, pregnancy, and amount of tracing element are presented.
http://www.spineuniverse.com/conditions/072400spin_bonescan.html

BRONCHOSCOPY

Atlas of Digital and Quantitative Bronchoscopy An overview of digital and quantitative bronchoscopy, information on virtual bronchoscopy, a complete bronchoscopic picture atlas with video clips, and example discussion and images of both benign and malignant disease are presented at this complete online tutorial.
http://everest.radiology.uiowa.edu/nlm/app/atlas/welcome2.html

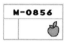

MDAdvice.com: Bronchoscopy At this online fact sheet, visitors will find summarized information on test preparation, purpose of the test, what to expect, and postcare information. Details on normal and abnormal values of the bronchoscopy are outlined.
http://www.mdadvice.com/library/test/medtest115.html

COLONOSCOPY

Society of American Gastrointestinal Endoscopic Surgeons: Colonoscopy This clinical guideline provides clinicians with information on the appropriate use of colonoscopy in the surveillance of patients at increased risk of colorectal cancer development. Discussions of several risk factors are found, and a summary of recommendations for screening is presented in table format.
http://www.sages.org/sg_asgepub1030.html

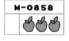

University of Alabama: Colonoscopy Clinical Resources A collection of authoritative resources is offered at this site of the Clinical Digital Libraries Project. Visitors can choose to access online textbook chapters, pathology resources, clinical guidelines, and clinical trials related to colonoscopy.
http://www.slis.ua.edu/cdlp/WebDLCore/
clinical/gastroenterology/procedures/colonoscopy.htm

COMPLETE BLOOD COUNT (CBC)

Family Practice Notebook.com: Complete Blood Count An outline of specimen details and individual cell counts is found at this online textbook

page. Links at the site bring visitors to further information on specific blood cell counts that include reference ranges and conditions indicated with increased and decreased values.
http://www.fpnotebook.com/HEM65.htm

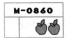

Ontario Medical Association: Introduction to Hematology A tutorial on the complete blood count is presented at this electronic outline, as well as information on reference intervals and significant abnormal values. Key definitions of terms can be accessed throughout the text, which is accompanied by photomicrographs and illustrations.
http://www.lptp.on.ca/services/education/cbc.html

COMPUTED TOMOGRAPHY

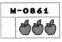

MEDLINEplus Medical Encyclopedia: Abdominal CT As a service of the National Library of Medicine, this site offers a collection of enlargeable CT images used in the diagnosis of various metastatic diseases. An overview of the test, risks, and a large listing of links to a variety of conditions discovered with computed tomography are available.
http://www.nlm.nih.gov/medlineplus/ency/article/003789.htm

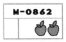

National Cancer Institute (NCI): Computed Tomography A description of computed tomography procedure, its advantages over simple X-ray techniques, and details on the latest innovations in computed tomography, such as spiral CT scanners, are introduced at this cancer information resource.
http://cis.nci.nih.gov/fact/5_2.htm

LIVER AND SPLEEN SCAN

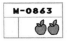

American Foundation for Early Detection: Liver-Spleen Scanning Excerpted from the *Complete Guide to Medical Tests,* this page offers general information and basic components of the procedure. Conditions that abnormal results may indicate are listed.
http://www.afed.org/mdx/MDX-3135

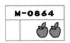

MEDLINEplus Medical Encyclopedia: Liver Scan An overview of how this test is performed, as well as risks and results are discussed on this National Library of Medicine site. Links to further information on disorders associated with abnormal results are provided.
http://www.nlm.nih.gov/medlineplus/ency/article/003825.htm

MAGNETIC RESONANCE IMAGING (MRI)

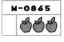

Magnetic Resonance Imaging in Oncology: An Overview This educational update from the University of Aberdeen offers information on

magnetic resonance imaging, including its original conception, its evolution, and basics of MRI technology. The use of MRI as a staging modality, example images, and MRI in tumor angiogenesis are presented. Lymph node evaluation and its applications in recurrent disease are examined.
http://www.rcsed.ac.uk/journal/vol44_2/4420013.htm

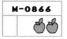

Memorial Sloan-Kettering Cancer Center: Laboratory of Functional MRI   Courtesy of both Cornell University Medical College and Memorial Sloan-Kettering Cancer Center, this page offers an in-depth discussion about functional MRI imaging methods, recent publications, current projects of the laboratory, and links to several additional sites specializing in diagnostic imaging. http://www.fmri.org/

Mammogram

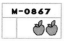

Imaginis: General Information on Mammography   From breast compression during mammography to specialized techniques, this printable, online brochure offers visitors information on key concepts. Steps necessary for an optimal picture, understanding the mammography report, and information on locating a mammography facility are provided.
http://www.imaginis.com/breasthealth/mammography.asp

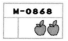

Mammography Basic Principles   More than 15 chapters dedicated to providing complete information on mammography modalities are presented at this breast cancer awareness article. Details on quality control in mammography are stressed, including correct positioning, apparatus, and other techniques to ensure accurate diagnosis. http://www.ozemail.com.au/~glensan/mamnotes.htm

Positron Emission Tomography (PET)

UHrad: Positron Emission Tomography Teaching Files   Provided by Case Western Reserve University, this Web site offers links to five case presentations in PET imaging. Several images, clinical history, findings, and diagnosis are presented for metastatic lung cancer, Ewing's sarcoma, metastatic disease to the liver, and suspicious lesions. Discussions of special considerations for each clinical scenario and references are available.
http://www.uhrad.com/petarc.htm

University of California Los Angeles (UCLA): Clinical PET—Oncology
Information on applications of the PET scan in oncology, including details on a standard protocol for whole-body scanning, is presented at this site. Scanning of the abdomen and pelvis, brain tumors, the head and neck, musculoskeletal system, and thorax is addressed in individual chapters of this tutorial. By accessing the main menu of the site, visitors gain access to an overview of PET imaging and isotopes used, as well as several case examples in oncology.
http://www.crump.ucla.edu/lpp/clinpetonco/oncoeval.html

TISSUE BIOPSY, GENERAL

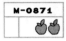

Biopsy Report: A Patient's Guide   This informative discussion addresses patient concerns about the biopsy report, distinguishing various biopsy types. Steps in specimen processing are reviewed, as well as descriptions of the macroscopic and microscopic examinations. A glossary of important terms is included.   http://cancerguide.org/pathology.html

OncoLog: From Biopsy to Diagnosis   The University of Texas M.D. Anderson Cancer Center provides this question and answer sheet offering basic information on types of biopsies and what to expect before, during, and after the procedure. A summary of the pathology examination is presented.   http://www3.mdanderson.org/~oncolog/housecalljan00.html

TUMOR MARKERS, GENERAL

National Cancer Institute (NCI): Tumor Markers   A fact sheet on tumor markers is presented on this site, including their role in cancer diagnosis, as well as in monitoring a patient's response to treatment. Common tumor markers are described such as prostate-specific antigen, CA 125, alpha-fetoprotein, and neuron-specific enolase. Links are provided for additional information resources.   http://cis.nci.nih.gov/fact/5_18.htm

Virtual Hospital: Tumor Marker Tests   Several tumor markers are described at this site, provided by the Holden Comprehensive Cancer Center of University of Iowa Health Care. An abbreviations guide assists with interpretation of more than 10 tumor marker listings, arranged and identified by primary and secondary cancer sites, associated false positives, benign diseases detected, and normal values.   http://www.vh.org/Patients/IHB/Cancer/Tumormarker.html

ULTRASOUND

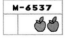

Endoscopic Ultrasonography   EUS Online, sponsored by a collaboration of European, French, and German endoscopic ultrasound organizations, presents a current literature review and facilitates exchange of information among its users. The site offers information on current research in the field and guidelines for endoscopic ultrasonography, including techniques for the upper gastrointestinal tract, retroperitoneum, and large bowel.   http://www.eus-online.org/

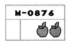

Society of Radiologists in Ultrasound   Detailed annual meeting information, an online version of the latest newsletter, and patient information on ultrasound exams and procedures are provided at the home page of the Society of Radiologists in Ultrasound. Links to other organizations in radiology are offered. A table at the patient site outlines types of ultrasound examinations and reasons for their prescription. http://www.sru.org/

10.10 OTOLARYNGOLOGY DIAGNOSTICS

HEARING TESTS, GENERAL

American Academy of Audiology News, professional and consumer guides and resources, the online Academy store, and an audiologist locator are all found within this organization's Web site. Discussion lists and *Audiology Today* are available to member viewers.

(some features fee-based) http://www.audiology.org/

University of Washington: Hearing Tests A review of basic hearing tests, including the audiogram, tympanogram, auditory brain stem response, and electronystagmogram, is presented at this informational brochure. Basic components of these tests are discussed, as a service of the Department of Otolaryngology at the University of Washington.

http://depts.washington.edu/otoweb/audiogram.html

HEARING TESTS (AUDIOMETRY)

American Academy of Audiology: Understanding Your Audiogram A description of the audiogram and information on interpreting its results are presented at this colorful, online brochure. Meanings of vertical and horizontal lines on an audiogram, frequency and intensity, and a representative audiogram are presented.

http://www.audiology.org/consumer/guides/uya.php

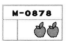

Pure-Tone Audiometry Provided by Audiophone Hearing Instruments, this page focuses primarily on the interpretation of the audiogram. Threshold measurement versus screening, function of the pure-tone audiometer, procedures for measurement, and a scale classifying the degree of hearing loss are included. Audiometric rules to determine the type of hearing loss and values for normal hearing, conductive loss, and sensorineural loss are listed.

http://www.audiphone.com/audiomet.htm

HEARING TUNING FORK

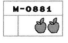

Family Practice Notebook.com: Tuning Fork Tests An outline of tuning fork tests is presented at this site, courtesy of Family Practice's Family Medicine Resource. Technique and normal and abnormal findings for both the

Weber and Rinne techniques are reviewed. Visitors can access further information on various types of hearing loss.
http://www.fpnotebook.com/ENT40.htm

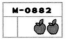

How to Perform and Interpret Weber and Rinne Tests Authored and reviewed by physicians of Dalhousie University, this article presents a simple description of performance techniques for both the Weber and Rinne tests. Their purpose, usefulness, and interpretation of abnormal results are clearly described. http://icarus.med.utoronto.ca/carr/manual/tuningfork.html

LARYNGOSCOPY

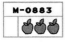

Virtual Laryngoscopy The article at this site, sponsored by Brigham and Women's Hospital and Harvard University, discusses work presented at an American Laryngological Association annual meeting regarding current methods of virtual endoscopy, their limitations, and results with the addition of three-dimensional anatomical reconstruction.
http://splweb.bwh.harvard.edu:8000/pages/papers/vik/virlar/virlar3.html

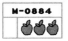

Voice Center at Eastern Virginia Medical School: Examining the Larynx Information on indirect laryngoscopy, flexible and rigid endoscopes, images of optical instruments, and discussion of a stroboscopic examination are provided at this fact sheet, intended for professional readers. Direct laryngoscopy is, additionally, reviewed, with an image at the site demonstrating positioning. Links to microlaryngeal surgery and a movie showing a stroboscopic exam are included.
http://www.voice-center.com/exam_larynx.html

OTOSCOPY

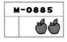

Family Practice Notebook.com: Otoscope Exam Preparation, technique of otoscopy, and procedures associated with pneumatic otoscopy are outlined at this online textbook chapter. Visitors can directly access related information on tympanometry and otitis media.
http://www.fpnotebook.com/ENT37.htm

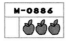

University of Texas Medical Branch: Tympanometer Patient evaluation for acute otitis media is discussed at this page, which provides information on the tympanometer, physics of the tympanogram, a normal tympanogram reading, and case examples of abnormal results. Connections are offered to additional portions of the site that address various aspects of patient evaluation, tympanic membrane anatomy, and a novel grading system approach to acute otitis media.
http://atc.utmb.edu/aom/tympanometry/default.htm

RAPID STREP TEST

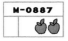

Harvard Medical School Family Health Guide: Rapid Strep Test The *Harvard Medical School Family Health Guide* offers visitors basic information on the rapid strep test that includes test preparation, an explanation of its performance, and waiting time for results. Viewers can easily access related tests within the guide. http://www.health.harvard.edu/fhg/diagnostics/strep/strepWhat.shtml

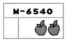

Virtual Hospital: Rapid Strep ID Testing Internally peer-reviewed, this University of Iowa Health Care site discusses the etiological agent of streptococcal pharyngitis, proper throat swab specimen collection, and principles and procedures for interpretation in an office setting. Sensitivity and specificity are stated, and the importance of follow-up procedures after a negative test is emphasized. http://www.vh.org/Providers/CME/CLIA/Microbiology/2RapidStrep.html

SCRATCH TEST FOR ALLERGIES

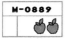

Harvard Medical School Family Health Guide: Scratch Test for Allergies Scratch tests for allergies are the focus of this chapter of Harvard's Family Health Guide. Pages on test preparations and what to expect during the procedure are provided.
http://www.health.harvard.edu/fhg/diagnostics/allergies/allergies.shtml

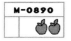

MEDLINEplus Medical Encyclopedia: Allergy Testing Alternative names, an image of skin testing, and a description of how the test is performed are provided at this site of the National Library of Medicine. Hyperlinks throughout the site bring visitors to further information on related terminology. Conditions under which the test is performed are listed, with connections available to related disorders.
http://www.nlm.nih.gov/medlineplus/ency/article/003519.htm

SINUS IMAGING

drkoop.com: Sinuses X-ray A summary of how this X-ray test is performed and special instructions for infants and children are provided at this encyclopedic reference of drkoop and the adam.com. Visitors can also access related pages on test results and an illustration of the sinus cavities.
http://umm.drkoop.com/conditions/ency/article/003803.htm

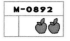

University of Michigan: Sinus CT May be Better Than X-ray This evidence-based pediatrics Web site offers a discussion of the advantages of computed tomography imaging of the sinuses over simple X-ray procedures for diagnosis of sinusitis, for distinguishing between allergic and non-allergic conditions, and for antibiotic selection. Clinical bottom lines and a summary of key evidence and conclusions are offered.
http://www.med.umich.edu/pediatrics/ebm/cats/sinusct.htm

THROAT CULTURE

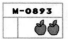

College of Physicians and Surgeons of Manitoba: Throat Culture
Providing information on the diagnostic value of culture and sensitivity of the throat, this article highlights recommendations of laboratory confirmation of group A streptococcal identification. Its use as the diagnostic test of choice and discussion of specificity and sensitivity are provided.
http://www.umanitoba.ca/cgi-bin/colleges/cps/college.cgi/1404.html

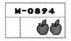

WebMDHealth: Throat Swab Culture   Reasons for performing a throat culture are explained at this online fact sheet in easy-to-understand terms. Normal values, special considerations, and links to further information on abnormal results are provided in adam.com's reader-friendly format.
http://my.webmd.com/content/asset/adam_test_throat_c_and_s

TYMPANOMETRY

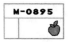

Family Practice Notebook.com: Tympanometry   Presented in outline format, this page offers a concise review of indications for otoscopy and links to information on pneumatic otoscopy and specific disorders.
http://www.fpnotebook.com/ENT38.htm

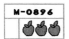

Tympanometry in Just Seconds   The diagnostic advantages of tympanometry over traditional methods of ear function assessment are introduced at this online article. Sponsored by Grason-Stadler, Inc., this page addresses key components of the procedure and test results. Figures at the site illustrate the normal ear, in addition to several abnormal findings.
http://www.grason-stadler.com/tymp.html#introduction

10.11 PSYCHIATRIC DIAGNOSTICS

DIAGNOSIS AND MANAGEMENT, GENERAL

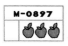

California Psychiatric Association: Prescribing Guidelines for Primary Care Physicians   Diagnosis and treatment of psychiatric conditions in the primary care setting is the focus of these online standards. Prescription and monitoring of psychotropic medication, accurate diagnosis, addressing the psychosocial components of illnesses, and determining accurate course of management are discussed.
http://www.calpsych.org/primarycare.html

Eastern Virginia Medical School: DSM-IV Disorders in Primary Care
Authored by S. Margaret Davies, M.D., and Olafur S. Palsson, Psy.D., this slide tutorial reviews some of the more common psychiatric problems encountered in

primary care practice. Intended to be a self-study module, the connections guide visitors through information on anxiety, depression, substance abuse, eating disorders, and somatoform disorders. Prevalence, recognition, statistics, screening recommendations, and diagnostic requirements are included. Visitors have the option of viewing the site in plain or graphic formats.

http://www.behavioralmedicine.net/tsld001.htm

DIAGNOSTIC CRITERIA/DSM-IV

American Family Physician: Using DSM-IV Primary Care Version

Published by the American Academy of Family Physicians, this *American Family Physician* document reviews the *Diagnostic and Statistical Manual of Mental Disorders* and emphasizes its usefulness in the primary care setting. Diagnostic algorithms, similarities between DSM-IV and the primary care version, and an illustrative case report are included.

http://www.aafp.org/afp/981015ap/pingitor.html

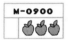

Internet Mental Health: Diagnosis

Offering an online diagnosis program, Internet Mental Health allows visitors to access information on any anxiety disorder, eating disorder, mood disorder, personality disorder, psychotic disorder, or substance-related condition from this page. Online, interactive programs that assist in diagnosis are found, with both patient self-assessment and therapist assessment questionnaires provided.

http://www.mentalhealth.com/fr71.html

MENTAL STATUS EXAMINATION

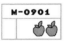

Indiana University School of Medicine: Mental Status Examination

Areas evaluated and assessment techniques are outlined at this page, which addresses the observation of a patient's behavior and interpretation of statements. Assessments of thinking, orientation, form of thought, assessment in children, perceptual-motor assessment, abstract thinking, thought content, affect, and behavior are reviewed.

http://php.iupui.edu/~flip/g505mse.html

UTMed.com: Mental Status Examination

Background on the mental status examination and summary information on general appearance, speech, thought processes and content, perception, and mood are presented. Formal cognitive screening and components of the basic examination are reviewed.

http://utmed.com/wmanuel/psyc/mse.html

10.12 RESPIRATORY AND PULMONARY MEDICINE

ARTERIAL BLOOD GAS ANALYSIS

Mount Sinai Medical Center: What's New in Blood Gas Interpretation   Excerpted from *All You Need to Know to Interpret Arterial Blood Gases,* this educational site offers access to chapter summaries on acid-base disorders and measurement, simple lung function measurement, and venous blood gas measurement. Each link provides users with a discussion of the particular assessment and utility of the information.
http://www.mtsinai.org/pulmonary/noninvasive/intro.htm

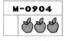

Virtual Hospital: Arterial Blood Gas Analysis   Sponsored by the University of Iowa College of Medicine, this page provides visitor with an introduction and basic concepts associated with arterial blood gas analysis. A systematic approach to analysis and a variety of case examples and discussions are found at this interactive teaching module.
http://www.vh.org/Providers/TeachingFiles/abg/ABGHome.html

AUSCULTATION AND RESPIRATORY ACOUSTICS

Loyola University Medical Education Network: Auscultation of Lungs   Method of lung exam is reviewed at this page, with links provided to Windows Media Player breath sounds. Connections at the bottom of the site bring readers to information on several categories of abnormal findings and a self-evaluation in lung auscultation screening techniques.
http://www.meddean.luc.edu/lumen/MedEd/medicine/pulmonar/pd/pstep29.htm

Loyola University Stritch School of Medicine: Auditory Findings   Provided, in part, by Dr. David Cugell and the American College of Chest Physicians, this site offers links to more than a dozen audio files via Windows Media Player. Visitors can easily listen to normal breath sounds, as well as rhonchus, crackles, and additional abnormal auditory findings.
http://www.meddean.luc.edu/lumen/MedEd/medicine/pulmonar/pd/auditory.htm

BRONCHOSCOPY

American College of Chest Physicians: Bronchoscopy   A patient education guide is found at this site, presenting reasons for performing bronchoscopy and advice on preparation. A description of the procedure and what to expect following the test are reviewed and provide basic information for consumer audiences.
http://www.chestnet.org/health.science.policy/
patient.education.guides/bronchoscopy.pted.html

Virtual Hospital: Bronchoscopy Atlas   This internally peer-reviewed site offers several bronchoscopy image links that provide appearance and general information on normal anatomy and anatomical variances and disorders of the larynx, trachea, bronchi, and distal airways.
http://www.vh.org/Providers/TeachingFiles/Bronchoscopy/BronchoscopyHome.html

Chest Imaging, General

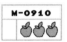

Society of Thoracic Radiology: Chest Imaging in the 21st Century
Moderated by Edward F. Patz, Jr, M.D., and Andre Duerinckx, M.D., Ph.D, this document provides chapters addressing digital imaging of the chest, computer-aided diagnosis, future directions in lung cancer imaging, and a new diagnostic approach to pulmonary embolism. Several additional chapters addressing recent innovations in pulmonary magnetic resonance (MR) angiography, and oxygen-enhanced MR of the lung are found, along with a scientific poster listing and abstracts. Adobe Acrobat Reader is required to open and print documents.
http://www.thoracicrad.org/str99/TI2000/thursday.htm

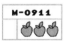

Virtual Hospital: A Multilingual Chest Imaging Database   Including a complete spectrum of chest diseases, this teaching file offers multiple examples of disease processes and presents inherent variations in appearance and severity of disease with a regularly updated image database. Contributions from around the world are found and supported by the University of Iowa Health Science Colleges. Clinical scenarios, etiology, images, and discussions are provided for each pathological entity. http://www.vh.org/Providers/TeachingFiles/ITTR/ITTR.html

Chest X-ray

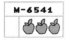

Loyola University Medical Education Network: Chest X-ray   Connections at this Loyola University site include the diagnostic value of chest X-ray, various pathologic images, and views of normal lung anatomy. Visitors can access a complete lecture outline, which includes how to evaluate sequential stages of abnormality. General principles of the chest X-ray, structure identification, and the pathological basis for abnormal shadows are reviewed.
http://www.meddean.luc.edu/lumen/MedEd/medicine/pulmonar/cxr/cxr.htm

Virtual Hospital: Introduction to Clinical Radiology: Chest   A module on chest imaging is provided as a service of University of Iowa Health Care at this address. Basic principles, normal anatomy, method for film analysis, and basic pulmonary pathologies are introduced. Various radiologic views, anatomic images, and patterns noticed with atelectasis, pleural effusions, pneumonia, cavitation, pulmonary nodules, pneumothorax, chronic obstructive pulmonary disease (COPD), and cardiac abnormalities are presented at this comprehensive tutorial.
http://www.vh.org/Providers/Lectures/icmrad/chest/01BasicPrinciples.html

PEAK FLOW MONITORING

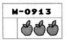

Loyola University: Home Peak Flow Monitoring Intended to provide a physician guide to supervising peak flow monitoring, this page describes the advantages of home monitoring of peak expiratory flow. Necessary materials, recommendations on describing the peak flow meter and its correct use to patients, and additional educational advice are presented. Worksheet connections provide further guidelines for clinicians that identify best uses, provide an asthma peak flow diary, and outline benefits of the technique.
http://www.meddean.luc.edu/lumen/MedEd/medicine/Allergy/Asthma/asthu6.html

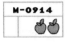

Medfacts: Peak Flow Monitoring The rationale for using a peak flow meter is explained at this Colorado site, sponsored by Denver's National Jewish Hospital. Determining one's personal best values, recognizing warning signs, and additional basic information on the use of peak flow monitoring in self-care are addressed. http://nationaljewish.org/medfacts/peak.html

PULMONARY ANGIOGRAPHY

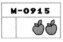

HealthCentral: Pulmonary Angiography The Pediatric Health Encyclopedia of HealthCentral includes this discussion of test preparation, risks, test performance, and normal and abnormal results of the pulmonary angiography. Hyperlinks throughout the text allow access to additional information on related disorders and other diagnostic concepts.
http://www.healthcentral.com/peds/top/003813.cfm

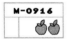

Virtual Hospital: Pulmonary Angiography Internally peer-reviewed, this site of the University of Iowa offers a description of pulmonary angiography procedures, accompanied by enlargeable, thumbnail images. Signs of pulmonary embolism are illustrated, and the safety and utility of pulmonary angiography in this diagnosis is emphasized.
http://www.vh.org/Providers/Textbooks/ElectricPE/Text/Angiography.html

PULMONARY FUNCTION TESTS

Merck Manual of Diagnosis and Therapy: Pulmonary Function Testing Simple spirometric techniques and physiologic testing procedures are described at this chapter of the online Merck reference. Static lung volumes and capacities are defined, as well as dynamic lung volumes and flow rates. Within the text, users can access a variety of tables and figures illustrating normal and abnormal spirogram and lung volumes and pulmonary function abbreviations. Information on lung mechanics, diffusing capacity, small airway studies, and other pertinent topics is provided, including the ordering and interpretation of pulmonary function tests and procedures for arterial blood gas analysis.
http://www.merck.com/pubs/mmanual/section6/chapter64/64a.htm

Virtual Hospital: Interpretation of Pulmonary Function Tests: Spirometry The Division of Pulmonary, Critical Care, and Occupational Medicine of the University of Iowa offers this presentation on requirements for optimal pulmonary function testing. Interpreting spirometry, a practice test for physicians, and other CME materials are available at this illustrated site.
http://www.vh.org/Providers/Simulations/Spirometry/SpirometryHome.html

RESPIRATORY EXAMINATION

Loyola University: Screening Physical Exam From this page, vistors can access several different pulmonary examination tutorials, as well as physical examination techniques across all medical specialties. Evaluation of respiratory rate, trachea position, voice transmission, chest percussion, and lung ausculation and chest observation are included among the accessible "Lungs" pages. Each chapter offers methods, a related image, links to definitions of related terminology, abnormal findings, and a self-evaluation quiz.
http://www.meddean.luc.edu/lumen/MedEd/medicine/pulmonar/pd/contents.htm

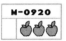

University of Florida: Respiratory Examination This physical exam study guide covers equipment needed, inspection, palpation, percussion, auscultation, and diagnostic tests that comprise the complete respiratory examination. Proper techniques, a table outlining percussion notes and their meaning, and steps in the examination of the posterior and anterior chest are reviewed.
http://www.medinfo.ufl.edu/year1/bcs/xclist/resp.html

SPUTUM CULTURE

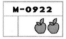

drkoop.com: Routine Sputum Culture Offered for consumer reference by drkoop, this adam.com site provides details on the sputum culture procedure and a connection to information on results. Links to various disorders associated with a report of a positive culture are found.
http://umm.drkoop.com/conditions/ency/article/003723.htm

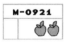

Royal College of Pathologists of Australia: Sputum Microscopy and Culture Specimen information and applications for sputum examination are discussed at this Web site. A reference interval and in-depth, clinical information on test interpretation are provided at this online *Manual of Use and Interpretation of Pathology Tests.*
http://www.rcpa.edu.au/pathman/sputum_m.htm

10.13 RHEUMATOLOGY DIAGNOSTICS

ANTINUCLEAR ANTIBODY (ANA) TEST

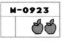

Antinuclear Antibody Test (ANA)   This AboutArthritis.com site discusses diseases associated with ANA, information on how the test is designed, what conditions cause ANAs to be produced, and ANA patterns. Visitors can also access an ANA forum, which features articles on topics such as ANA and lupus, pregnancy, and ulcerative colitis.
http://www.aboutarthritis.com/script/main/art.asp?li=ART&d=218&articlekey=7083

Royal College of Pathologists of Australia: Antinuclear Antibodies
The application of ANA testing in the diagnosis of systemic lupus erythematosus and other diseases is the focus of this page, part of an online handbook in laboratory medicine. Sensitivity and specificity, as well as other diagnostic considerations, are reviewed.
http://www.rcpa.edu.au/pathman/antinucl.htm

ARTHROSCOPY

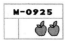

Arthroscopy   Hosted by AboutArthritis.com, information on arthroscopy includes discussion of conditions and diseases for which arthroscopy is considered, preparation, the procedure, and recovery information.
http://www.aboutarthritis.com/script/main/art.asp?li=ART&d=218&articlekey=283

YourSurgery.Com: Arthroscopy of the Knee   The anatomy and function of the knee, the pathology of diseases of the knee amenable to arthroscopic diagnosis and treatment, the arthroscopic procedure, possible complications of surgery, and numerous arthroscopic images are presented at this site of Your-Surgery.com.
http://www.yoursurgery.com/data/Procedures/knee/p_knee.cfm

C-REACTIVE PROTEIN

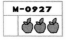

Laboratory Testing in the Rheumatic Diseases: C-Reactive Protein (CRP)   The University of Washington offer this discussion of the discovery of C-reactive protein, methodology for testing, and this particular acute phase reactant's ability to reflect inflammation directly. C-reactive protein versus erythrocyte sedimentation rate, reference range, and test utility are discussed.
http://uwcme.org/courses/rheumatology/rheumlab/crp.html

MEDLINEplus Medical Encyclopedia: C-reactive Protein   Reasons for performing the test for C-reactive protein are available for viewing from this site of adam.com and the National Library of Medicine. A link to further information on result information yields a listing of diseases implicated with a positive CRP. http://www.nlm.nih.gov/medlineplus/ency/article/003356.htm

COMPLEMENT

Complement   Information on complement proteins and their range of activities is found at this page, which includes nomenclature, complement pathways, and regulation of the complement cascade. The biological functions of complement and an outline of complement deficiencies are provided, courtesy of Kirksville College of Osteopathic Medicine.
http://www.kcom.edu/faculty/chamberlain/Website/MSTUART/lect9.htm

Family Practice Notebook.com: Complement   This family medicine resource offers an outline of complement physiology; C3, C4, and CH50 markers; and low complement level indications and causes.
http://www.fpnotebook.com/HEM93.htm

ERYTHROCYTE SEDIMENTATION RATE (ESR)

American Family Physician: Clinical Utility of the Erythrocyte Sedimentation Rate (ESR)   The use of the ESR in diagnosis of temporal arteritis, polymylagia rheumatica, and other diseases is the focus of this American Academy of Family Physicians publication. Physiologic basis for the test, reference ranges, factors that may influence ESR, and its use as a monitoring tool are explored, with comparisons among the ESR and related assessments addressed.
http://www.aafp.org/afp/991001ap/1443.html

ThriveOnline: Erythrocyte Sedimentation Rate   A consumer-oriented fact sheet explains the usefulness and indications for measurement of erythrocyte sedimentation rate (ESR). Visitors to this site will find a description of the test and some details on what high and low values indicate.
http://www.thriveonline.com/medical/library/article/003638.html

JOINT FLUOROSCOPY (ARTHROGRAM)

Center for Diagnostic Imaging: Arthrography   A description of the purpose and procedures involved in arthrogram of the joint are presented, along with patient preparations and restrictions. Links to similar pages on related diagnostic injections and pain management procedures, such as MRI arthrography and discography, are found. http://www.cdiradiology.com/d_artho.htm

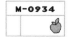

McGill University: Arthrogram   A description of joint fluoroscopy is offered at this page, with details on patient preparation included. Special considerations prior to testing with regard to medications, allergies, and heart disease are introduced.   http://www.car.ca/patients/arthrogram.htm

LABORATORY TESTING, GENERAL

Postgraduate Medicine: Laboratory Testing for Systemic Rheumatic Diseases An electronic reprint of an article discussing several tests available for diagnostic and follow-up evaluation in rheumatologic illness is presented, with specificity, sensitivity, and predictive values of numerous tests and their particular applications presented. Autoantibody tests, tests of inflammation, and the conditions associated with a positive rheumatoid factor test, antinuclear antibody screen, and other autoimmune antibodies are reviewed.
http://www.postgradmed.com/issues/1998/02_98/ward.htm

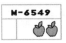

University of Wasington: About Laboratory Tests and Arthritis
Information on laboratory tests used in rheumatologic diagnosis is provided by the University of Washington Department of Orthopaedics at this page and its links. Goals of laboratory tests and their effectiveness are discussed, as well as the clinical utility of a variety of specific blood tests, immunologic blood tests, urine tests, joint fluid analyses, biopsies, and X-ray procedures.
http://www.orthop.washington.edu/Bone%20and%20Joint%20Sources/xzzzzzlz1_2.html

LUPUS BLOOD TESTS

Joanne's Lupus Site: Blood Tests Written in easy-to-understand terms, this personal page offers visitors a review of more than 25 blood tests used to diagnose, monitor disease activity, and evaluate side effects of drugs in lupus. A synopsis of each test presents a normal range and brief discussions of problems associated with abnormal results.
http://www.geocities.com/Heartland/Acres/7228/tests.html

Lupus Around the World: Laboratory Tests Common for Lupus This detailed site from Lupus Around the World offers an alphabetical list of blood tests common for lupus. The information, presented in table format, includes the name of the test, the normal ranges, and comments that include definitions and lists of conditions associated with an increase or decrease in the selected test values. http://www.mtio.com/lupus/lfalt1.htm

LYME DISEASE SEROLOGY

WebMD Health: Lyme Disease Antibody Test WebMD Health provides general information about the Lyme disease antibody test, with a quick reference table illustrating expectations and a discussion of test purpose, interpretation, factors that may affect results, and advantages and disadvantages.
http://my.webmd.com/content/asset/yale_
lab_tests_test_name_lyme_disease_antibody.html

MUSCLE ENZYME TESTS

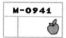

Family Practice Notebook.com: Serum Aldolase Normal aldolase value and a listing of diseases in which abnormal results may occur is provided at this online family medicine resource. Connections to dermatomyositis and polymyositis present pathophysiology, signs, and their related laboratory data. http://www.fpnotebook.com/REN56.htm

MDA Publications: Creatine Kinase Test This volume of the Muscular Dystrophy Association's *Quest* newsletter discusses the relevance of the creatine kinase (CK) test to muscular damage and offers general information on CK level measurement. Five basic ways that CK tests are used to evaluate disease are presented. http://www.mdausa.org/publications/Quest/q71ss-cktest.html

RHEUMATOID FACTOR

Laboratory Testing in the Rheumatic Diseases: Rheumatoid Factor A history of the development of rheumatoid factor testing, along with methodology, range, and test utility, is presented in this online publication of diagnostic testing in rheumatic disease. Visitors will encounter a use of disease associations, both rheumatologic and non-rheumatologic, and a literature review on the test's predictive value. http://uwcme.org/courses/rheumatology/rheumlab/rafactor.html

Northern Illinois University: Rheumatoid Factor (Rf) A slide tutorial offers visitors information on rheumatoid factor (Rf), rheumatoid arthritis, affected individuals, diagnostic criteria, and Rf characteristics. Additional conditions associated with an increased Rf level and principles of detection are summarized. http://www.ahp.hhsweb.com/cearlock/AHLS301/week1a/

SYNOVIAL FLUID ANALYSIS (ARTHROCENTESIS)

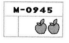

MEDLINEplus Medical Encyclopedia: Synovial Fluid Analysis An overview of synovial fluid analysis, along with risks and result information, is presented at this MEDLINEplus reference. An enlargeable illustration of needle insertion is accessible. http://www.nlm.nih.gov/medlineplus/ency/article/003629.htm

Virtual Hospital: Office and Hospital Procedures: Arthrocentesis Indications, contraindications, and general principles of technique involved in arthrocentesis are outlined at this site of the University of Iowa's Virtual Hospital. Specific positioning and preparation for the shoulder, wrist, elbow, and knee are presented, accompanied by related illustrations for practice. Use of intra-articular steroids is mentioned. http://www.vh.org/Providers/ClinRef/FPHandbook/Chapter17/02-17.html

URIC ACID (GOUT)

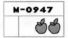

Arthritis Research Campaign: Gout: An Information Booklet An explanation of gout, with particular attention to the role of uric acid and its abnormal deposition, is found at this publication of the Arthritis Research Campaign. Disease specifics and diagnostic information, including plasma urate measurement, are presented.

http://www.arc.org.uk/about_arth/booklets/6015/6015.htm

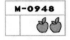

Uric Acid Tests The purpose of uric acid testing and certain drugs that may affect test results are discussed at this AllHealth Web page. Normal reference values for both blood and urine and the critical value for the blood test is stated. Causes of abnormal production of uric acid, including gout, are summarized and presented, along with key terms and references for further reading.

http://www.ahealthyme.com/article/gale/100084845

11

PRINCIPLES OF CLINICAL PHARMACOLOGY

11.1 GENERAL RESOURCES

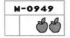

American Society for Clinical Pharmacology and Therapeutics
Founded to promote and advance the science of human pharmacology and therapeutics, this professional organization site supplies information on its annual meeting and other lectures and invites visitors to view their press room and grants and awards information. A secure member area includes an online membership directory.
(some features fee-based) http://www.ascpt.org/

Clinical Pharmacology 2000 With a free membership to Clinical Pharmacology 2000, members can access information on prescription, over-the-counter, investigational drugs, and herbal products, as well as photographs of drugs and product identification information. Also available in an encyclopedic format is a listing of details on drug comparisons, interactions and adverse reactions, intravenous compatibility reports, patient specific profiles and clinical alerts, electronic prescription writing, and advanced searching.
(free registration) http://cp.gsm.com

11.2 ADVERSE REACTIONS AND DRUG SAFETY

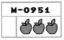

Adverse Reactions The Adverse Reactions Source offers an online forum and information to healthcare professionals and other interested viewers who want to share their knowledge about drug reactions, blood products, and other administered substances. Links to the Food and Drug Administration for adverse drug event reporting, a slide show about adverse drug reactions, therapy for treating anaphylaxis, and article summaries from leading experts in the field are provided. http://adversereactions.com/

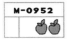

Center for Adverse Reactions Monitoring: Adverse Reactions of Current Concern This Medicines Awareness Reactions Committee's list offers reports on cases of adverse reactions of current concern. A list of medicines, their adverse reactions, and date of addition to the list are found, as well as further information on recent additions and deletions.
http://www.medsafe.govt.nz/Profs/adverse/cc.htm

MedWatch: FDA Medical Products Reporting Program The U.S. Food and Drug Administration sponsors this site to provide safety information to healthcare professionals. Features of the site include safety notifications on biologics, dietary supplements, and drugs, as well as labeling changes on drugs, recall reports, and food and drug interactions reports.
http://www.fda.gov/medwatch/safety.htm

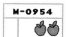

Merck Manual of Diagnosis and Therapy: Adverse Drug Reactions A brief discussion of adverse drug reactions, procedures for reporting them, incidence, causes, and treatment are offered at this site. Categories of reactions, including side effects, overdosage toxicity, drug allergies, and unexpected adverse reactions are addressed.
http://www.merck.com/pubs/mmanual/section22/chapter302/302b.htm

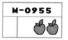

Yahoo! Health: Drug Safety Ratings Created to provide information on drug safety in pregnancy, this site provides an alphabetical listing of drugs and their FDA safety rating.
http://health.yahoo.com/health/drugsafety/

11.3 CLASSES OF DRUGS

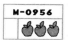

Clinical Formulary and Prescribing Guidelines Extensive details regarding clinical formulary and prescribing guidelines for clinicians are provided at this site for antimicrobials and antiinfective agents; antineoplastics and immunosuppressants; neurological drugs; anticoagulants and hematopoietics; cardiovascular agents; pain and anti-inflammatory medications; psychotropic medications; eye, ear, nose, and throat medicines; gastrointestinal drugs; diabetes mellitus medications; hormones; topical preparations; respiratory drugs; and supplements.
http://www.druglist.com/

DrugClasses A brief directory of drugs under review by the U.S. Food and Drug Administration, organized by drug classification, is available on this site. Names and numbers of principal investigators are provided.
http://www.fda.gov/cder/rdmt/drugclasses.htm

Medication Information Index The Cheshire Medical Center offers a medication information index to visitors of this site. More than 70 classes of medications such as antihistamines, beta-blockers, calcium channel blockers, nonsteroidal anti-inflammatory drugs, and penicillin are presented with links to details about their uses, administration methods, side effects, precautions, drug interactions, and storage.
http://www.cheshire-med.com/services/pharm/medindex.html

11.4 DRUG INTERACTIONS

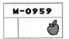

Adverse Medication Reactions Caused by Drug-Drug Interactions and Food-Drug Interactions Brief overviews of adverse medication reactions resulting from interactions between different drugs and from food and drug interactions are presented at this page, created by the Ohio Department of Aging at Ohio State University. In addition, potential warning signs of harmful drug reactions such as fatigue, constipation, incontinence, depression, hallucinations, and dizziness are outlined.
http://www.ag.ohio-state.edu/~ohioline/ss-fact/0129.html

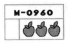

American Family Physician: Clinically Significant Drug Interactions Originally published by the American Academy of Family Physicians, this online article in clinical pharmacology describes interactions between medications, with special attention to multiple drug regimens and drugs that are more likely to cause problems. An overview of selected serious interactions are discussed, along with illustrative tables.
http://www.aafp.org/afp/20000315/1745.html

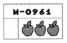

Drug Store News: A Common Sense Approach to Drug Interactions As its name implies, this article, presented as a courtesy of Findarticles.com, offers practitioners a guide to prediction, identification, and management of potential drug-drug interactions. Major mechanisms involved, common techniques for minimizing drug-drug interaction potential, and information on prediction based upon known routes of metabolism are examined.
http://www.findarticles.com/m3374/13_21/55693815/p1/article.jhtml

11.5 DRUG TOXICITY

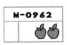

CliniWeb International: Drug Toxicity Visitors to this site will find links to PubMed queries related to drug eruptions, drug-induced dyskinesia, neuroleptic malignant syndrome, and serotonin syndrome. Related articles from the University of Iowa are accessible.
http://www.ohsu.edu/cliniweb/C21/C21.613.276.html

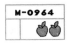

Merck Manual of Diagnosis and Therapy: Evaluation of Drug Toxicity Discussions of acute, subchronic, and chronic toxicity studies are presented at this online *Merck* chapter. Visitors can also browse information on in vitro toxicity studies and Phase One through Phase Four drug safety and efficacy studies.
http://www.merck.com/pubs/mmanual/section22/chapter302/302a.htm

Texas Cancer Online: Preventing Chemotherapy Drug Toxicity With a focus on information and support, this Web site discusses common toxic effects of chemotherapy, including nausea and vomiting, blood dyscrasias, neu-

ropathies, and hypersensitivity reactions. Cardiac toxicity and infertility are, additionally, addressed, as well as efforts to reduce these complications.
http://www.jasper-web.com/texascanceronline/prevention.htm

11.6 PHARMACOKINETICS/PHARMACODYNAMICS

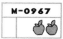

American Association of Pharmaceutical Scientists: Pharmacokinetics, Pharmacodynamics, and Drug Metabolism Section This section of the association, whose goal is to unite interested investigators, offers a professional forum for exchange of ideas and deliberation of issues in the field. News, focus groups, an online expo, and information about the organization's annual meetings are provided, as well as membership details.
(some features fee-based) http://www.aapspharmaceutica.com/resources/sections/ppdm/

Creighton University: Basic Pharmacokinetics Featured at this site is a complete, downloadable version of textbook for an introductory course in pharmacokinetics. Visitors can access information from the electronic text by chapter. Chapter topics include pharmacological response, biopharmaceutical factors, oral dosing, bioavailability, clearance, dosage, the multicompartment model, protein binding, non-linear kinetics, and online exams.
http://pharmacy.creighton.edu/pha443/pdf/Default.asp

Pharmacokinetics and Biopharmaceutics Authored by David Bourne, Ph.D., this searchable site offers a pharmacokinetic introduction, as well as chapters on background material and calculations, analysis of urine data, intravenous infusion information, and routes of drug administration. Pharmacokinetics of oral administration, calculation of bioavailablility principles, formulation factors, routes of excretion, and several related topics are covered in their entirety at this complete, online tutorial.
http://gaps.cpb.uokhsc.edu/gaps/pkbio/

RegSource Pharmacokinetics This site features a variety of resources related to pharmacokinetics on the Web, including access to software developed by University of California for analysis of pharmacokinetic data, pharmacokinetic equations, research and development, and a virtual library.
http://www.regsource.com/European_Page/Pharmacokinetics/pharmacokinetics.html

University of Kansas School of Medicine: Medical Pharmacology Units Medical students and physicians visiting this site will find access to general principles of medical pharmacology, as well as units on the endocrine system, central nervous system, cardiovascular drugs, chemotherapy, and additional pharmacology topics. The link to general principles in the field offers educational units on both pharmacokinetics and pharmacodynamics.
http://www.pharmacology2000.com/learning2.htm

TOPICAL RESOURCES FOR INTERNAL MEDICINE

12.1 ABUSE/NEGLECT/VIOLENCE

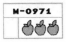

National Center on Elder Abuse This Web site features a fact sheet describing abuse of the elderly, access to center publications, adult protective services statistics, information on the National Elder Abuse Incidence Study, details about federal and state statutes regarding elderly abuse, the research agenda of the center, and access to current and archived newsletters.
http://www.elderabusecenter.org/

National Clearinghouse on Child Abuse and Neglect Information
The National Clearinghouse on Child Abuse and Neglect Information provides visitors with access to its various publications, including fact sheets on child maltreatment, child abuse and neglect national statistics, child fatalities, and child abuse and neglect prevention. The user manual series, statistical information, bibliographies, prevention resources, and listings for various areas, such as adult survivors, child advocacy, and child fatalities, are provided.
http://www.calib.com/nccanch

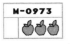

National Coalition Against Domestic Violence Visitors to the National Coalition Against Domestic Violence Web site will find descriptions, statistics, and more than 50 links regarding domestic violence, along with guidelines for starting a domestic violence shelter. Links include the Batterer Intervention Services Coalition, the Bryant Program on Domestic Violence, the Family Violence Prevention Fund, and the National Clearinghouse on Marital and Date Rape.
http://www.ncadv.org

12.2 ADOLESCENT HEALTH

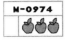

American Medical Association (AMA): Adolescent Health On-Line
Answers to FAQs, the AMA's Scientific Update on adolescent health, Internet adolescent health resources, and an assortment of special topics related to child and adolescent health are addressed. Tips for successful navigation of the site are provided, as well as information on adolescent-related health observances.
http://www.ama-assn.org/ama/pub/category/1947.html

Centers for Disease Control and Prevention (CDC): Adolescent and School Health Statistics on pregnancies, abortions, and sexually transmitted diseases; state profiles; and trends dealing with adolescent and school health are presented at this site from the National Center for Chronic Disease Prevention and Health Promotion. Information on national school health strategies, research and evaluation, risk behaviors and health topics, and additional resources and tools are featured as well.
http://www.cdc.gov/nccdphp/dash/ahson/ahson.htm

MEDLINEplus Health Information: Child and Teen Health Topics MEDLINEplus is the host of this extensive site dealing with child and teen health topics. 50 children's health topics are presented, including learning disorders, measles, attention deficit disorder with hyperactivity, rubella, teen violence, alcohol and youth, and teenage pregnancy. Various resources providing general information, as well as information on topics such as prevention and screening, specific conditions, related news, laws, clinical trials, and organizations dealing with each featured area of teen health are provided.
http://www.nlm.nih.gov/medlineplus/childandteenhealth.html

National Women's Health Information Center: Adolescent Health Questions regarding critical issues in adolescent health today and what parents can do to promote and improve a teen's health and lifestyle habits are addressed at this site, created by the National Women's Health Information Center. Links to various resources, including the National Center for Chronic Disease Prevention and Health Promotion, the Department of Adolescent Health, Girls Incorporated, the Youth Services Bureau, and the American Academy of Child and Adolescent Psychiatry, are provided along with articles on HIV/AIDS, sexually transmitted diseases, substance abuse and treatment, eating disorders, diet and nutrition, exercise, stress, and teen pregnancy.
http://www.4woman.gov/faq/adoles.htm

12.3 ALTERNATIVE MEDICINE

Alternative Medicine Foundation Highlighted at the Alternative Medicine Foundation is "HerbMed," an interactive herbal database with links to scientific data regarding the use of various herbal remedies in healthcare. Also featured at this site is the *Journal of Alternative and Complementary Medicine* and resource guides in the areas of acupuncture, herbal medicine, manual therapies, mind/body medicine, traditional Chinese medicine, and ayurveda.
http://www.amfoundation.org/

HerbMed The Alternative Medicine Foundation, Inc. hosts HerbMed, a scientific database devoted to the use of herbs for health purposes. The evidence for activity, warnings, preparations, mixtures, and mechanism of action for an extensive list of herbs are presented.
http://www.herbmed.org/

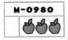

National Center for Complementary and Alternative Medicine (NCCAM) The National Center for Complementary and Alternative Medicine, part of the National Institutes of Health, offers this Web page to provide consumers, practitioners, and investigators with information on this growing field. Practitioners will find the fact sheets, consensus reports, and complementary and alternative medicine databases useful. A special section of the site is dedicated to funding opportunities and deadlines for investigators.
http://nccam.nih.gov/

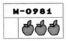

New York Online Access to Health (NOAH): Alternative (Complementary) Medicine Links to information and resources regarding various types of alternative medicine, including acupuncture, the Alexander Technique, ayurvedic medicine, electrical therapies, herbal medicine, homeopathy, macrobiotics, massage, naturopathic medicine, and reflexology are offered by New York Online Access to Health (NOAH).
http://www.noah-health.org/english/alternative/alternative.html

12.4 BLOOD DONATIONS/BLOOD BANKS

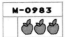

America's Blood Centers America's Blood Centers (ABC) is a national network of independent community blood centers, which provides information on its members, blood banking philosophy, and research and development. News releases for America's blood centers, legislative advocacy, and medical topic coverage in the form of online bulletins are provided. Publications from *ABC BloodNews* are viewable from links at the site, as are archived issues of *ABC Blood Bulletin,* the *ABC Newsletter,* and position papers of the organization. http://4.21.230.152/sitemap/default.htm

American Association of Blood Banks The home page of the American Association of Blood Banks (AABB) provides details to visitors about membership, legislative programs, educational programs, publications, and other services, including the AABB's special interest groups, the question and answer services, the autologous blood transfusion resources, the National Blood Exchange, and a section for professionals about the AABB's annual meeting, audio conferences, and computer-assisted conferences.
http://www.aabb.org

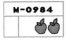

American Red Cross: Give Blood This portion of the American Red Cross Web site offers information to visitors on blood donation, and a search engine allows visitors to locate their nearest chapter. Additional departments of the site provide publications, news, answers to FAQs, and details of other services of the organization.
http://www.redcross.org/donate/give/

12.5 CAREER RESOURCES

American College of Physicians-American Society of Internal Medicine (ACP-ASIM): Career Resource Center Hosted by the American College of Physicians - American Society of Internal Medicine, visitors will find job openings, CME opportunities, and a schedule of chapter meetings. Residents and fellows will find a series of full-text articles designed to assist in career planning, organized by month for the last year of residency or fellowship training. The site also contains a residency database and information on the physician renewal project, which is aimed at countering physician burnout.
http://www.acponline.org/careers/

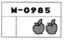

InternalMedicineJobs.com Two databases related to internal medicine jobs are featured on this site—one offers job openings, and the other advertises jobs wanted. http://www.internalmedicinejobs.com/

Jobscience.com Job openings in the healthcare industry are featured on this Web page. The jobs are organized under categories such as nursing, physicians, dental, allied health, pharmaceuticals, management, and diagnostics. The site also features educational seminars; career tools, such as a salary calculator; career counseling; and related resources. A catalog of career-related books is also available on the site.
http://www.jobscience.com/

12.6 CHRONIC DISEASE AND DISABILITY

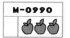

Department of Justice: Americans with Disabilities Act (ADA) Home Page Hosted by the Department of Justice, this Web page on the Americans with Disabilities Act (ADA) features a wealth of information on complying with the law. The site contains the latest enforcement reports, ADA settlements and consent agreements, and technical assistance publications for the public, businesses, and government agencies.
http://www.usdoj.gov/crt/ada/adahom1.htm

Medscout: Chronic Disease and Disability A comprehensive bibliographical listing of chronic disease and disability publications, associations, and related resources can be found on this site.
http://www.medscout.com/diseases/chronic/index.htm

12.7 COMMUNITY HEALTH

Health Resources and Services Administration: Community Health Status Indicators Visitors to this Web page can look up a *Community Health Status Report* for their county. The reports offer demographic information, along with life expectancy, number of unhealthy days, leading causes of

death, access to care, and overall health status relative to other similar communities. Reports can also be produced by state, county population size, or race.
http://www.communityhealth.hrsa.gov/

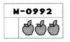

National Association of Community Health Centers   Dedicated to serving the interests of community, migrant, and homeless health centers, the association offers community health centers a broad array of resources. Services target health center operations, such as finance and capital assistance programs, leadership training, and technical assistance. In addition, the site offers information on federal and state policy issues, meetings, training opportunities, and association programs, such as the Adolescent and School Health Initiative.
http://www.nachc.com/

12.8 DIPLOMATS IN INTERNAL MEDICINE

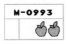

American Board of Internal Medicine (ABIM): Directory of Diplomats   A directory of diplomats in internal medicine is featured on this site. The directory can be searched by city, region, country, zip code, or physician's name. http://www.abim.org/dp/apps/physdir.htm

12.9 ENVIRONMENTAL AND OCCUPATIONAL HEALTH

American College of Occupational and Environmental Medicine   A general overview of the American College of Occupational and Environmental Medicine is offered at this Web site, along with resources regarding federal relations, state relations, the Legislative Action Center, members forums, and news. The latest news releases regarding environmental medicine, various position statements and guidelines, and the Code of Ethical Conduct for physicians are also included.
http://www.acoem.org/

Centers for Disease Control and Prevention (CDC): Occupational Health   Occupational Health is the focus of this site, provided by the Centers for Disease Control and Prevention. Topics include accident causes and prevention, effects of workplace hazards on male reproductive health, latex allergies, occupational injuries, and violence in the workplace. Access to information on topics in the areas of adolescent and teen health, foodborne illnesses, men's health, senior health, traveler's health, and women's health are offered.
http://www.cdc.gov/health/occupati.htm

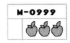

Environmental Protection Agency (EPA)   The United States Environmental Protection Agency provides daily news coverage of topics related to the environment and its effect on the nation's health. An interactive map of the United States provides visitors with regional coverage of environmental issues.

Sections on laws and regulations, current legislation, and numerous additional features and related sites are provided.
http://www.epa.gov

Health, Environment, and Work: Occupational and Environmental Health Links A directory of sites regarding occupational and environmental health is provided by the Health, Environment and Work site. Hundreds of connections dealing with current topics, news sites, educational resources, toxicology databases, pollution, resources and directories, journals and books, societies and lobby groups, and Internet navigation are offered.
http://www.agius.com/hew/links/

New York Online Access to Health (NOAH): Environmental Health Articles and information on various environmental health topics are made available through links at this well-known, non-profit portal. Topics presented include asbestos, biological contaminants, combustion, appliances, ozone, pollution, lead, radiation, water quality, and secondhand smoke. Visitors to this site will also find links to environmental health advocacy groups, general resources, technical/professional resources, and legal resources.
http://www.noah-health.org/english/illness/environment/environ.html

Occupational Safety and Health Administration (OSHA) Resources for healthcare professionals, as well as for workers, are offered at this site from the Occupational Safety and Health Administration, including technical links and resources for training, consultation, construction, ergonomics, small businesses, compliance, federal registrars, standards, and interpretations. News releases, OSHA regulations, congressional testimonies, fact sheets, and reports are provided. Publications on key topics may be downloaded directly from the site.
http://www.osha.gov

12.10 EPIDEMIOLOGY

Centers for Disease Control and Prevention (CDC) The home page of the CDC, the leading federal agency for protecting health and safety, contains an A-to-Z listing of health topics, data and statistics, and current news headlines. The CDC's mission, access to several online publications and reports, and CDC's vision for the 21st century are presented. http://www.cdc.gov/

National Center for Infectious Diseases The National Center for Infectious Diseases of the Centers for Disease Control and Prevention (CDC) offers details about its divisions and programs in the areas of AIDS, bacterial and mycotic diseases, hospital infections, parasitic diseases, quarantine, scientific resources, vector-borne infectious diseases, and viral and rickettsial diseases. For each infectious disease, an extensive listing and write-up drawn from the CDC database are found. Current health-related news articles are featured at this site, as well as links to related resources.
http://www.cdc.gov/ncidod/index.htm

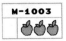

World Health Organization (WHO): Statistical Information System
Health-related statistical information from the WHO Global Programme on Evidence for Health Policy is found at this collection of links. Health surveys, mortality data, the *Weekly Epidemiological Record*, additional WHO publications and library information services, and health-related demographic impacts are examined. Numerous connections to disease-oriented epidemiological data are accessible, as well as additional learning opportunities at the WHO home page link. http://www.who.int/whosis/

WWW Virtual Library: Epidemiology   Links to epidemiology resources are provided in various subject areas, including government agencies, infectious diseases, reproductive epidemiology, newsgroups and mailing lists, university sites, hospitals, quantitative epidemiology, employment opportunities, and professional societies in the field. Additional topics include molecular epidemiology, epidemiology of cancer, behavioral epidemiology, cardiovascular epidemiology, environmental epidemiology, and diabetes-related information.
http://www.epibiostat.ucsf.edu/epidem/epidem.html

12.11 EXERCISE AND PHYSICAL FITNESS

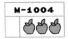

American Council on Exercise   Visitors to this site can access a database of qualified fitness professionals, subscribe to *ACE FitnessMatters*, and sign up to receive free monthly health and fitness newsletters. Details on ACE certification, practical training programs, online articles on fitness, and a certified professional section area are available.
(some features fee-based) http://www.acefitness.org/

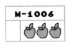

MEDLINEplus Health Information: Exercise/Physical Fitness   Various areas of exercise and physical fitness are covered by MEDLINEplus links available at this site. In addition, news articles about physical fitness, links to the American Running Association and Shape Up America, and exercise and health statistics are provided.
http://www.nlm.nih.gov/medlineplus/exercisephysicalfitness.html

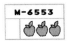

National Center for Chronic Disease Prevention and Health Promotion: Physical Activity and Health   A report of the U.S. Surgeon General is available at this site, stating the evolution of its recommendations, adaptations to exercise, and the effects of exercise on both health and disease. An entire chapter of the publication is devoted to the understanding and promotion of physical activity, and a complete list of illustrative tables and figures is provided.
http://www.cdc.gov/nccdphp/sgr/sgr.htm

12.12 FIRST AID, INJURIES, AND WOUNDS

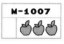

First Aid with PARASOL EMT An Internet version of a first aid book created for emergency medical personnel is available at this site, in addition to downloadable brochures and a first aid kit description. Visitors can order a full range of first aid supplies and medical equipment or gain access to information on educational seminars.

http://www.parasolemt.com.au/

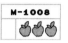

MEDLINEplus Health Information: First Aid/Emergencies This site created by MEDLINEplus, a federal information program, provides a useful assortment of links to general first aid information. Details on clinical trials, diagnostic criteria and symptoms, prevention and screening, first aid for specific conditions, treatment options, and news articles are ready accessible. First aid information specific to children is presented, as well as links to the American College of Emergency Physicians, the American Red Cross, and The National Institute for Occupational Safety and Health.

http://www.nlm.nih.gov/medlineplus/firstaidemergencies.html

MEDLINEplus Health Information: Injuries and Wounds Topics This site on injury and wound topics contains links to extensive information on such topics as bites and bee stings, radiation exposure, rape, spinal cord injuries, and other conditions requiring immediate attention. With each link, patients are able to access organizations, news articles, clinical trial information, treatment options, and fact sheets on the condition.

http://www.nlm.nih.gov/medlineplus/injuriesandwounds.html

12.13 GENETICS AND GENOMICS

National Center for Biotechnology Information (NCBI) Molecular databases, literature databases, genomic biology related resources, tools for data mining, teaching resources and online tutorials, and downloadable data and software can be accessed through this site from the National Center for Biotechnology Information. Details regarding research conducted at the Computational Biology Branch is also presented.

http://www.ncbi.nlm.nih.gov

Online Mendelian Inheritance in Man (OMIM) Dedicated to human genes and genetic disorders, the OMIM database contains in-depth articles regarding an A-to-Z listing of genetic conditions and supported by reference information. A catalog of genetic diseases and their cytogenetic map locations is also available from the site. Information on browsing the OMIM database, gene map, or morbid map is provided, as well as links to OMIM allied resources.

http://www.ncbi.nlm.nih.gov/Omim/

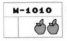

World of Genetics Societies Links to several genetics societies, as well as information on genetics education, certification, and other related sites are featured at this Web page.

http://www.faseb.org/genetics/mainmenu.htm

12.14 GERIATRIC MEDICINE

American Geriatrics Society (AGS) Features of the American Geriatrics Society (AGS) Web site include links to eight AGS publications; general, consumer, and professional educational materials; current news articles; and health links to over 75 sources, including Healthfinder, MEDLINE, the Society of General Internal Medicine, the National Center for Health Statistics, the American Medical Association, and the American Society on Aging. Readers can also access a section on public policy and a members-only area.

(some features fee-based) http://www.americangeriatrics.org

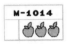

MedBioWorld: Geriatrics and Gerontology Journals Access to more than 35 journals in the field of geriatrics and gerontology is provided by MedBioWorld at this site. Journals include *Age and Aging, Drugs & Aging, The Gerontologist, Reviews in Clinical Gerontology,* and *Psychology and Aging.* A variety of online content, abstracts, and full-text articles are available on the Web from individual publishers.

http://www.medbioworld.com/journals/medicine/geriatrics.html

MEDLINEplus Health Information: Seniors' Health Topics Senior health resources are provided at this site from MEDLINEplus. Visitors can gain access to basic information, symptoms and diagnostic measures, aspects of specific conditions, treatment options, organizations, and statistics dealing with various topics regarding senior health. Coverage of stroke, cataract, elder abuse, glaucoma, menopause, Alzheimer's, urinary incontinence, and osteoporosis is provided, as well as drug information searchable by generic or brand name.

http://www.nlm.nih.gov/medlineplus/seniorshealth.html

12.15 IMMUNIZATION

Centers for Disease Control and Prevention (CDC): National Immunization Program An overview of vaccine safety is presented at this site from the Centers for Disease Control and Prevention. Topics discussed include the importance of vaccinations, the National Childhood Vaccine Injury Act, monitoring vaccine safety, the Vaccine Injury Compensation Program, improvements in vaccination, risk communication, and the future of vaccination safety.

http://www.cdc.gov/nip/vacsafe/default.htm

Medscout: Immunizations Various sources of information regarding immunization are presented for patients at this site from Medscout. Access to

brochures, immunization schedules for numerous conditions, journals, online resources, research information, and vaccine companies is provided.
http://www.medscout.com/immunizations/index.htm

National Network for Immunization Information Featured news, a vaccine information database, and immunization newsbriefs are all part of the Internet location for this scientifically-based organization. A resource kit, available in Adobe Acrobat PDF format, can be downloaded from the site, which facilitates communication with patients about immunization. Feature archives are available, covering childhood immunization schedules and evidence-based research. http://www.immunizationinfo.org/

12.16 INSURANCE AND MANAGED CARE

American College of Physicians-American Society of Internal Medicine Online: Effective Medical Practice and Managed Care (EMPMC) The Effective Medical Practice and Managed Care Web site allows visitors to gain a greater understanding of the management of current healthcare delivery systems. Links to information on products and services for practicing medicine in today's managed care environment, basic review of the managed care setting, and links to guidelines, journal articles, position papers, and external resources related to managed care are offered as a service of the American College of Physicians-American Society of Internal Medicine.
http://www.acponline.org/mgdcare/

Medscape: Managed Care Following a free and simple registration process, users have access to professional resources addressing the complex issues associated with the managed care system. Managed care news, journal articles, and conference coverage are available.
(free registration)
http://managedcare.medscape.com/Home/Topics/ManagedCare/ManagedCare.html

12.17 INTERNATIONAL HEALTH

National Center for Infectious Diseases: Division of Global Migration and Quarantine To prevent transmission of communicable diseases, the Division of Quarantine at the National Center for Infectious Diseases provides the United States Code and the Code of Federal Regulations regarding travel. Requirements for animal transportation from the U.S. Public Health Service are listed, as well as information about foreign quarantine and the duties of quarantine inspectors.
http://www.cdc.gov/ncidod/dq/index.htm

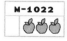

Pan American Health Organization The Pan American Health Organization provides visitors to this site with health data resources, information on

health topics, including disasters, diseases, environmental health, epidemiology, research, vaccines, and immunization. Informative resources, such as technical documents, books, periodicals, and announcements, as well as featured health-related articles are presented.
http://www.paho.org

World Health Organization (WHO)   Current health news on disease outbreaks and emergencies, as well as recently published health news from the World Health Organization are made available to visitors at this site. Visitors can search for articles about specific health conditions and information about communicable diseases, tropical diseases, vaccine-preventable illness, the environment, family and reproductive health, health policies, health technology, lifestyle, and non-communicable diseases. Additional information sources include the *Bulletin of the World Health Organization, World Health Report,* and the *International Digest of Health Legislation.*
http://www.who.int

12.18 LEGISLATION AND PUBLIC POLICY

American Hospital Association Policy Forum   For those interested in healthcare policy, this site offers a variety of policy resources. There are live chat events with healthcare leaders and policy makers, American Hospital Association policy briefs and reports, and a quarterly report on hospital and health system trends entitled *TrendWatch*. Members have access to a message board for online policy discussion.
http://www.ahapolicyforum.org/trendwatch_home.asp

American Medical Association (AMA): AMA in Washington   Information on the AMA's legislative and regulatory priorities; its interactions with Congress, the White House, and federal agencies; political education programs; and its Grassroots Action Center are found at this action-oriented site. The AMA offers patients a page on patients' rights legislative information, containing testimony, letters, and details about current issues in healthcare policy.
http://www.ama-assn.org/ama/pub/category/4015.html

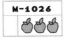

Medical Laws and Legislation   Important online government resources, including the Agency for Healthcare Research and Quality, FEDWORLD Information Network, and the National Science Foundation Office of Legislative and Public Affairs, are accessible through this site, which is dedicated to offer various pages addressing medical laws, legislation, and policy. Additional resources for government-health issues and interface include the Centers for Disease Control and Prevention, the Department of Health and Human Services, the Food and Drug Administration, the Office of Disease Prevention and Health Promotion, and the Occupational Safety and Health Administration.
http://www.libsci.sc.edu/bob/class/clis734/webguides/Medical.htm

12.19 MEN'S HEALTH

Harvard Health Online: Harvard Men's Health Watch The doctors of Harvard Medical School present this Harvard Health publication, which offers special reports related to men's health. Readers will find answers to commonly asked questions about men and their experience with depression, cancer, and heart disease. The current issue of the *Harvard Men's Health Watch* is available online. (some features fee-based) http://www.health.harvard.edu/aboutmens.shtml

MEDLINEplus Health Information: Men's Health General information on men's health can be accessed from this collection of links, which includes the latest news in men's treatment and health research, links to general sites that focus on men's health, prevention and screening tests for men, an online men's health newsletter, and information from the National Center for Health Statistics. Links also include a listing of men's health topics, including prostate disease and reproductive health.
http://www.nlm.nih.gov/medlineplus/menshealthgeneral.html

Men's Health Network Based in Washington, D.C., this men's health organization offers information about its strategy, goals, and programs at this site. Several nationwide men's health initiatives are described, and access to feature events of Men's Health TV webcasts are available. Programming at this site addresses mental health, diet, sexual health, fitness, and medical conditions. The reference library of the site connects to a multitude of related links and documents. http://www.menshealthnetwork.org/

12.20 MINORITY AND CROSS-CULTURAL HEALTH

Center for Cross-Cultural Health Upcoming events, answers to FAQs, conference details, the *CrossWinds* newsletter are provided at this site, in addition to links to the National Center for Education in Maternal and Child Health, the Office of Minority Health Resource Center, and the Ethnic Health Improvement Project. Information about training units, staff members, and volunteer opportunities are provided.
http://www.crosshealth.com/

EthnoMed EthnoMed, an ethnic medical guide sponsored by Harborview Medical Center and the University of Washington offers cultural profiles and medical topics regarding Chinese, Vietnamese, and other cultures. Cross-cultural health topics and clinical pearls are presented, as well as immigration issues and research challenges. Related Web sites, including Tribal Connections in the Pacific Northwest, Asian Pacific Islanders Women's Health, Multicultural Health Communication, the Cross Cultural Health Care Program, and the Office of Minority Health are accessible through this site.
http://healthlinks.washington.edu/clinical/ethnomed

Initiative to Eliminate Racial and Ethnic Disparities in Health   The U.S. Department of Health and Human Services hosts this page, which provides departments on infant mortality, cancer management, cardiovascular disease, diabetes, HIV infection, and immunizations in minority populations. Details regarding organizational activities, grants, and funding are offered, as well as related resources provided by the Centers for Disease Control and Prevention, the National Immunization Program, various FDA Web sites, and the National Coalition for Adult Immunization.
http://www.raceandhealth.omhrc.gov

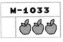 **National Institutes of Health (NIH): Office of Minority Health**   Access to the Office of Minority Health publications is provided at this Web site, as well as access to federal and non-federal publications. Visitors to this site will also find statistical information regarding minority health and links to related health sites, such as the NIH Research Training Opportunities for Minorities, the Office of Minority Health Resource Center (OMHRC) Health Materials Database, and the CDC's Diabetes Racial and Ethnic Health Disparities Initiative. http://www.omhrc.gov

 University of California San Francisco (UCSF): Cross-Cultural Resources   Curriculum links, articles addressing cross-cultural issues, and connections to sites dedicated to cross-cultural healthcare issues are provided. Access to organizations such as the Minority Affairs Consortium, the Office of Multicultural Health, and the National MultiCultural Institute are offered, as well as a link to clinical guidelines for health topics included within more than 20 health categories.
http://medicine.ucsf.edu/resources/guidelines/culture.html

12.21 NUTRITION

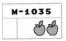 **American Dietetic Association**   The site map for the American Dietetic Association provides access to information on healthy lifestyles, books and nutrition resources designed for both consumers and professionals, meetings and events, press releases and kits, policy initiatives and advocacy, and details on becoming a member.
http://www.eatright.org/

 Information About Nutrition   Nineteen links to information on nutrition from the Center for Food Safety and Applied Nutrition and the U.S. FDA are offered at this site. Information is provided on topics such as fiber intake, healthful snacks, pregnancy, medical foods, infant formula, dietary guidelines, soy, fat, calcium, and vegetarian diets.
http://vm.cfsan.fda.gov/~dms/wh-nutr.html

 International Food Information Council   The Nutrition International Food Information Council Foundation provides food safety and nutrition information regarding sweeteners, food labeling, food biotechnology, adult nutri-

tion, health and physical activity, food additives, food safety, international food issues and resources, fats and fat replacers, food allergy and asthma, and food irradiation and technologies. In addition, the council's publications are made available in PDF format from governmental agencies.
http://ificinfo.health.org

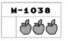

MEDLINEplus Health Information: Nutrition   General information sources, clinical trial details, information on specific conditions, law and policy information, and news articles focused on nutrition are provided at this site from MEDLINEplus. Information specific to seniors, teenagers, and women regarding nutrition is also offered.
http://www.nlm.nih.gov/medlineplus/nutrition.html

12.22 PATIENT EDUCATION AND SUPPORT

Checkup on Health Insurance Choices   When thinking about health insurance choice, consumers may wish to consult this Internet guide, provided by the Agency for Health Care Policy and Research. Information about health insurance types, managed care, and a checklist and worksheet to assist in the buying process are provided.
http://www.ahcpr.gov/consumer/insuranc.htm

Healthfinder   News articles are featured at this government site, as well as coverage of numerous areas of health. Consumer information on AIDS, influenza, hepatitis, Medicare, tobacco, and government health resources are provided. This site also provides special coverage of health issues specific to infants, children, teens, adults, seniors, the Spanish speaking community, families, men, women, minority groups, and professionals.
http://www.healthfinder.gov

MedicineNet.com   MedicineNet.com is a comprehensive source of medical information, featuring current health news, doctor's views, health facts, and links to organizations such the American College of Surgeons, the National Cancer Institute, and the Virtual Hospital. Patients can access information about the symptoms, risk factors, diagnosis, and treatment options for hundreds of disorders, as well as information on hundreds of medications.
http://www.medicinenet.com/Script/Main/hp.asp?li=MNI&d=222&cu=16583&w=1&

MedicineNet.com: Medications Index   An alphabetical index of medications is made available by MedicineNet.com at this site. Consumers will find hundreds of links to detailed information about both generic and brand name medications. Drug class and mechanism, indications for use, dosage, interactions, use during pregnancy, and possible side effects of each are addressed.
http://www.medicinenet.com/Script/Main/AlphaIdx.asp?li=MNI&p=A_PHARM

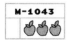

MedicineNet.com: Procedures and Tests Index   A procedure and tests index covering hundreds of diagnostic tools is available at MedicineNet.com.

For each procedure, the visitor will learn about why the procedure is conducted, the design of the procedure, what conditions various tests can diagnose, other surgical options, and basic facts about various conditions.
http://www.medicinenet.com/Script/Main/AlphaIdx.asp?li=MNI&p=A_PROC

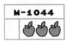

MEDLINEplus Health Information   MEDLINEplus provides extensive information through off-site links on hundreds of conditions, diseases, and general health issues. At this page, visitors have access to a medical encyclopedia; descriptions of general and brand name medications; medical dictionaries; directories of physician, dentists, and hospitals locators; and access to numerous organizations, consumer health libraries, and medical publications. Links to the U.S. National Library of Medicine, the National Institutes of Health, the Department of Health and Human Services, and the Freedom of Information Act are provided. http://medlineplus.nlm.nih.gov/medlineplus

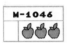

New York Online Access to Health (NOAH): Support Groups Support group information specific to a variety of diseases can be found at this site from NOAH. Over 40 representative Internet connections are offered, including links to Web sites concerning asthma, cancer, diabetes, mental health, rare diseases, and sexual abuse.
http://www.noah-health.org/english/support.html

SupportPath.com   Over two-hundred support-oriented bulletin boards are offered at SupportPath.com, as well as numerous links providing Internet and local chapter support group information. More than 200 conditions and health-related topics are presented alphabetically, with details and links to related organizations, government Web sites, and general information links on specific conditions. http://www.supportpath.com/

12.23 PATIENT RIGHTS

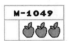

Center for Patient Advocacy   Working toward reform of the healthcare system, the home page of the Center for Patient Advocacy provides access to the Cancer Care Alliance; details about healthcare debates in Washington concerning Medicare, managed care, and other healthcare issues; a patient resource center offering healthcare headlines; and ordering information for organization publications. The organization stresses healthcare advocacy and access to quality patient care. (free registration) http://www.patientadvocacy.org

Consumer.gov: Patient Rights and Responsibilities   The Consumer Bill of Rights and Responsibilities, a Patient's Bill of Rights, and links to information on prescription medicines, the Agency for Healthcare Research and Quality, and answers to questions about recent changes in healthcare law are provided at this site's connections.
http://www.consumer.gov/qualityhealth/rights.htm

National Coalition for Patients' Rights Details about current news topics regarding patient's rights are provided by the National Coalition for Patient Rights, at this Web site. Patients can get answers to questions about genetic privacy, patient privacy on the Web, and updates from Washington. Congressional contact information, as well as information about current issues and legislation are provided. http://www.nationalcpr.org

New York Online Access to Health (NOAH): Patients' Rights and Resources Patients' rights and resources regarding death, health care proxy information, medical records and privacy, Medicare, and nursing homes can be found at this site. In addition, physician information in the areas of misconduct/disciplinary action and verification is made available. Sources of information include the American Medical Association and the Centers for Medicare & Medicaid Services, formerly the Health Care Financing Administration. http://www.noah-health.org/english/patients.html

12.24 POISONING AND TOXICOLOGY

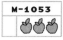

American Association of Poison Control Centers The American Association of Poison Control Centers' Web page offers a search engine for visitors to locate the nearest poison control center by zip code. Of further value is the Toxic Exposure Surveillance System Database, along with details on poison prevention and education and information on legislation regarding poison control. http://www.aapcc.org/

MEDLINEplus Health Information: Poisoning, Toxicology, Environmental Health Topics MEDLINEplus offers this extensive link listing covering various poisoning, toxicology, and environmental health topics. Documents on air pollution, asbestos, carbon monoxide poisoning, pesticides, radiation, and food contamination are accessible, as well as links to research information and related organizations. http://www.nlm.nih.gov/medlineplus/poisoningtoxicologyenvironmentalhealth.html

TOXNET Sponsored by the National Library of Medicine, TOXNET, the Toxicology Data Network, contains databases for toxicology data, literature, toxic release information, and chemical nomenclature and identification. The databases are drawn from such agencies as the Environmental Protection Agency and the National Cancer Institute. http://toxnet.nlm.nih.gov/

12.25 PREVENTION

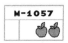

Agency for Healthcare Research and Quality (AHRQ): Put Prevention into Practice This Personal Health Guide publication provides patients with a way to keep track of their health needs and records. Covering preventive

care from immunizations to lifestyle choices, the guide is intended to be used in cooperation with a healthcare provider.
http://www.ahcpr.gov/ppip/ppadult.htm

American College of Preventive Medicine   The American College of Preventive Medicine (ACPM) is a professional society for physicians committed to disease prevention. Visitors will find policy statements, resources for further education, links to clinical and community preventive services, and recent news from ACPM at this site.
http://www.acpm.org/

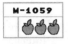

MedMark: Preventive Medicine   This site offers more than 100 links on preventive medicine in categories such as associations, education/training, sites for consumers, clinical guidelines, journals, and research programs.
http://www.medmark.org/prevent/

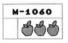

National Center for Chronic Disease Prevention and Health Promotion   The National Center for Chronic Disease Prevention and Health Promotion hosts this site, providing links to numerous sources of information on more than 30 health-related topics, including maternal and infant health, smoking, school health, epilepsy, disease prevention, cancer, and diabetes. The organization's five databases include the Health Promotion and Education Database, the Comprehensive School Health Database, and the Cancer Prevention and Control Database.
http://www.cdc.gov/nccdphp/index.htm

12.26 RESIDENCY

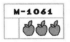

American College of Physicians-American Society of Internal Medicine (ACP-ASIM): Career Counseling Timeline   A series of career counseling articles is featured on this Web page for residents and fellows. The articles are organized by month for the last year of a residency or fellowship.
http://www.acponline.org/counseling/index.html

American College of Physicians-American Society of Internal Medicine (ACP-ASIM): Internal Medicine Residency Database   Maintained by the American College of Physicians - American Society of Internal Medicine, this site features an internal medicine residency database for the United States and Canada. Search results return contact information, a link to the program's Web site, and information on subspecialty tracks.
http://www.acponline.org/residency/

12.27 REVIEW AND CERTIFICATION

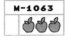

American Board of Internal Medicine (ABIM): Certification and Recertification   Information on certification and recertification with the

American Board of Internal Medicine is provided on this site. Examination dates, sample examination questions, and a summary of content on the examinations are provided. There is also a diplomate directory, and visitors can verify their physician's certification.
http://www.abim.org/info/default.htm

American Board of Internal Medicine (ABIM): Verification of Certification Status This site offers a verification of certification status service. Users enter the physician's name and the results indicate if they are currently certified by the American Board of Internal Medicine.
http://www.abim.org/dp/apps/physver.htm

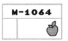

Exam Master: Internal Medicine This site offers information on the Exam Master CD-ROM for use in reviewing for the American Board of Internal Medicine certification exam.
(fee-based) http://www.exammaster.com/Certification-Review/internal-medicine.htm

Internal Medicine Board Review Course An internal medicine board review course for American Board of Internal Medicine and United States Medical Licensing Examining is featured on this Web page. A few quizzes and clinical tutorials are available on the site for free, although most of the site requires membership. Members can also access a chat room.
(fee-based) http://www.usmlecourse.com/

12.28 SAFETY

American Red Cross Dedicated to providing a range of health and safety services, the American Red Cross offers descriptions of its programs at this page. Disaster services, biomedical services, and health and safety commitments are discussed. News presentations and Spotlight information are found, including school safety tips, the safety of the nation's blood supply, and the rapid responses initiated by the organization to national and international disasters.
http://www.redcross.org/

MEDLINEplus Health Information: Safety Topics A listing of links on a variety of safety topics, such as motor vehicle safety, child safety, and fire safety are provided, on this site. By clicking on a topic, visitors are led to relevant publications, organizations, and related resources, courtesy of the National Library of Medicine. http://www.nlm.nih.gov/medlineplus/safety.html

12.29 SUBSTANCE ABUSE AND SMOKING

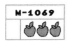

Center for Substance Abuse Treatment: Treatment Improvement Protocol Series The Treatment Improvement Protocol Series features guidelines that deal with pregnant, substance-using women; intensive outpatient treatment for alcohol and drug abuse; detoxification from alcohol and other

drugs; substance abuse among older adults; and treatments of adolescents with substance use disorders. A table of contents for each searchable guideline is supplied, as a service of the Health Services/Technology Assessment Text of the National Institutes of Health.
http://text.nlm.nih.gov/ftrs/pick?collect=tip&dbName=0&cc=1&t=971969662

MEDLINEplus Health Information: Alcohol and Youth Information on alcohol and youth is featured on this Web page, hosted by the National Library of Medicine. Topics covered include patterns of alcohol abuse, the effect of alcoholism on children, and talking to children about alcohol abuse. Statistics on alcohol abuse are provided, along with links to related organizational resources.
http://www.nlm.nih.gov/medlineplus/alcoholandyouth.html

MEDLINEplus Health Information: Smoking A collection of links on smoking-related news and health information is found at this site, hosted by the National Library of Medicine. Connections to details about clinical trials dealing with smoking, as well as prevention/screening, specific conditions, organizations, statistics, and news articles are featured.
http://www.nlm.nih.gov/medlineplus/smoking.html

National Clearinghouse for Alcohol and Drug Information: PREV-LINE PREVLINE provides visitors to its site with basic facts on different drugs of abuse, as well as facts on drug use related to various groups within the population. As a service of the Substance Abuse and Mental Health Services Administration, this site offers news regarding substance abuse, research information, statistics, and links to related databases. http://www.health.org

National Digestive Diseases Information Clearinghouse: Smoking and Your Digestive System The link between smoking and heartburn, peptic ulcers, liver disease, Crohn's Disease, and gallstones is discussed at this page from the National Digestive Diseases Information Clearinghouse. Visitors will also find information about damage reversal and additional information sources. http://www.niddk.nih.gov/health/digest/pubs/smoke/smoking.htm#reversed

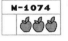

Tobacco Information and Prevention Source: Cigarette Smoking-Related Mortality An article on cigarette smoking-related mortality is presented at this site by the National Center for Chronic Disease Prevention and Health Promotion of the Centers for Disease Control and Prevention (CDC). A table presenting various statistics that illustrate cigarette smoking's relation to chronic diseases is also provided, in addition to links to other citations, individualized state information, and recent campaigns and events against tobacco use. http://www.cdc.gov/tobacco/research_data/health_consequences/mortali.htm

12.30 TRAVEL MEDICINE

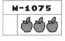

MedicinePlanet: Travel Health.com Online travel health centers for men, women, seniors, and those with special needs are found at this Mobile Health

Resource, in addition to health travel planning, disease risk and vaccination information, and up-to-date information on regional and global health.
(free registration) http://www.travelhealth.com/home/

National Center for Infectious Diseases: Traveler's Health A page about traveler's health is presented by this division of the Centers for Disease Control and Prevention. This site features information dealing with international outbreaks, traveling with children, special needs travelers, diseases, vaccinations, safe food and water, and cruise ships and air travel. Additional resources from the World Health Organization, current news items related to traveler's health, and a traveler checklist are presented at this site.
http://www.cdc.gov/travel/

Travel Health ONLINE Sponsored by Shoreland, this useful site provides visitors with access to information about various illnesses around the globe and recommendations regarding both health and safety. Details on travel-related illnesses, guides to safety in more than 200 countries, and contact information for providers of pretravel health services are offered. http://www.tripprep.com/

12.31 WELLNESS

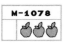

MEDLINEplus Health Information: Wellness and Lifestyle Topics A broad array of wellness and lifestyle topics is featured on this site, including exercise, nutrition, mental health, occupational health, and sports injuries. Each topic leads to additional resources such as the latest news, overviews, clinical trials, research, and specific conditions. Information specific to women, children, and seniors is also provided. Many resources are also available in Spanish.
http://www.nlm.nih.gov/medlineplus/wellnessandlifestyle.html

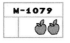

WellnessWeb Dedicated to wellness, this site offers a wide variety of articles and information on books by Donald B. Ardell, Ph.D. In addition, there are interviews with presenters from wellness conferences. A message board is also available. http://www.wellnessweb.com/

12.32 WOMEN'S HEALTH

Centers for Disease Control and Prevention (CDC): Women's Health In the form of national summaries, surveys, health program information, and fact sheets, this site contains coverage of women's health topics as a service of the Centers for Disease Control and Prevention (CDC). Assisted reproductive technology, cancer, maternal health, ectopic pregnancy, hysterectomy, and women and heart disease are a selection of the topics addressed. In addition, health related news, CDC publications and software, and data and statistics regarding women's health are made available.
http://www.cdc.gov/health/womensmenu.htm

Department of Health and Human Services: Office on Women's Health   Visitors to this site will find access to brochures of the division, its briefings, guides, and more than 30 fact sheets on topics such as eating disorders, older women's health, young women and smoking, lupus and women, and breast cancer. Details are provided regarding health initiatives of the organization, communication and outreach programs, and education and leadership. Additional topics addressed include healthcare access, HIV and women's health, international health, minority women's health, reproductive health, violence against women, and women and the environment.
http://www.4woman.gov/owh/index.htm

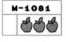

JAMA: Women's Health Information Center   Intended as a resource for physicians and other healthcare professionals, this page includes a Sexually Transmitted Diseases (STD) Information Center, a Contraception Information Center, and an archive of literature and commentaries on women's health, courtesy of the *Journal of the American Medical Association*. Access to searchable, peer-reviewed resources in women's health is provided.
http://www.ama-assn.org/special/womh/womh.htm

13

MAJOR DISORDERS
ENCOUNTERED IN
INTERNAL MEDICINE

13.1 ALLERGIC DISORDERS

GENERAL RESOURCES

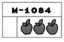

Allergy Internet Resources A comprehensive directory of allergy Internet resources is featured on this site. The links are organized under categories such as general allergy information, asthma, food allergies, children's allergies, latex allergy, and hay fever. Additional categories include skin allergies, insect stings, e-mail lists, and newsgroups.
http://www.immune.com/allergy/allabc.html

Allergy Report The full text of a report entitled *Allergic Disorders: Promoting Best Practice* is featured on this Web page, written by the American Academy of Allergy, Asthma, and Immunology. The report offers an overview of allergic diseases, including diagnostic testing and management of the diseases. Diseases of the atopic diathesis are also discussed, such as rhinitis, asthma, and atopic dermatitis. Conditions with an allergic component, including drug reactions, insect sting reactions, and latex reactions, are examined. A glossary is available, along with links to related resources.
http://www.theallergyreport.org/reportindex.html

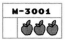

Johns Hopkins Asthma & Allergy The Johns Hopkins Asthma and Allergy Case Study Database can be searched from this page by entering either symptom or diagnostic information. Additional features of this Johns Hopkins specialty site include individual home pages for rhinitis, asthma, and sinusitis, with each of these links providing details on triggers, disease mechanisms, therapeutics, and environmental control.
http://www.hopkins-allergy.org/

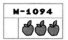

MEDLINEplus Health Information: Allergy Presenting the latest news, general overviews in the field, clinical trials, and documents on prevention, this collection of links offers something for all viewers searching for information on

allergic disorders. Research, documents on specific conditions, treatment, organizations, and Spanish language publications can be accessed.
http://www.nlm.nih.gov/medlineplus/allergy.html

 NYC - Allergy and Immunology and On-line Resources The list at this site offers professional and consumer-oriented links to a variety of Web sites on allergy and immunology topics, including a Web directory, treatment documents for allergists, current opinions in the field, and basic fact sheets on various allergic disorders. http://www.allny.com/health/allergy.html

ANAPHYLAXIS

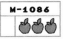 **eMedicine: Anaphylaxis** Richard S. Krause, M.D., of Buffalo General Hospital describes the causes, symptoms, and treatment for anaphylaxis on this site. Detailed information is provided on laboratory tests and procedures, as well as drugs used for emergency intervention. Hyperlinks are provided for differential diagnosis.
http://www.emedicine.com/emerg/topic25.htm

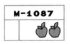 **Medfacts: Anaphylaxis** The National Jewish Medical and Research Center provides this fact sheet on anaphylaxis. The site contains a short discussion of symptoms, triggers, prevention, and treatment.
http://www.nationaljewish.org/medfacts/anaphalaxis.html

ASTHMA

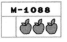 **American College of Allergy, Asthma, & Immunology (ACAAI): Asthma Disease Management Resource Manual** Created to assist clinicians in the assessment, diagnosis, and management of asthma, this document, available in Adobe Acrobat format, offers guidelines, checklists for care, treatment algorithms, and specific recommendations for therapy. Chapters of the manual are listed and briefly described, with easy access provided to any individual section.
http://www.allergy.mcg.edu/physicians/manual/manual.html

 American College of Allergy, Asthma, & Immunology (ACAAI): Immunotherapy in Allergic Asthma Dedicated specifically to allergic asthma, this online CME module explores immunotherapy from an historical perspective. Viewers can listen to, as well as read, chapters on epidemiology and heterogeneity of asthma and the best management options at this site, which includes RealPlayer audio files. Portions of an online test follow each module.
http://www.audio-digest.org/cgi-bin/start/acaai/immunotherapy/main.html

Drug Reactions

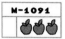

Allergy Society of South Africa: Drug Allergy   Incidence, types, risk factors, and important features of allergic drug reactions are discussed at this neatly organized online guideline. Additional sections of the document address the immunological basis of drug reactions, drugs associated with anaphylaxis, diagnosis, and treatment approach.
http://allergysa.org/drugallergy.htm

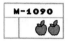

drkoop.com: Drug Allergies   Intended for consumers, this site focuses on the presentation, symptoms, and treatment of drug allergies, with hyperlinks provided throughout the text to further explanation of related terminology. A variety of enlargeable images of various dermatologic reactions are displayed.
http://www.drkoop.com/conditions/ency/article/000819.htm

Food Allergy

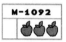

Food Allergy and Anaphylaxis Network   Working in conjunction with the American Academy of Allergy, Asthma, and Immunology (AAAAI), this online resource offers awareness of the issues surrounding food allergy and sensitivities. Featured topics, breaking news in the field, advocacy, and research departments are provided at the site.
http://www.foodallergy.org/

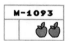

National Institute of Allergy and Infectious Diseases (NIAID): Food Allergy and Intolerances   The National Institute of Health offers this fact sheet on food allergy and intolerance. Topics covered include common allergies, cross-reactivity, diagnosis, treatment, and controversial methods of diagnosis and treatment. Links to related resources on the Web are provided.
http://www.niaid.nih.gov/factsheets/food.htm

House Dust Allergy

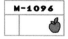

Allergy Society of South Africa: The Control Measures of Housedust Mites   Authored by Dr. Adrian Morris, this article examines measures aimed at reducing levels of the mite in and around the home and offers suggestions for house dust- mite-free living. Allergy treatment is briefly addressed at this online information sheet.
http://www.allergysa.org/hdm.htm

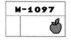

American College of Allergy, Asthma, & Immunology (ACAAI): House Dust Allergy   Advice regarding the control of house dust and allergic symptoms is outlined at this informative brochure of the American College of Allergy, Asthma, and Immunology. Allergens in dust mites and mold and strategies for prevention are discussed, including those for reducing dust mites in the

bedroom, reducing surface dust, and special products available for inactivation of dust mite allergens.
http://www.allergy.mcg.edu/advice/dust.html

INSECT ALLERGY

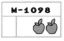

American College of Allergy, Asthma, & Immunology (ACAAI): Insect Allergy In addition to the "Three A's of Allergy Management," this page provides access to physician information on insect sting anaphylaxis, a patient link, facts about stinging insects, and a connection emphasizing avoidance.
http://www.allergy.mcg.edu/ALK/insect.html

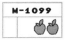

National Allergy and Asthma Newsletter: Stinging Insect Allergy This educational brochure, prepared by Dr. Robert Heddle and Dr. Raymond Mullins, addresses problem insects and their natural history. Diagnosis of allergic reaction to stings, and risk of anaphylaxis to future stings are discussed. Management strategies and immunotherapy are introduced.
http://www.allergy.org.au/gpnews/vol1_no4/editor.htm

LATEX ALLERGY

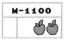

American College of Allergy, Asthma, & Immunology (ACAAI): Latex Allergy Home Page Professional resources available at this site include a latex allergy position statement, guidelines for the management of latex allergies, and information on risks posed especially to medical personnel. Useful external links are provided, including an additional management page, courtesy of the Cleveland Clinic. http://allergy.mcg.edu/physicians/ltxhome.html

National Latex Allergy Network: Latex Allergy Links A comprehensive listing of latex allergy-related material on the Internet is found at this resource, brought to visitors by the National Latex Allergy Network and ELASTIC, Inc. Links by category include connections for clinicians, legislative material, tutorials, position statements, and news. An alternative table of contents is provided, which provides direct connections and mentions page sources and sponsors. http://latexallergylinks.tripod.com/

RHINITIS

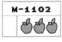

eMedicine: Allergic Rhinitis Pathophysiology, demographic information, and clinical picture of the allergic patient are reviewed at this online textbook page. Causes, appropriate laboratory testing, and complete treatment information are reviewed, with an emphasis on pharmacologic intervention.
http://www.eMedicine.com/ENT/topic194.htm

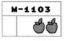 **Medfacts: Allergic and Non-Allergic Rhinitis** Primarily for patients who suffer from allergic and non-allergic rhinitis, this site explains the most common forms of rhinitis, their symptoms, the need to avoid triggers of allergic rhinitis, and treatment options, provided as a service of the National Jewish Medical and Research Center.
http://www.njc.org/medfacts/allergic_rhinitis.html

URTICARIA

 American College of Allergy, Asthma, & Immunology (ACAAI): Urticaria The American College of Allergy, Asthma and Immunology sponsors this patient guide to urticaria. Identification of triggers, types of urticaria, and treatment options are examined.
http://www.allergy.mcg.edu/advice/urtic.html

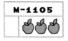 **eMedicine: Urticaria** Presented by the Emergency Medicine/Dermatology publication of eMedicine, this page offers practitioners details on the clinical presentation, diagnostic work-up, and pharmacologic and medical management of urticaria. Diagnostic differential links are offered at the site, including angioedema and anaphylaxis.
http://www.eMedicine.com/emerg/topic628.htm

13.2 BLOOD DISORDERS/HEMATOLOGY

GENERAL RESOURCES

 Karolinska Institutet: Hemic and Lymphatic Diseases A comprehensive listing of links on hemic and lymphatic diseases is available at this site connecting to Web sites in the United States and abroad. Links are categorized by disease and include a variety of fact sheets, pathology sites, clinical guidelines, and support resources.
http://www.mic.ki.se/Diseases/c15.html

 MEDLINEplus Health Information: Bleeding Disorders Created to provide information about bleeding disorders, this comprehensive Web site provides hyperlinks to clinical trials, diagnosis, research, specific blood disorders, and treatment. Other links include a blood bank locator, law and policy information, organizations, and information on special considerations for women.
http://www.nlm.nih.gov/medlineplus/bleedingdisorders.html

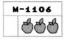 **MEDLINEplus Health Information: Blood/Lymphatic System** A broad array of blood and lymphatic system topics are listed on this site, including bleeding disorders, bone marrow diseases, leukemia, lymphatic diseases, and multiple myeloma. Each topic offers additional resources such as news, over-

views, clinical trials, treatment, and related organizations. Some of the resources are available in Spanish.
http://www.nlm.nih.gov/medlineplus/bloodlymphaticsystem.html

ANEMIA, APLASTIC

MEdIC: Aplastic Anemia: Introduction for the General Physician A concise description of aplastic anemia is presented at this site, maintained by the University of Texas Houston Medical School. The summary includes information on diagnosis, treatment, the need for blood transfusions, and prognosis and is presented by the Medical Education Information Center.
http://medic.med.uth.tmc.edu/ptnt/00001040.htm

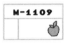

Merck Manual of Diagnosis and Therapy: Aplastic Anemia Information on aplastic anemia, including etiology, symptoms, and treatment is found in this subsection of a larger *Merck* publication chapter. Symptoms, laboratory diagnosis, and management are discussed.
http://www.merck.com/pubs/mmanual/section11/chapter127/127c.htm#A011-127-0124

ANEMIA, IRON DEFICIENCY

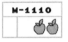

Family Practice Notebook.com: Iron Deficiency Anemia This resource provides a concise outline of causes, symptoms, laboratory work-up, and management of iron deficiency anemia. Hematologic images are available, as well as hyperlinks throughout the text to related parts of this Family Medicine Resource. http://www.fpnotebook.com/HEM6.htm

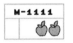

Oregon Health Sciences University: Diagnosing Iron Deficiency Written by Thomas DeLoughery of Oregon Health Sciences University, this site explores the common problem of misdiagnosis of iron deficiency and presents recommended methods for diagnosis.
http://www.ohsu.edu/som-hemonc/handouts/deloughery/fe.shtml

ANEMIA, PERNICIOUS

Healthwell: Pernicious Anemia This article, intended for a variety of audiences, defines pernicious anemia, explains symptoms, and provides suggestions for dietary and lifestyle changes. Hyperlinks are provided throughout the text to definitions of related terminology.
http://www.healthwell.com/healthnotes/Concern/Pernicious_Anemia.cfm

RxMed: Anemia, Pernicious A short definition of pernicious anemia, its causes, risk factors, and treatment are addressed at this consumer-oriented site.
http://www.rxmed.com/illnesses/anemia,_pernicious.html

HEMOCHROMATOSIS

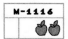

American Hemochromatosis Society   Created to educate the medical community and support those dealing with this disease, the American Hemochromatosis Society site provides information for patients, treatment guidelines, an electronic newsletter, support group access, and information on genetic screening facilities. http://www.americanhs.org/

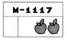

National Institute of Diabetes and Digestive and Kidney Diseases (NIDDK): Hemochromatosis   Sponsored by the National Institutes of Health, this site offers an online brochure on hemochromatosis, including causes, risk factors, symptoms, diagnosis, and treatment. A short description of current research of the disease and links to other organizations for more information are provided.
http://www.niddk.nih.gov/health/digest/pubs/hemochrom/hemochromatosis.htm

HEMOPHILIA

Hemophilia Galaxy   The Hemophilia Galaxy Web site provides healthcare professionals with information on CME courses, including online modules, teaching tools, and a comprehensive list of related links. Patients have access to fact sheets, a hemophilia glossary, a directory of treatment centers, and assistance programs. http://www.hemophiliagalaxy.com

National Hemophilia Foundation   The home page of the National Hemophilia Foundation offers sections on bleeding disorders, the latest research, programs and services, a marketplace for consumers, and links to related Internet sources. An online education workshop series is available for providers and consumers after a free registration. Of particular interest to physicians are the numerous research grants and fellowships available for the study of bleeding disorders. (free registration) http://www.hemophilia.org/

INFECTIOUS MONONUCLEOSIS

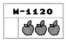

MEDLINEplus Health Information: Infectious Mononucleosis   This resource contains links for information on all aspects of infectious mononucleosis. General overviews, links to related organizations, and articles that focus on the disorder in children and adolescents can be accessed at this compilation of the National Library of Medicine.
http://www.nlm.nih.gov/medlineplus/infectiousmononucleosis.html

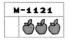

Postgraduate Medicine: Infectious Mononucleosis   Created to educate physicians, this article on infectious mononucleosis discusses the complexities of the disease, as well as recommendations for diagnosis and management.

Clinical manifestations, useful laboratory tests, differential diagnosis, and potential complications are described and accompanied by a site bibliography.
http://www.postgradmed.com/issues/2000/06_00/godshall.htm

MULTIPLE MYELOMA

International Myeloma Foundation Webcasts of myeloma educational material, research grant application, and an information packet that may be ordered online are just a few of the features of this disease-oriented Web page. The site can be explored by way of its Guided Tour or Quick Start features.
http://www.myeloma.org/index.html

MEDLINEplus Health Information: Multiple Myeloma Visitors will find comprehensive information on multiple myeloma by accessing this site's assortment of links. Categorized as general overviews, clinical trials, diagnosis, prevention, and treatment, the connections offer a variety of information and also address the latest from the National Institutes of Health, journals, organizations, and statistical information.
http://www.nlm.nih.gov/medlineplus/multiplemyeloma.html

MYELOPROLIFERATIVE DISORDERS

CancerNet: Myeloproliferative Disorders PDQ Supported by the National Cancer Institute, complete information is provided on myeloproliferative disorders, including polycythemia vera and essential thrombocythemia. Symptoms and treatment options for the diseases are discussed, and references are available through site hyperlinks.
http://cancernet.nci.nih.gov/cgi-bin/srchcgi.exe?DBID=pdq&TYPE=search&
UID=208+01983&ZFILE=professional&SFMT=pdq_treatment/1/0/0

Myeloproliferative Disorders An informational source for myeloproliferative disorders (MPD), this Web site provides a newsletter, online support groups, answers to frequently asked questions, reports from past MPD medical conferences, and many links to medical and other support information sources, citations, abstracts, and articles. http://www.acor.org/diseases/hematology/MPD

PLATELET DISORDERS

Merck Manual of Diagnosis and Therapy: Platelet Dysfunction
Examining platelet dysfunction, this site, a chapter of the online *Merck* reference, features a detailed discussion of Von Willebrand's disease, including symptoms, diagnosis, and treatment. Shorter descriptions of hereditary, intrinsic platelet disorders and acquired platelet dysfunction are also included.
http://www.merck.com/pubs/mmanual/section11/chapter133/133c.htm

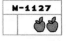 **Temple University: Platelets and Platelet Disorders**   Created to provide information about platelets and platelet disorders, this site provides a brief discussion on platelet structure and production and both congenital and acquired platelet disorders. Symptoms and treatment for thrombocytopenia, thrombocytosis, and von Willebrand disease are examined.
http://blue.temple.edu/~pathphys/hematology/platelet.html

PORPHYRIAS

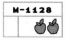 **Merck Manual Home Edition: Porphyrias**   Presented by Merck, this site describes the symptoms, diagnosis, and treatment for porphyria cutanea tarda, acute intermittent porphyria, and erythropoietic protoporphyria.
http://www.merck.com/pubs/mmanual_home/sec12/141.htm

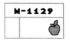 **Oregon Health Sciences University: Diagnosing the Porphyrias**   A concise explanation on the diagnosis of porphyrias is presented by Thomas G. DeLoughery of the Oregon Health Sciences University. Diagnosis of acute intermitted porphyria, hereditary coproporphyria, variegate porphyria, and porphyria cutanea tarda are discussed.
http://www.ohsu.edu/som-hemonc/handouts/deloughery/por.shtml

SICKLE CELL ANEMIA

 Family Practice Notebook.com: Sickle Cell Anemia   A concise outline of the sickle cell trait and disease is found at this site, which reviews the pathophysiology, types, precipitating factors, symptoms, labs, and management of sickle cell disease. Links are offered to additional, related chapters of this online Family Medicine Resource.
http://www.fpnotebook.com/HEM39.htm

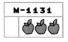 **Sickle Cell Information Center**   The Sickle Cell Information Center site offers a comprehensive link section, divided into categories intended for healthcare providers, administrators, patients and families, teachers, students, and employers. Visitors to this site will find information on blood banks, newborn screening, and pharmaceutical research.
http://www.cc.emory.edu/PEDS/SICKLE/

THALASSEMIA

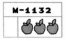 **Cooley's Anemia Foundation Inc.**   Dedicated solely to thalassemia, this site has sections for both physician and patient viewers. By clicking on the "Medical News and Information" link, physicians will find management guidelines, research updates, fellowship awards, and a discussion group. At the pa-

tients section, answers to FAQs, support group information, and scholarship details are found. An extensive list of related links is provided.
http://www.thalassemia.org/

Thalassemia.com Information on thalassemia is offered at this site for both healthcare providers and patients. Medical management, genetics, psychosocial aspects, and transfusion therapy are explained. A comprehensive links section provides additional resources of medical information, cordblood and bone marrow transplants, and support groups.
http://www.thalassemia.com/home.shtml

13.3 CANCER

GENERAL RESOURCES

American Cancer Society: Cancer Reference Information More than 50 forms of cancer can be reviewed through profiles at this site. Visitors to the site can select or enter the type of cancer for which information is desired, and the database provides a description, incidence information, causes, tests and diagnostic data, treatment options, staging information, and other relevant material. http://www.cancer.org/eprise/main/docroot/CRI/CRI_0

CancerNet: Cancer Disorder Profiles, Alphabetical Listing More than 100 types of cancer are profiled in Physician Data Query (PDQ), the comprehensive cancer database of the National Cancer Institute. Each profile contains an extensive general description of the disorder, cell classification, stages of the disease, treatment options, subclassifications of the disease, and bibliographic references. http://cancernet.nci.nih.gov/alphalist.html

OncoLink: Disease-Oriented Menus for Oncology The University of Pennsylvania Cancer Center has provided comprehensive disease-oriented menus for adult and pediatric cancers, including pathology images, technical articles, and case studies. Adult cancers covered include bone cancers, brain tumors, breast cancer, endocrine system cancers, gastrointestinal cancers, genitourinary (male) cancers, gynecologic cancers, head and neck cancers, adult leukemia, lung cancers, lymphomas, metastases, myelomas, sarcomas, skin cancers, and urinary tract cancers. Pediatric cancers covered include pediatric brain tumors, pediatric leukemias and lymphomas, pediatric liver cancer, neuroblastoma, retinoblastoma, rhabdomyosarcoma and other sarcomas, other pediatric cancers, and Wilms' tumor.
http://www.oncolink.upenn.edu/disease

BLADDER CANCER

CancerNet: Bladder Cancer Comprehensive information on bladder cancer, including incidence, treatment, clinical trials, causes, and diagnosis, is available at this site, sponsored by the National Cancer Institute. Of interest to patients is a collection of links on coping with bladder cancer, which covers issues ranging from side effects of treatment to emotional concerns.
http://www.cancernet.nci.nih.gov/Cancer_Types/Bladder_Cancer.shtml

OncoLink: Bladder Cancer Provided as a service of the University of Pennsylvania Cancer Center, this OncoLink site offers visitors links to a bladder cancer support and information group, as well as the opportunity to subscribe to a professional urology network. OncoLink documents on bladder cancer evaluation, diagnosis, and management are accessible, in addition to related Reuters news releases and medication updates. Information from the National Cancer Institute, geared toward both physicians and patients, can be easily obtained, in addition to CancerLit citations and a useful bladder cancer patient guide. http://cancer.med.upenn.edu/disease/bladder/index.html

BREAST CANCER

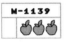

Doctor's Guide: Breast Cancer This detailed Web site directs visitors to a comprehensive listing of links that offer up-to-date medical news and information concerning breast cancer and other breast-related disorders. The links are presented topically as medical news and alerts, general information, discussion groups, and related sites.
http://www.pslgroup.com/BREASTCANCER.HTM

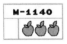

OncoLink: Breast Cancer General Information This section of University of Pennsylvania OncoLink directory offers comprehensive information about breast cancer screening, risk factors and prevention, treatment options, genetics, support, and other topics. Visitors can find answers to frequently asked questions and news stories related to breast cancer at this comprehensive online cancer center.
http://cancer.med.upenn.edu/disease/breast

CERVICAL CANCER

CancerNet: Cervical Cancer The National Cancer Institute sponsors this comprehensive site on cervical cancer that includes causes, prevention, treatment, clinical trials, and testing. A wide variety of patient guides covering physical and emotional effects of cervical cancer are available in a section on coping with cancer.
http://www.cancernet.nci.nih.gov/Cancer_Types/Cervical_Cancer.shtml

MEDLINEplus Health Information: Cervical Cancer Information on cervical cancer, excerpted from a variety of sources, is displayed at this comprehensive site. Hyperlinks take visitors to information on clinical trials, documents on detection and symptoms, prevention information, treatment protocols, and the latest news on cervical cancer management.
http://www.nlm.nih.gov/medlineplus/cervicalcancer.html

DIGESTIVE CANCER

CancerBACUP: Digestive System Cancers By clicking on any one of eight specific cancerous conditions, visitors are offered access to CancerBACUP factsheets. Each document addresses causes, symptoms, diagnosis, and various treatment options and provides hyperlinks to further information on related terminology. http://www.cancerbacup.org.uk/info/digest.htm

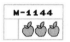

CancerNet: Cancer by Body Location/System: Digestive This resource offers information on a variety of gastrointestinal cancers, including cancer of the colon, esophagus, gallbladder, liver, pancreas, small intestine, and stomach. Links provided for each type of cancer offer information on causes, symptoms, treatment, and patient resources. Several resources are found for the prevention of colon and rectal cancer.
http://www.cancernet.nci.nih.gov/location.html#digestive

ENDOCRINE CANCER

Cancereducation.com: Endocrine Cancer This site features audio and video educational programs for coping with cancer, as well as World Wide Web connections specific to endocrine cancer. Visitors can click on one of the categories under "Medical Links" and retrieve related Internet connections associated with disease risk factors, symptoms, diagnosis, and treatment options.
(free registration)
http://www.cancereducation.com/cancersyspages/
index.cfm?ct=1&CFID=14653&CFTOKEN=65085211

CancerNet: Cancer by Body Location/System: Endocrine Information on several types of endocrine cancer, including adrenocortical carcinoma, carcinoid tumor, parathyroid cancer, and thyroid cancer, are available at this comprehensive site, hosted by the National Cancer Institute. Connections to the various types of endocrine cancers provide information on symptoms, causes, clinical studies, treatment, and patient resources.
http://www.cancernet.nci.nih.gov/location.html#endocrine

HEAD AND NECK CANCER

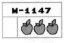

CancerNet: Cancer by Body Location/System: Head and Neck
Created by the National Cancer Institute, this site features information on head and neck cancers, such as hypopharyngeal cancer, laryngeal cancer, lip and oral cavity cancer, and salivary gland cancer. Both physicians and patients will find a variety of links at this site, useful for detailed discussions of causes, symptoms, clinical studies, and treatment.
http://www.cancernet.nci.nih.gov/location.html#head

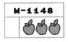

Oncologychannel: Head and Neck Cancers An overview of head and neck cancers is offered at this site. Links to additional information on symptoms, staging, types of head and neck cancers, and new treatments available are found, offering a comprehensive overview of interest to both patients and professionals. http://www.oncologychannel.com/headneck/

HODGKIN'S DISEASE

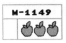

CancerNet: Hodgkin's Disease Dedicated to Hodgkin's disease, this Web site provides information on statistics, treatment, clinical studies, causes, prevention, and coping with the illness.
http://www.cancernet.nci.nih.gov/Cancer_Types/Hodgkin's_Disease.shtml

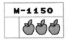

Lymphoma Information Network: Hodgkin's Disease Detailed information resources on Hodgkin's disease are featured on this Web page. Visitors will find information on diagnosis, treatment, incidence, chemotherapy, and related resources. Each section offers links to other Web sites for additional information. There is also information specific to childhood Hodgkin's disease.
http://www.lymphomainfo.net/hodgkins/

LEUKEMIA

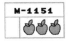

CancerNet: Leukemia A broad range of information on leukemia is available at this National Cancer Institute site, including causes, symptoms, prevention, treatment, and coping resources. Within the treatment, causes, and coping sections, individual connections are provided for both patients and healthcare professionals.
http://www.cancernet.nci.nih.gov/Cancer_Types/Leukemia.shtml

MEDLINEplus Health Information: Leukemia, Adult Chronic Dedicated to adult chronic leukemia, this site contains an assortment of links, including disorder overviews, clinical trials, coping, diagnosis, and prevention sites. Also of interest are links to the latest research, specific aspects of leukemia, and treatment information.
http://www.nlm.nih.gov/medlineplus/leukemiaadultchronic.html

LUNG CANCER

CancerNet: Lung Cancer Provided by the National Cancer Institute, this site offers statistics, symptoms, and treatment options for patients with lung cancer. The causes and prevention subsections feature detailed information targeted toward consumers.
http://www.cancernet.nci.nih.gov/Cancer_Types/Lung_Cancer.shtml

Lung Cancer Online Resources for patients with lung cancer and their physicians are provided at this site, including links to general information on the disease, treatment options, complications, and diagnostic tests. Fact sheets are presented in clinical terms, and a comprehensive listing of related resources is provided. http://www.lungcanceronline.org

LYMPHOMA

CancerNet: Cancer by Body Location/System: Lymphomas This Web site has links to information on several kinds of lymphoma, including AIDS-related lymphoma, cutaneous T-cell lymphoma, Hodgkin's disease, non-Hodgkin's disease, and T-cell lymphoma. A disease overview, causes, and treatments are presented on each disease, as well as general information on coping with cancer. http://www.cancernet.nci.nih.gov/location.html#lymphomas

Lymphoma Research Foundation of America This organization promotes research, offers support programs, conducts advocacy activities, and raises community awareness of lymphoma. Healthcare professionals will discover an assortment of CME programs, research grants, and patient education materials. The site also offers patient fact sheets and an online bookstore.
http://www.lymphoma.org/pages/index.html

NEUROLOGIC CANCER

CancerNet: Cancer by Body Location/System: Neurologic Cancer Hosted by the National Cancer Institute, this resource presents information on neurologic cancers, including brain tumors, neuroblastoma, pituitary tumors, and primary central nervous system lymphoma. Each primary link connect visitors to information in several categories, including clinical trials, causes, testing, support, and literature. http://www.cancernet.nci.nih.gov/location.html#neurologic

MEDLINEplus Health Information: Brain Cancer Visitors to this site can access information on brain cancer, offering everything from discussion of causes to labeled diagrams from Harvard Medical School. Other valuable resources include diagnosis and symptom information, clinical trials, and treatment options, with a special section dedicated to treatment of children.
http://www.nlm.nih.gov/medlineplus/braincancer.html

Ovarian Cancer

CancerNet: Ovarian Cancer   Maintained at the National Cancer Institute, this site offers a large variety of documents addressing the causes and treatment options for ovarian cancer. Both physicians and patients will benefit from in-depth coverage of genetics, other causes, and diagnosis, as well as review of the current literature.
http://www.cancernet.nci.nih.gov/Cancer_Types/Ovarian_Cancer.shtml

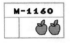

National Ovarian Cancer Coalition   A large collection of ovarian cancer information, written for consumers, is available here. The Resources section provides an opportunity to ask questions of experts in the field; supplies information about state resources; and contains a database, organized by state, of more than 600 gynecologic oncologists.
http://www.ovarian.org

Paraneoplastic Syndrome

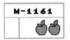

10 Most Commonly Asked Questions About Paraneoplastic Syndromes   Answered by Jerome B. Posner, M.D., this question and answer format provides a concise discussion on the types of paraneoplastic syndromes, causes, incidence, symptoms, diagnosis, and treatment. This is one of a series of articles offered by the online journal, *The Neurologist*.
http://lww.com/theneurologist/articles/paraneoplastic.html

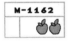

Merck Manual Home Edition: Paraneoplastic Syndromes   Drawn from a *Merck* publication, this chapter explains paraneoplastic syndromes and includes a table illustrating the various effects and cancers responsible. Brief descriptions of cancer emergencies, such as cardiac tamponade, pleural effusion, superior vena cava syndrome, spinal cord compression, and hypercalcemic syndrome, are provided.
http://www.merck.com/pubs/mmanual_home/sec15/165.htm

Prostate Cancer

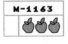

CancerNet: Prostate Cancer   For those interested in learning more about prostate cancer, this site provides detailed information on causes, clinical trials, prevention, testing, and treatment for the disease at a variety of patient and clinically-oriented links.
http://www.cancernet.nci.nih.gov/Cancer_Types/Prostate_Cancer.shtml

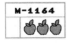

MEDLINEplus Health Information: Prostate Cancer   Drawn from a variety of sources, this Web site offers links to a variety of information on prostate cancer, including a general overview, clinical trials, symptoms, and treatment. Of interest to patients and physicians are connections to recent research from the Mayo Clinic, as well as the latest news articles on prostate cancer Spanish-language publications.

http://www.nlm.nih.gov/medlineplus/prostatecancer.html

SARCOMAS OF SOFT TISSUE AND BONE

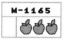

CancerBACUP: Understanding Soft Tissue Sarcomas   Designed as an online booklet for patients, this site provides a review of soft tissue sarcomas, with links available to information on causes, symptoms, tests, treatment, and research. Related organizations and books are also included.

http://www.cancerbacup.org.uk/info/sarcomas.htm

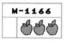

CancerNet: Cancer by Body Location/System: Sarcomas   Information is accessible to an assortment of both consumer and professionally-oriented documents on Ewing's sarcoma and osteosarcoma. Each link provides statistical papers, treatment information, clinical trial details, coping resources, and current cancer literature, as a service of the National Cancer Institute.

http://www.cancernet.nci.nih.gov/location.html#aids

SKIN CANCER

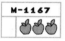

CancerNet: Cancer by Body Location/System: Skin   Detailed information on skin cancers such as cutaneous T-cell lymphoma, Kaposi's sarcoma, melanoma, and nonmelanomatous skin cancers are provided by the National Cancer Institute from this site. General overviews, treatment, causes, and clinical trial information are presented for each type of cancer, with individual documents geared toward both patient and professional audiences.

http://www.cancernet.nci.nih.gov/location.html#skin

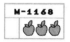

MEDLINEplus Health Information: Skin Cancer   Organized by topic, this collection of links offers visitors access to fact sheets, organization sites, general overviews, the latest news, clinical trials, diagnosis information, and coverage of specific aspects of skin cancer.

http://www.nlm.nih.gov/medlineplus/skincancer.html

TESTICULAR CANCER

CancerNet: Testicular Cancer   Examining testicular cancer, this National Cancer Institute Web site provides complete information for both practitioners and the public, with an overview of the disease, treatment, and diagnosis documents. General resources for coping with cancer, participating in clinical trials, and in support groups are available for patients.

http://www.cancernet.nci.nih.gov/Cancer_Types/Testicular_Cancer.shtml

MEDLINEplus Health Information: Testicular Cancer Primarily for patients with testicular cancer, this site provides a number of sources for general information on testicular cancer, symptoms, and treatment. Several articles on early detection are also available through hyperlinks.
http://www.nlm.nih.gov/medlineplus/testicularcancer.html

Uterine Cancer

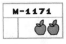

CancerNet: Uterine Sarcoma A patient-oriented overview of uterine cancer is featured at this site, as well as a description of treatment options. General information on cancer is also available, including statistical data sources, clinical trials, and coping with cancer.
http://www.cancernet.nci.nih.gov/Cancer_Types/Uterine_Sarcoma.shtml

MEDLINEplus Health Information: Uterine Cancer The purpose of this site is to provide resources, in terms understandable to the public, pertaining to uterine cancer, its causes, symptoms, and treatment. Prevention and risk factor information, as well as specific conditions, such as cervical stenosis and gestational trophoblastic tumors, are addressed at the site's links.
http://www.nlm.nih.gov/medlineplus/uterinecancer.html

13.4 Cardiovascular Disorders

General Resources

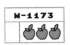

American Heart Association (AHA): Heart and Stroke Guide The AHA provides an extensive list of hundreds of cardiovascular disorders. Included for each disorder is a description and links to other pages on the site that contain related information about the disorder.
http://www.americanheart.org/Heart_and_Stroke_A_Z_Guide

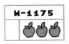

Merck Manual of Diagnosis and Therapy: Cardiovascular Disorders Section 16 of the online *Merck Manual of Diagnosis and Therapy* offers 17 searchable chapters on diseases of the cardiovascular system, including arrhythmias, endocarditis, and pericardial disease. By accessing a specific chapter, visitors arrive at a comprehensive overview of included disorders accompanied by several additional connections to specific disorders within the classification and details regarding pathophysiology, diagnosis, and treatment.
http://www.merck.com/pubs/mmanual/section16/sec16.htm

ANGINA PECTORIS

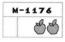

American Heart Association (AHA): Angina Pectoris Treatments
Part of the Heart and Stroke Guide published by the AHA, this site details with the treatment of angina pectoris. It includes a discussion of drugs, procedures, warning signs, and variant angina. Hyperlinks to related topics within the guide are also provided.

http://www.americanheart.org/Heart_and_Stroke_A_Z_Guide/anginat.html

Merck Manual of Diagnosis and Therapy: Angina Pectoris   The etiology, pathogenesis, symptoms and signs, diagnosis, prognosis, and treatment of angina pectoris are discussed at this address. Discussions of unstable angina and variant angina are also provided.

http://www.merck.com/pubs/mmanual/section16/chapter202/202c.htm

AORTIC ANEURYSMS

Merck Manual Home Edition: Aortic Aneurysms and Dissection   This site, drawn from an authoritative *Merck* reference, describes symptoms, diagnosis, and treatment of aortic aneurysms and dissection. Aneurysms in general are defined, as well as abdominal and thoracic aortic aneurysms.

http://www.merck.com/pubs/mmanual_home/sec3/29.htm

University of Iowa: Aortic Aneurysms: 3D Visualization and Measurement   A valuable tool for professionals, the site contains an overview of abdominal aortic aneurysm and its analysis with basic volumetric techniques, including oblique sectioning, region of interest analysis, geometric analysis of outer aortic boundaries and vessel tortuosity, volume rendering, and surface rendering. The site examines imaging techniques and features a collection of case studies with images. Abstracts of related literature are included.

http://everest.radiology.uiowa.edu/nlm/app/aorta/aorta.html

ARRHYTHMIAS

American Heart Association (AHA): Arrhythmia   Offering a starting point for research on arrhythmias for both consumer and professional readers, this site includes comprehensive overviews of a variety of arrhythmias. Details on diagnosis, treatment, and long-term management are included at a series of online articles. Additional professional resources include AHA monographs, lifestyle information sheets, pharmaceutical roundtable proceedings, and related articles from *Circulation* and other noteworthy sources. A consumer education department includes discussion of important risk factors, medications, and self-care measures.

http://www.americanheart.org/arrhythmia/index.html

Texas Arrhythmia Institute: Specific Arrhythmias Premature beats, tachycardias, and the bradycardias are reviewed at this educational page, with common forms seen in daily practice, related ECG readings, and therapies that ECG focus on defining and correcting the underlying problems. The discussion is accompanied by colorful images that illustrate atrial fibrillation, atrial flutter, atrioventricular (AV) nodal reentry tachycardia, and ventricular tachycardia.
http://www.txai.org/spec.html

ATHEROSCLEROSIS

Merck Manual of Diagnosis and Therapy: Atherosclerosis The pathology and pathogenesis, risk factors, symptoms and signs, diagnosis, prevention, and treatment of atherosclerosis are discussed in this comprehensive textbook chapter. Two hypotheses explaining pathogenesis and reversible risk factors are described in detail.
http://www.merck.com/pubs/mmanual/section16/chapter201/201b.htm

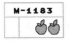

University of Alabama: Atherosclerosis Clinical Resources Visitors to this address will find links to general information, pathology images, clinical guidelines, scientific statements, and other miscellaneous resources related to atherosclerosis. Links to directories devoted to related topics are also available.
http://www.slis.ua.edu/cdlp/WebDLCore/
clinical/cardiology/cardiovascular/atherosclerosis.html

ATRIAL FIBRILLATION

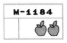

Atrial Fibrillation Page Developed to provide accurate information about atrial fibrillation (AF) and the Maze procedure, this site helps patients make informed decisions with the help of their healthcare providers. A glossary of AF-related terms and a message board are provided.
http://members.aol.com/mazern

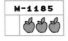

eMedicine: Atrial Fibrillation From eMedicine, this site gives an overview of atrial fibrillation. Clinical information about patient history, physical findings, and causes; a workup review, including laboratory studies, imaging studies, and other tests; treatment modalities; medication profiles; and follow-up procedures are recommended.
http://www.eMedicine.com/emerg/topic46.htm

CARDIOMYOPATHIES

Cardiomyopathy Association The purpose of this site is to explain the background, diagnosis, and treatment of cardiomyopathy using common medi-

cal terms. The site provides discussions of each of four recognized conditions of cardiomyopathy, accompanied by illustrations.
http://www.cardiomyopathy.org

Johns Hopkins Medical Institutions: Cardiomyopathy and Heart Transplant Service   Created by the Johns Hopkins Cardiomyopathy and Heart Transplant Service, this site describes the clinical developments in the fight against cardiomyopathy and heart failure. The site includes a discussion of pressure-volume loops, causes, patient evaluation, new treatments and procedures, and heart transplantation. A listing of heart failure studies is also available.   http://www.hopkinsmedicine.org/cardiology/heart/

CLAUDICATION

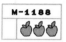

American Family Physician: A Primary Care Approach to the Patient with Claudication   Presented by the American Academy of Family Physicians and authored by Teresa L. Carman, M.D., and Bernardo B. Fernandex, Jr., M.D., of the Cleveland Clinic Florida, this article describes a primary care approach to treating patients with claudication. Discussion of a prognosis for patients with the condition, as well as recommendations for evaluation criteria and treatment are presented.
http://www.aafp.org/afp/20000215/1027.html

Familydoctor.org: Claudication   Presented in easy-to-understand terms, the American Academy of Family Physicians gives this general overview of claudication, including causes, risk factors, and treatment of the condition.
http://www.familydoctor.org/handouts/008.html

CONGENITAL HEART DISEASE

Three-Dimensional Visualization of Congenital Heart Disease   This site provides an overview of three-dimensional magnetic resonance imaging of congenital heart disease. Patient scan protocols, case studies, and examples in literature are offered, including right aortic arch, hypoplastic aorta, and vascular rings. Graphics and links to online video images are found, along with links to related Web sites.
http://everest.radiology.uiowa.edu/nlm/app/cnjheart/cnjheart.html

University of Alabama: Congenital Heart Disease Clinical Resources
Professionals can browse through links to related Internet documents on congenital heart anomalies by subtopics that include aortic stenosis, atrial septal defect, patent ductus arteriosus, pulmonary stenosis, and ventricular septal defect. A link for patients provides educational materials.
http://www.slis.ua.edu/cdlp/unthsc/clinical/cardiology/congenital/index.htm

CONGESTIVE HEART FAILURE

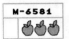

American Heart Association (AHA): Living with Heart Failure
Intended to provide support to patients, their families, and caregivers, this Web site directs visitors to fact sheets on the symptoms, causes, diagnosis, and treatment options for heart failure. Additional departments offer dietary guidance, lifestyle and exercise recommendations, and complete information on treatment alternatives. A caregivers guide is provided, allowing concerned friends and family members to locate coping and planning resources.
http://www.americanheart.org/chf/

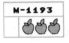

University of Alabama: Congestive Heart Failure   Peer-reviewed congestive heart failure resources, courtesy of the Clinical Digital Libraries Project, are available from this online directory, including clinical fact sheets, CME articles, pathology images, clinical guidelines, and consumer resources. Links are available to related disorders, as a service of the University of Alabama.
http://www.slis.ua.edu/cdlp/WebDLCore/clinical/cardiology/cardiovascular/chf.html

COR PULMONALE

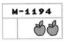

Family Practice Notebook.com: Cor Pulmonale   A concise outline at this address offers a technical overview of cor pulmonale. Topics include pathophysiology, causes, symptoms, differential diagnosis, appropriate laboratory tests and diagnostic imaging, and therapeutic management. Links are available to related pages with this Family Medicine Resource.
http://www.fpnotebook.com/CV125.htm

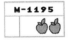

Merck Manual of Diagnosis and Therapy: Cor Pulmonale   The authoritative *Merck* publication offers this chapter on cor pulmonale, which addresses the etiology, causes, symptoms, and treatment of the disease. A brief description of primary pulmonary hypertension, a rare disease of unknown cause, is also addressed.
http://www.merck.com/pubs/mmanual/section16/chapter203/203c.htm

DEEP VEIN THROMBOSIS (DVT) AND THROMBOPHLEBITIS

American Heart Association (AHA): Management of Deep Vein Thrombosis   The American Heart Association's medical/scientific statement on the management of deep vein thrombosis and pulmonary embolism provides healthcare professionals with the clinical information needed to manage common venous thromboembolic problems. Symptoms, diagnosis, and treatment options are described. Special cases of venous thromboembolism in pregnant women and children are also examined.
http://www.americanheart.org/Scientific/statements/1996/069601.html

eMedicine: Deep Vein Thrombosis and Thrombophlebitis Deep venous thrombosis and thrombophlebitis are discussed at this site, which provides a complete clinical guidelines to management. A discussion of causes, incidence, symptoms, imaging studies and other diagnostics, and treatment is found, as well as detailed medication profiles.
http://www.eMedicine.com/emerg/topic122.htm

HYPERTENSION

 Heart Information Network: Hypertension Guide Comprehensive information about hypertension at this page includes a description of hypertension, risk factors, symptoms, and details on the distinctions between primary and secondary hypertension. Information about screening, complications, treatment, prevention, and links to related articles are provided.
http://www.heartinfo.org/search/display.asp?Id=429&header=T_pat.gif&caller=458

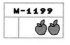 **Hypertension-Info.com** Provided by MEDIVISION, this site is dedicated to providing patients and healthcare professionals with up-to-date resources for the treatment of hypertension. The site contains multimedia educational activities and information on the latest in hypertension diagnostics and therapeutics. Clinical trial details, research, and links to related organizations are offered.
http://www.hypertension-info.com

INFECTIVE ENDOCARDITIS

 eMedicine: Endocarditis Authored by a physician from New York University Bellevue Medical Center, this eMedicine site contains frequently updated information about the disorder. Background information, including statistics on pathophysiology, frequency, mortality, sex, and age, and a clinical discussion of the illness, including symptoms, causes, and variations, are provided. Diagnostic differential links, guidelines for diagnosis, and information on drug treatment and follow-up management are included.
http://www.eMedicine.com/emerg/topic164.htm

 Vanderbilt Medical Center: Infective Endocarditis Courtesy of the Cardiology Department of Vanderbilt Medical Center, this site offers an informative online brochure addressing the symptoms, diagnostic procedures, and treatment of infective endocarditis. A list of references is also displayed.
http://www.mc.vanderbilt.edu/peds/pidl/cardio/sbe.htm

MITRAL VALVE PROLAPSE

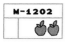 **Heart Information Network: Mitral Valve Prolapse: A Patient Guide**
The Heart Information Network presents an overview of mitral valve prolapse

including symptoms, problems associated with the condition, use of antibiotics, and the potential need for surgery. Related articles can be reached through hyperlinks included at the site.
http://www.heartinfo.org/news97/mvp82697.htm

Physician and Sports Medicine: Mitral Valve Prolapse Courtesy of *The Physician and Sportsmedicine,* this site presents information on pathophysiology and epidemiology, symptoms, key diagnostic findings, management, and exercise guidelines for mitral valve prolapse. Included is a table on evaluation and management of the disorder and a section addressing complications of the disorder.
http://www.physsportsmed.com/issues/jul_96/joy.htm

MYOCARDIAL INFARCTION

ACC/AHA Guidelines for the Management of Patients with Acute Myocardial Infarction The American College of Cardiology/American Heart Association Task Force created this comprehensive guideline for the management of patients with acute myocardial infarction. The document addresses prehospital issues, management in the emergency room, hospital treatment, pharmacotherapy, discharge evaluation, and long-term management recommendations. http://www.americanheart.org/Scientific/statements/1999/AMI/edits/

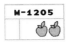

Internet Medical Education, Inc.: Myocardial Infarction (Heart Attacks) The Internet Medical Education site offers a description of myocardial infarction, including what to do in an emergency situation. Common problems associated with the condition, tests, and treatments are also covered.
http://www.med-edu.com/patient/cad/infarct.html

MYOCARDITIS

eMedicine: Myocarditis A detailed description of myocarditis is presented at this clinical presentation, with background on the condition, symptoms, causes, laboratory tests and procedures, and treatment. A hyperlink section on differentials is provided, as well as sample CME test questions relating to the condition and a bibliography.
http://www.emedicine.com/emerg/topic326.htm

University of Nebraska Medical Center: Coxsackie Virus and Viral Myocarditis This laboratory studies the role of non-poliovirus enteroviruses in human disease and focuses primarily on their role in inflammatory heart disease. The site offers a description of current research, articles about inflammatory heart disease, and links to related sites.
http://www.unmc.edu/Pathology/Myocarditis

PERICARDIAL DISEASE

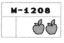

Merck Manual Home Edition: Pericardial Disease Provided by Merck, this Web site explains pericardial disease, both in its acute and chronic forms. Information on causes, symptoms, diagnosis, prognosis, and treatment are provided. http://www.merck.com/pubs/mmanual_home/sec3/22.htm

University of Medicine and Dentistry of New Jersey: Diseases of the Pericardium This site links visitors to summaries of a variety of pericardial diseases. The discussions includes etiology, symptoms, diagnosis, and treatment options. http://www2.umdnj.edu/~shindler/pericardium.html

PERIPHERAL ARTERIAL DISEASE

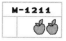

American Heart Association (AHA): Peripheral Vascular Disease A fact sheet on peripheral vascular disease and peripheral arterial disease is provided at this online guide of the AHA. Diagnosis, treatment, and several related chapters in the guide are available. Visitors also have access to scientific statements of the AHA on diagnosis, treatment, and peripheral percutaneous transluminal angioplasty of extremity vessels.
http://www.americanheart.org/Heart_and_Stroke_A_Z_Guide/pvd.html

Medscape: Management of Peripheral Artery Disease CME The report at this page, provided by the American College of Cardiology, examines symptoms and provides a detailed description of risk factor modifications, such as smoking cessation, exercise, hypolipidemic therapy, control of diabetes and hypertension, antiplatelet therapy, revascularization, and prescription drugs.
(free registration)
http://pulmonarymedicine.medscape.com/
Medscape/CNO/1999/ACC/eng/03.08/0202.mich/0202.mich.html

RHEUMATIC FEVER

eMedicine: Rheumatic Fever Information on this cardiologic sequela of previous group-A streptococcal infection is presented in a clinical, tutorial format at this address. In addition to background details, clinical presentation and diagnostic workup, visitors are afforded direct access to diagnostic differentials of the eMedicine database and pharmacologic profiles on antimicrobials, anti-inflammatories, and other prescribed treatments.
http://www.eMedicine.com/emerg/topic509.htm

WebMDHealth: Rheumatic Fever Intended for consumers, a concise tutorial on rheumatic fever is presented at this site. Topics include causes, symptoms, diagnostic tests, treatment, and prognosis.
http://my.webmd.com/content/asset/adam_disease_rheumatic_fever

STROKE

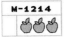

Acute Stroke Toolbox   Created by the Brain Attack Coalition, this site provides tools for healthcare professionals working to develop systems for rapid diagnosis and treatment of acute stroke. Management guidelines, the Stroke Coding Guide of the American Academy of Neurology, and Stroke Prevention Guidelines of the National Stroke Association are available. Patient education materials are also provided.
http://www.stroke-site.org

Washington University: Internet Stroke Center   The Internet Stroke Center site provides healthcare professionals with current research findings and connections to consensus statements, pharmacologic profiles, diagnostic procedures, images, teaching links, and brain anatomy. In addition, there are links available for training and employment opportunities. General stroke information for patients is provided.
http://www.neuro.wustl.edu/stroke

VALVULAR HEART DISEASE

About.com: Valvular Heart Disease   More than a dozen sites on valvular heart disease are featured on this Web page. Visitors will find information on topics such as valvular heart lesions, an overview of valvular heart disease from the *Merck Manual of Diagnosis and Therapy,* and information on artificial valves.   http://heartdisease.about.com/cs/valvulardisease/index.htm?once=true&

ACC/AHA Guidelines for the Management of Patients with Valvular Heart Disease   Presented as the Executive Summary of a report by the American College of Cardiology/American Heart Association task force, this site offers indications and recommendations for patients with cardiac murmur, several types of specific valve lesions, and infective endocarditis. An in-depth discussion is presented on pregnant women, adolescents, and patients with prosthetic heart valves. The full text of the report is available through a hyperlink.   http://www.americanheart.org/Scientific/statements/1998/119801.html

VARICOSE VEINS

MedicineNet.com: Varicose Veins   Designed for patients, this site answers commonly asked questions about varicose and spider veins, including symptoms, causes, and procedures available for treatment. Links are provided to related conditions, procedures, and medications.
http://www.medicinenet.com/script/main/Art.asp?li=MNI&ArticleKey=514

MEDLINEplus Health Information: Varicose Veins   Information on varicose veins is provided at this site of the National Library of Medicine

through a series of links that contain general overviews of the condition, clinical trials, and treatment details. Consumers may find the self-care flowcharts available under the "Diagnosis/Symptoms" section to be especially useful. http://www.nlm.nih.gov/medlineplus/varicoseveins.html

13.5 DERMATOLOGICAL DISORDERS

GENERAL RESOURCES

Karolinska Institutet: Skin and Connective Tissue Diseases A directory of hundreds of sites related to skin and connective tissue diseases is maintained on this Web page. The links are organized under headings such as skin diseases, nail diseases, hair diseases, acne rosacea, and erythema. Connective tissue diseases include cellulitis, panniculitis, and systemic lupus erythematosus. http://www.mic.ki.se/Diseases/c17.html

LookSmart: Skin Diseases and Conditions Resources related to skin diseases and conditions are featured on this site. The directory's topics include acne, albinism, birthmarks, dermatitis, head lice, leprosy, and skin parasites. More than 60 conditions are listed. Each link has a brief description of the site. http://www.looksmart.com/eus317837/eus317920/eus53948/eus89134/r?l&

ACNE VULGARIS

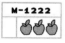

AcneNet Described as a comprehensive online acne information resource, AcneNet offers patients basic facts about acne, including social impact, causes, types of lesions, and treatment for the condition. Answers to FAQs, a glossary, and a link to an acne site just for teens are also provided. http://www.skincarephysicians.com/acnenet/index.html

Family Practice Notebook.com: Acne Vulgaris Management The management of mild acne vulgaris is featured at this physician-oriented site, which addresses exacerbating factors, common myths, and recommendations for treatment. Links related to management of moderate and severe conditions are found. http://www.fpnotebook.com/DER4.htm

ALOPECIA

DermWeb: Practical Management of Hair Loss Three common hair loss disorders and their respective course, appearance, and age of onset are outlined at this online table. By advancing to the next page, visitors will find treatment options for androgenetic alopecia in males and females, telogen effluvium, and alopecia areata. http://dermweb.org/hairinfo/10.html

University of Texas Medical Branch: Management of Alopecia This introduction to alopecia in both men and women reviews etiology and its progressive presentation in all types. Patient evaluation for potential hair replacement therapies, medications that affect hair growth, and hair transplantation methods are presented.
http://www2.utmb.edu/otoref/Grnds/Alopecia-9809/Alopecia-9809.ppt

Burns

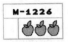

MEDLINEplus Health Information: Burns Resources on burns are provided at this site's link listing, which is organized topically. Overviews, clinical trials, coping, prevention, rehabilitation, and treatment material are offered, as well as additional links for children, seniors, and Spanish-speaking individuals. http://www.nlm.nih.gov/medlineplus/burns.html

Merck Manual of Diagnosis and Therapy: Burns Part of the online *Merck Manual of Diagnosis and Therapy,* this chapter provides assessment, diagnostic, and treatment information for thermal, radiation, chemical, and electrical burns. Emergency care, burn wound care, related respiratory care, fluid replacement, infection prevention, and follow-up care are addressed.
http://www.merck.com/pubs/mmanual/section20/chapter276/276a.htm

Calluses and Corns

Foot Talk Place on the Net Authored by Ron LeDoux, doctor of podiatric medicine, visitors to this site will find information on either corns or calluses by clicking on the respective hyperlink. Patients can learn about the causes, symptoms, and treatment for their condition. Links at the bottom of each description take visitors to related images as well as treatment procedure details.
http://www.foottalk.com/ftdisord.htm

Merck Manual of Diagnosis and Therapy: Calluses and Corns Sponsored by the online *Merck* reference, this site provides general information on superficial, circumscribed hyperkeratosis and painful, conical keratosis. Causes, locations, symptoms, and diagnosis, as well as prophylaxis and treatment information are found.
http://www.merck.com/pubs/mmanual/section10/chapter121/121c.htm

Candidiasis/Fungal Infections

Candida Many links to sites about candida albicans/candidiasis are described and organized into category headings. Sites operated by individuals, educational institutions, associations, companies, and sites for books and mailing lists are all found at this all-inclusive collection.
http://www.panix.com/~candida/#top

MEDLINEplus Health Information: Candidiasis Resources on candidiasis can be accessed from this site, including an overview, information on specific kinds of infections, and treatment options. Separate sections for the special cases of children and teenagers are found, as well as links to the latest news and research. http://www.nlm.nih.gov/medlineplus/candidiasis.html

CELLULITIS

eMedicine: Cellulitis Cellulitis is described in terms of demographic information and clinical presentation at this clinically-oriented site. Bacterial and fungal causes of infection, diagnostic differential links, laboratory studies, and treatment information are presented. Visitors will find photographs depicting mild to severe cases of cellulitis.
http://www.eMedicine.com/emerg/topic88.htm

Merck Manual of Diagnosis and Therapy: Cellulitis Superficial cellulitis is presented at this online Merck reference. A variety of bacterial sources, symptoms, diagnosis, and antibiotic intervention are reviewed, in addition to an overview of preventative measures.
http://www.merck.com/pubs/mmanual/section10/chapter112/112b.htm

DRUG ERUPTIONS

Handbook of Dermatology and Venereology: Cutaneous Drug Eruptions This portion of an online textbook offers a review of cutaneous drug reactions, describing presentations, causes, and diagnosis. A detailed table at the site outlines the morphological classification of drug eruptions along with the many drugs that cause them.
http://www.hkmj.org.hk/skin/drugerup.htm

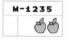

Merck Manual of Diagnosis and Therapy: Drug Eruptions Symptoms, diagnosis, and treatment of drug eruptions are featured at this site, courtesy of Merck. Links are available to information on drug hypersensitivity and adverse drug reaction information.
http://www.merck.com/pubs/mmanual/section10/chapter118/118b.htm

ECZEMA/ATOPIC DERMATITIS

MEDLINEplus Health Information: Dermatitis Providing a list of links to a variety of material on dermatitis, this site of the National Library of Medicine offers an overview, clinical trials, test allergens, prevention, and research information connections. Numerous resources on the different types of dermatitis and treatment are available.
http://www.nlm.nih.gov/medlineplus/dermatitis.html

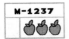

National Eczema Society Patients with eczema will find answers to FAQs that address causes, types, and management of the condition. A special section of the site is dedicated to eczema in schools and provides a guide for teachers and for children of various ages. Numerous links to related resources are provided. http://www.eczema.org/

IMPETIGO

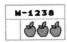

eMedicine: Impetigo *Impetigo contagiosa* is explained at this site, including the variations in clinical presentation, diagnostic tests, and medication profiles. Diagnostic differentials, prognosis, and possible complications are also offered. http://www.eMedicine.com/emerg/topic283.htm

MOLES (NEVI)

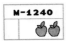

American Academy of Dermatology (AAD): Moles An online tutorial for consumers is offered at this organizational site, which addresses the lifecycle of moles, different types, the early warning signs of malignant melanoma, and medical treatment of moles. A link is provided to a national dermatologist locater. http://www.aad.org/pamphlets/Moles.html

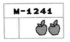

Skinsite: Moles The definition and causes of these usually harmless growths are explained at this Skin Site Web address and safe removal of moles for cosmetic reasons is examined. A link to the "Surgical Excision" site explains surgical risks, results of round and oval excisions, pathological investigation, and scar formation. http://www.skinsite.com/info_moles.htm

PEDICULOSIS (LICE)

Centers for Disease Control and Prevention (CDC): Division of Parasitic Diseases: Head Lice Infestation (Pediculosis) At this site, the Centers for Disease Control and Prevention (CDC) presents several patient and professional resources on pediculosis, including three online fact sheets and professional information on the life cycle, geographic distribution, clinical features, and treatment of the condition. Screening guidelines in the educational setting are provided. http://www.cdc.gov/ncidod/dpd/parasites/headlice/default.htm

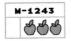

Handbook of Dermatology and Venereology: Pediculosis Pubis This chapter of the *Handbook of Dermatology and Venereology* describes *pediculosis pubis;* information on the etiological organism, the crab louse; clinical manifestations of the condition; and facts regarding the application of topical pediculocide. http://www.hkmj.org.hk/skin/pediculo.htm

PHOTOSENSITIVITY

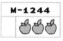

LiveAbled.com: Photosensitivity and Other Adverse Reactions to Sunlight Authored by a physician at the University of Virgina Health Systems, this article describes the physical factors and classifications of solar radiation, the skin's natural defenses, and disorders caused by sunlight in normal people. Photosensitizing reactions are introduced, as well as discussion of diseases aggravated or induced by sunlight and goals of photoprotection.
http://www.liveabled.com/manual/photosensitivity.htm

Merck Manual of Diagnosis and Therapy: Photosensitivity Physicians interested in photosensitivity will find a concise discussion of the condition, including causes, symptoms, and treatment at this online textbook chapter.
http://www.merck.com/pubs/mmanual/section10/chapter119/119d.htm

PSORIASIS

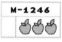

American Family Physician: Topical Psoriasis Therapy The clinical pharmacology section of the online *American Family Physician* provides a review of topical psoriasis therapy, including new vitamin D analogs, an anthralin preparation, and topical retinoids. The mechanism of disease in psoriasis and traditional therapies and their disadvantages are reviewed as a service of the American Academy of Family Physicians.
http://www.aafp.org/afp/990215ap/957.html

MEDLINEplus Health Information: Psoriasis Psoriasis links at this site contain question and answer sheets about the condition, clinical trial listings, and a diagnostic tool, the Severity of Psoriasis. Specific aspects of the disorder, statistical information, and a unique site on alternative therapies are offered.
http://medlineplus.nlm.nih.gov/medlineplus/psoriasis.html

ROSACEA

Dermatology Online Journal: Acne Rosacea A thorough discussion of acne rosacea, intended for physicians, is the focus of this site. Photographs of the condition complement the discussion of the dermatologic and ocular findings, diagnostic tests, therapy, and complications.
http://dermatology.cdlib.org/DOJvol1num2/review/rosacea.html

MEDLINEplus Health Information: Rosacea Resources on rosacea are provided at this site, including several overviews, coping, the relationship of rosacea to spicy food, and a photograph of the condition. Additional links to an online journal, statistics, and related organizations are found at this compilation, created by the National Library of Medicine.
http://medlineplus.nlm.nih.gov/medlineplus/rosacea.html

SCABIES

American Academy of Dermatology (AAD): Scabies This AAD patient pamphlet includes section on the causes of scabies, those at risk, symptoms, diagnosis, and treatment. Images of the scabies skin mite and patients with the condition are featured.
http://www.aad.org/pamphlets/Scabies.html

drkoop.com: Scabies Causes and risks of scabies, description of the condition, incidence, and preventative management information are offered at this site. This adam.com encyclopedic reference also contains several enlargeable images, courtesy of the Centers for Disease Control and adam.com sources, demonstrating extensive involvement of various body parts. Photomicrographs of the scabies mite are also displayed.
http://www.drkoop.com/conditions/ency/article/000830.htm

SHINGLES (HERPES ZOSTER)

American Academy of Dermatology (AAD): Herpes Zoster The information contained at this site explains the common reemergence of the virus that causes chicken pox in the form of herpes zoster. The symptoms of zoster, close-up images of zoster blisters and larger affected areas, post-herpetic neuralgia, and less frequent complications are described. Diagnosis and treatment options are reviewed.
http://www.aad.org/pamphlets/herpesZoster.html

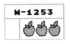

American Family Physician: Management of Herpes Zoster (Shingles) and Postherpetic Neuralgia This clinician's guideline offers management information on shingles, with the clinical presentation, explanation of rash distribution, images of shingles lesions and complicated cases, and details surrounding post-herpetic neuralgia. Treatment, pain management, and potential complications are presented, as well as a link to a related patient information handout.
http://www.aafp.org/afp/20000415/2437.html

SKIN CANCERS

CancerNet: Cancer by Body Location/System: Skin Detailed information on skin cancers, such as cutaneous T-cell lymphoma, Kaposi's sarcoma, melanoma, and nonmelanomatous skin cancer, are provided by the National Cancer Institute at links to this site. Special documents are geared toward both consumer and professional audiences, with general overviews, treatment, and causes presented for each type of cancer. Cancer literature and clinical trial details are presented.
http://www.cancernet.nci.nih.gov/location.html#skin

MEDLINEplus Health Information: Skin Cancer Skin cancer facts, including symptoms and treatment, can be accessed from the links of this National Library of Medicine collection. A wealth of information is available on skin cancer prevention, including specific fact sheets focused on children and teenagers. http://www.nlm.nih.gov/medlineplus/skincancer.html

TINEA

eMedicine: Tinea Offering nine sections on presentation, diagnosis, and management, this eMedicine chapter contains a complete guideline for practitioners. Causes, several diagnostic differential links, and antifungal medication profiles are provided and accompanied by related Medline abstract connections. http://www.eMedicine.com/EMERG/topic592.htm

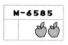

Familydoctor.org: Tinea Infections: Athlete's Foot, Jock Itch, and Ringworm A fact sheet at this page provides basic information to visitors on tinea infections and the ways that they can be acquired. Areas of the body infected, recognition of fungal infections, treatment, and prevention are addressed, courtesy of the American Academy of Family Physicians. http://familydoctor.org/handouts/316.html

TINEA VERSICOLOR

eMedicine: Tinea Versicolor For those interested in clinical information on tinea versicolor, this Web page offers an overview, complete with its pathophysiology and causes. Symptoms are described, and links to differentials are provided. Diagnostic tests are reviewed, and details are provided for topical antifungal and oral therapies. http://emedicine.com/derm/topic423.htm

Tinea Versicolor: A Case Study Dr. Peter R. Hull, a noted dermatologist, presents an online case study of tinea versicolor, including the patient history, diagnosis, treatment, and outcome. The typical hypopigmented patches of the patient's chest before treatment, as well as a direct microscopy image, are viewable at the image strip. Methods of recurrence prevention are explained. http://www.chronicle.org/tvers.htm

URTICARIA/HIVES

American Academy of Dermatology (AAD): Hives A brief patient primer on hives is provided on this site, including a definition, common triggers, and treatment. Images of the condition are included. http://www.aad.org/pamphlets/Urticaria.html

MEDLINEplus Health Information: Hives Visitors will find several accessible resources on hives at this site, such as an overview, clinical trials, self-care flowcharts, prevention, and treatment. Links to related information on mastocytosis, related organizations, and a Spanish brochure are offered.
http://www.nlm.nih.gov/medlineplus/hives.html

WARTS

Family Practice Notebook.com: Wart Treatment Examining wart treatment, this site offers physicians information on general precations, general home care measures, and management tutorials on management with medication, wart immune therapy, and cryotherapy technique.
http://www.fpnotebook.com/DER182.htm

MEDLINEplus Health Information: Warts Resources for information on wart identification and treatment are featured on this site. Links include an overview, clinical trials, information on plantar warts, and a description of removal of warts by freezing. Special information on warts in children and a Spanish language brochure are offered.
http://www.nlm.nih.gov/medlineplus/warts.html

13.6 DISEASES OF THE EYE

GENERAL RESOURCES

Karolinska Institutet: Eye Diseases Visitors to this site will find a comprehensive directory of links on eye diseases. In addition to general information on eye diseases, there are links specific to eyelid diseases, lacrimal apparatus diseases, eye abnormalities, eye hemorrhage, and optic nerve diseases. Additional topics include corneal diseases, conjuctival diseases, and eye infections. The sites are drawn primarily from the United States and Canada.
http://www.mic.ki.se/Diseases/c11.html

LookSmart: Eye Conditions Information on eye diseases and conditions, including treatment and surgery, is featured in this directory of Internet resources. Topics include astigmatism, diabetic retinopathy, optic neuritis, and uveitis. A brief description of each link is provided.
http://www.looksmart.com/eus317837/eus317920/eus53948/eus71238/r?l&

BLEPHARITIS

Handbook of Ocular Disease Management: Blepharitis Various forms of blepharitis are described at this eye management site, with the pathophysiology and mainstay of therapy described. Ocular preparations for use where excessive inflammation is present are discussed, and an image of blepharitis is displayed. http://www.revoptom.com/handbook/sect1a.htm

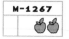

Harvard Medical School Family Health Guide: Blepharitis Consumer-oriented information is presented at this site of the Massachusetts Eye and Ear Infirmary of Harvard Medical School. A figure illustrating the condition and answers to frequently asked questions about blepharitis are provided, with information available on hygienic and antibiotic treatment. http://www.djo.harvard.edu/meei/PI/blepharitis/ptinfobleph.html

Cataract

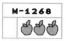

MEDLINEplus Health Information: Cataract A variety of information on cataracts is offered at this site's link listing, including patient information, clinical trials, and treatment details. Several diagrams and illustrations are accessible that demonstrate the anatomy of the eye and vision with a cataract. http://www.nlm.nih.gov/medlineplus/cataract.html

RxMed: Cataract A concise description of cataracts, their causes, symptoms, prevention, and treatment are provided at this peer-reviewed resource for family physicians. http://www.rxmed.com/illnesses/cataract.html

Conjunctivitis

eMedicine: Conjunctivitis A comprehensive presentation on conjunctivitis is offered at this article, authored by Michael A. Silverman, M.D., of Johns Hopkins Bayview Medical Center. Topics covered include pathophysiology, incidence, symptoms, causes, laboratory diagnoses are provided in order for visitors to contrast and compare conditions more easily. http://www.eMedicine.com/emerg/topic110.htm

Handbook of Ocular Disease Management: Bacterial Conjunctivitis Intended for physicians, this site describes the symptoms, pathophysiology, management of bacterial conjunctivitis, and clinical pearls in diagnosis. Links to related conditions are also provided in addition to a close-up image of the condition. http://www.revoptom.com/handbook/sect2c.htm

Corneal Abrasion

eMedicine: Corneal Abrasion Created to provide information for physicians on corneal abrasion, this Web site provides information on symptoms, causes, diagnostic procedures, and treatment of the condition. A detailed dis-

cussion on prescription drugs used to treat corneal abrasion, including dose, contraindications, and precautions, is found.
http://www.emedicine.com/emerg/topic828.htm

 M-1273

Physician and Sports Medicine: Treating Corneal Abrasions and Lacerations Drawn from an issue of *The Physician and Sportsmedicine,* this site features signs and symptoms, diagnosis, and treatment of corneal abrasions and lacerations. Images at the site illustrate identification of abrasions, procedures in diagnosis, and treatment. Distinctions between partial and full-thickness lacerations are introduced.
http://www.physsportsmed.com/issues/1997/03mar/zagel.htm

GLAUCOMA

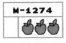 **M-1274**

Glaucoma Foundation General information about glaucoma for consumer viewing and back issues of the *Glaucoma Foundation Newsletter* are offered at this site. Visitors will also find a patient guide, Internet newsroom, and various research programs and resources of the Foundation presented.
http://www.glaucoma-foundation.org/index.htm

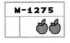 **M-1275**

National Eye Institute (NEI): Glaucoma The National Eye Institute has provided this informative guide for patients on glaucoma. Causes, symptoms, treatment, and related resources are provided, along with diagrams illustrating the condition.
http://www.nei.nih.gov/publications/glauc-pat.htm

IRITIS

 M-1276

eMedicine: Iritis and Uveitis Written from the perspective of the emergency medicine physician, this site addresses diagnosis and treatment of acute uveitis in the emergency room prior to referral to an ophthalmologist. Symptoms, causes, clinical diagnosis, differentials, and treatment are addressed.
http://www.emedicine.com/emerg/topic284.htm

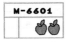 **M-6601**

HealthSquare: Iritis Supplied by the *PDR Family Guide Encyclopedia of Medical Care,* this page introduces causes, signs and symptoms, and care for iritis. Several self-treatment measures are listed, as well as information on when to seek professional treatment.
http://www.healthsquare.com/mc/fgmc1929.htm

MACULAR DEGENERATION

 M-1278

American Family Physician: Age-Related Macular Degeneration: Update for Primary Care Presented by the American Academy of Family Physicians, this article discusses the leading cause of vision loss among the eld-

erly and offers information on diagnosis, currently proven treatments, and vision rehabilitation. Tables at the site outline risk factors, and figures throughout the article illustrate macula-related changes. A variety of experimental treatments are introduced.
http://www.aafp.org/afp/20000515/3035.html

Macular Degeneration Foundation   The Macular Degeneration Foundation Web site offers a wealth of information on the condition. A portion of the site is devoted exclusively to physician use and contains an index of the latest in research findings. Patients can learn more about macular degeneration, current research, and surgical procedures through text and visual presentations provided at the site. http://www.eyesight.org/

OPTIC NEURITIS

National Eye Institute (NEI): Optic Neuritis   A site collecting information and links related to multiple sclerosis (MS) offers this discussion of optic neuritis, including new therapy as reported in the *New England Journal of Medicine.* The disorder's relationship to MS and the impact that vision research can have on a related medical discipline is emphasized at the article, courtesy of the National Institutes of Health.
http://members.aol.com/Firelady40/doc5.html

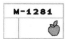

WebMDHealth: Optic Neuritis   Powered by adam.com, this site offers information to consumers on optic neuritis, with a brief description of its causes, symptoms, tests, treatment, and prognosis. Hyperlinks are provided throughout the text to further explanation of terms.
http://my.webmd.com/content/asset/adam_disease_optic_neuritis

13.7   ENDOCRINE AND METABOLIC DISORDERS

GENERAL RESOURCES

Healthtouch Online: Endocrine, Hormonal, and Metabolic Disorders
Endocrine disease profiles are provided by Healthtouch through the "Health Information" link at this home page. All health topics are listed alphabetically, including a section entitled "Endocrine, Hormonal, and Metabolic Disorders." This section provides reprints of articles from several NIH institutes and other sources on acromegaly, Addison's disease, Cushing's syndrome, hyperparathyroidism, prolactinoma, Gaucher's disease, familial multiple endocrine neoplasia type 1, and Tay-Sachs disease.
http://www.healthtouch.com/bin/EContent_HT/hdSubIndex.asp?goto_type=1x5-Grid&index=119052&title=Endocrine%2C+Hormonal+%26+Metabolic+Disorders&cid=HTHLTH

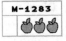

National Institute of Diabetes and Digestive and Kidney Diseases (NIDDK): Endocrine and Metabolic Diseases This site provides links to the institute's publications that describe a variety of endocrine disorders. Topics include acromegaly, Addison's disease, Cushing's syndrome, cystic fibrosis, familial multiple endocrine neoplasia, hyperparathyroidism, and prolactinoma. Other resources provided by this site include links to national endocrine organizations. Visitors can follow the "Health Information" link at this address to access a list of health topics by subject area, including diabetes, digestive diseases, kidney diseases, nutrition, urologic diseases, and weight loss and control. http://www.niddk.nih.gov/health/endo/endo.htm

Virtual Hospital: Hematologic, Electrolyte, and Metabolic Disorders Full profiles of many endocrine and metabolic diseases are available from this publication. Profiles include an overview and definition of the particular disorder and discussions of etiology, evaluation, and treatment. Diseases listed include hyperthyroidism, thyroid storm, hypothyroidism, myxedema coma, thyroid enlargement, adrenal disease, and acid-base disorders. The site also offers discussions of disorders in the metabolism of glucose, potassium, sodium, calcium, and magnesium. Electrolyte and metabolic formulas are also provided. http://www.vh.org/Providers/ClinRef/FPHandbook/05.html

ACROMEGALY

Clinical and Investigative Medicine: Diagnosis and Management of Acromegaly This scientific article begins by covering the prevalence, etiology, morphology, and clinical presentation of the disease. Related diagnostic studies, treatment objectives, and therapeutic monitoring are discussed, as are treatment options, such as surgery, drug therapies, and radiotherapy. http://www.cma.ca/cim/vol-19/0259.htm

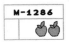

National Institute of Diabetes and Digestive and Kidney Diseases (NIDDK): Acromegaly This fact sheet, provided by the NIDDK, offers information about acromegaly, with an overview of the disease and discussions of causes, incidence, diagnosis, and treatment. Treatment options discussed include surgery, drug therapy, and radiation therapy. A list of suggested readings and additional resources is also provided. http://www.niddk.nih.gov/health/endo/pubs/acro/acro.htm

ADDISON'S DISEASE

eMedicine: Addison's Disease The clinical presentation of chronic and acute Addison's disease, in-depth information on causes, and links to several diagnostic differentials are presented at this eMedicine site. Laboratory and other diagnostic studies, medical and surgical care, and profiles of pharmacologic therapies are available. http://www.eMedicine.com/med/topic42.htm

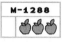

National Institute of Diabetes and Digestive and Kidney Diseases (NIDDK): Addison's Disease Sponsored by the National Institutes of Health, this online brochure introduces readers to the causes, symptoms, diagnosis, and treatment for Addison's disease. Hormone replacement or substitution, problems related to surgery and pregnancy, patient education, and suggested readings are offered.

http://www.niddk.nih.gov/health/endo/pubs/addison/addison.htm

Amyloidosis

Amyloidosis Support Network The Amyloidosis Support Network was created to provide education and resources to patients and the general public. Opportunities for patient and family networking, case histories, potential new treatments, and professional information links to published papers are provided.

http://amyloidosis.org

Weill Medical College of Cornell University: Amyloidosis Authored by Robert C. Mellors, M.D., Ph.D., this article discusses characteristics of amyloid, clinical disease classifications, pathogenesis of amyloidosis and systemic pathology. Photomicrographs of amyloid deposition are accessible, and clinical and laboratory manifestations are examined.

http://edcenter.med.cornell.edu/CUMC_PathNotes/Immunopathology/Immuno_04.html

Cushing's Syndrome

Cushing's Support and Research Foundation Founded in 1995, the Cushing's Support and Research Foundation is a resource for patients and healthcare professionals alike. The site provides a fact sheet on Cushing's syndrome, suggested readings, information about the foundation, current news and events, and contact information.

http://world.std.com/~csrf

EndocrineWeb: Cushing's Syndrome A core description of Cushing's syndrome and a thorough and illustrated guide to the disease are found at this online presentation. Common causes of excess steroids, tests for Cushing's syndrome, and treatment details are provided, as well as several links basic and clinical information on adrenal imaging.

http://www.endocrineweb.com/obesity.html

Diabetes Insipidus

Diabetes Insipidus Foundation, Inc. The Web site of the Diabetes Insipidus Foundation, Inc., with pages available in English, Spanish, or French,

contains several articles, facts sheets, and brochures on the symptoms, diagnostic tests, and medications for effective treatment of this disorder.
http://diabetesinsipidus.maxinter.net

Family Village: Diabetes Insipidus The Diabetes Insipidus and Related Disorders Network (DIARD), along with other major organizations dedicated to disease research provide ample opportunity for both professionals and patients to carry on further research of this disorder of insufficient vasopressin secretion. http://www.familyvillage.wisc.edu/lib_di.htm

DIABETES MELLITUS

American Diabetes Association In addition to current news from the association, articles from *Diabetes Forecast,* and nutrition information, this page addresses research goals and provides a variety of resources for professionals, including clinical practice recommendations, journal access, and professional education opportunities.
http://www.diabetes.org/

National Institute of Diabetes and Digestive and Kidney Diseases (NIDDK): Diabetes As a service of the National Institutes of Health, this NIDDK site sponsors a large variety of online publications covering every major aspect of diabetes. In addition, visitors are offered access to several other diabetes resources, such as the National Diabetes Information Clearinghouse, a directory of links to national diabetes organizations, and an assortment of bibliographic searches.
http://www.niddk.nih.gov/health/diabetes/diabetes.htm

DISORDERS OF FLUID, ELECTROLYTE, AND ACID-BASE METABOLISM

Postgraduate Medicine: A Stepwise Approach to Acid-Base Disorders A primer on acid-base disorders is found at this online journal site. Topics addressed include the physiologic processes involved in acid-base disorders, patient evaluation, and common associated clinical states. Calculations and an illustrative case are included.
http://www.postgradmed.com/issues/2000/03_00/fall.htm

Saladin Online Learning Center: Water, Electrolyte, and Acid-Base Balance Following an introduction to water, electrolyte, and acid-base balance, visitors will find links to several outlines, related Internet activities, and clinical applications and cases.
http://www.mhhe.com/biosci/ap/saladin/student/olc/chapterindex24.htm

Graves' Disease

National Graves' Disease Foundation The National Graves' Disease Foundation is a volunteer effort to provide education and support for Graves' patients. The site provides a bulletin board, contact list, and links to support groups. Answers to frequently asked questions, references to recommended readings, and links to related sites are offered.
http://www.ngdf.org

Postgraduate Medicine: The Many 'Faces' of Graves' Disease Important clues to diagnosis of Graves' disease are reviewed at this site of the *Postgraduate Medicine* publication. An analysis of these clinical manifestations, updated information on diagnostic testing, and clarifications regarding the merits of antithyroid pharmacologic regimens are presented.
http://www.postgradmed.com/issues/1999/10_01_99/felz.htm

Hashimoto's Thyroiditis

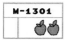

drkoop.com: Chronic Thyroiditis (Hashimoto's Disease) Adam.com's Web-based encyclopedic reference offers an overview of Hashimoto's thyroiditis at this site, with its symptoms, signs, and tests outlined, and its relation to other autoimmune endocrine disorders cited. Links to further information on related terminology are found, as well as an enlargeable image of a goiter.
http://www.drkoop.com/conditions/ency/article/000371.htm

Thyroid Disease Manager: Hashimoto's Thyroiditis The Thyroid Disease Manager presents pathogenesis, disease course, and diagnostic information for Hashimoto's thyroiditis. The autoimmune nature of the condition and a link to Chapter seven, which provides a review of the putative causes of the disease, are found. A discussion explores several unusual syndromes believed to be related to or a part of the clinical spectrum of the disorder are cited.
http://www.thyroidmanager.org/Chapter8/8-contents.htm

Hyperlipidemia

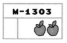

American Heart Association (AHA): Hyperlipidemia From the Heart and Stroke Guide of the AHA, this site provides a patient guide to hyperlipidemia, with a listing of five families of plasma lipoproteins and discussion of various types of hyperlipidemia. Related AHA publications and access to online guides regarding specific syndromes, pharmacotherapeutics, and diets are found. http://www.americanheart.org/Heart_and_Stroke_A_Z_Guide/hyp.html

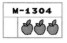

Stanford University: Management of Common Lipid Disorders Overviews of three categories of common lipid disorders, with example patient cases and in-depth discussions, are found at this site. Management procedures

for each are detailed, with drugs of choice, genetics, and gender-specific information provided. Screening recommendations are reviewed, and references on lipid disorder management are cited, courtesy of Stanford University Division of General Internal Medicine.
http://www.med.stanford.edu/fm/?/school/scrdp/&lipids.html

HYPOPITUITARISM, GENERAL

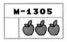

eMedicine: Hypopituitarism The pituitary's role in the endocrine system, details regarding the hormones it secretes, signs of anterior and posterior insufficiencies, and signs and symptoms of a variety of acute and insidious examples of hormone depletion are clinically described. Diagnostic differential links are provided, and laboratory studies for diagnosis, possible imaging studies, and agent profiles for hormone replacement therapy are reviewed in terms of their safety, administration, and contraindications.
http://www.eMedicine.com/EMERG/topic277.htm

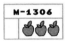

Postgraduate Medicine: How to Diagnose Hypopituitarism The features of a variety of secondary hormonal deficiencies caused by hypopituitarism are explored in this *Postgraduate Medicine* article. With an emphasis on the correct diagnosis of hypopituitarism, the authors present an illustrative case report of abnormal thyroid function values and possible causes. Clinical features and recognition of hormonal deficiencies in secondary hypothyroidism, adrenal insufficiency, and hypogonadism are reviewed, as well as management considerations. http://www.postgradmed.com/issues/1998/07_98/schmidt.htm

HYPOTHYROIDISM, GENERAL

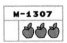

EndocrineWeb: Hypothyroidism: Too Little Thyroid Hormone An overview of hypothyroidism, its symptoms, and the potential dangers of the disorder, as well as links to information on diagnosis and treatment, thyroid gland function, diagnostic testing, and goiter formation, are all found at this EndocrineWeb location.
http://www.endocrineweb.com/hypo1.html

Hospital Practice: Recognizing the Faces of Hypothyroidism Diverging from the stereotypical picture of hypothyroidism, the author of this article offers four case examples with strikingly diverse clinical pictures. For each study, details regarding the physical exam and laboratory tests are discussed, in conjunction with the author's individually tailored diagnostic algorithms. Details regarding the physician's conclusions, information on thyroid function testing, and a table outlining the common signs and symptoms of mild and severe disease are presented.
http://www.hosppract.com/issues/1999/03/dmmmazz.htm

KLINEFELTER'S SYNDROME

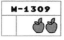

drkoop.com: Klinefelter's Syndrome   The failure of development of secondary sexual characteristics in boys and other symptoms of Klinefelter's syndrome are reviewed at this site of the adam.com encyclopedic reference. Treatment, prognosis, and complications are introduced, with links to definitions of related terms offered.

http://www.drkoop.com/conditions/ency/article/000382.htm

Hospital Practice: Diagnosis and Treatment of Klinefelter Syndrome   A case presentation provides practitioners and other interested readers information on the prevalence of Klinefelter's syndrome, its most common features, and the impact that the disease has on the physical and social development of those it affects. Treatment regimens, related disorders, and CME credit opportunity are offered as part of this presentation.

http://www.hosppract.com/issues/1999/0915/cesmyth.htm

OBESITY

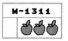

American Obesity Association   The American Obesity Association (AOA) offers answers to FAQs, facts and statistics about obesity, publications discussing current and future therapies, and an online version of the *AOA Report* newsletter at its site. Discussions of health conditions associated with obesity, information on insurance-related issues and initiatives, and an interactive Weight Wellness Profile are available.

http://www.obesity.org

Merck Manual of Diagnosis and Therapy: Obesity   The epidemiology, etiology, and signs of overweight and obesity are reviewed at this text of the online Merck Reference. Diagnosis, complications, prognosis and treatment, and details on surgical and behavioral intervention are provided.

http://www.merck.com/pubs/mmanual/section1/chapter5/5a.htm

OSTEOPOROSIS

National Osteoporosis Foundation   The National Osteoporosis Foundation features informative books for consumers and physicians at their Web site. News, statistics, reports on current research, and information about the disorder are found, including disease facts and sections on bone health, bone density, and osteoporosis in men. Information for professionals includes clinical guidelines, research grants, and clinical symposia.   http://www.nof.org

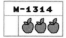

University of Washington: Osteoporosis and Bone Physiology   An educational site intended for both physicians and patients is presented at address, which offers an A-to-Z listing of osteoporosis-related hyperlinks, treat-

ment algorithms, and images of X-ray findings and other diagnostic measures. Cases, evidence, and reference connections are provided.
http://courses.washington.edu/bonephys/

PHEOMCHROMOCYTOMA

EndocrineWeb: Pheochromocytoma Intended for professional review or consumer education, this page presents classical symptoms of pheochromocytomas attributable to excess adrenaline and includes information on diagnosis, surgical intervention, and links to minimally invasive procedure details.
http://www.endocrineweb.com/pheo.html

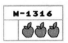

OncoLink: NCI/PDQ Physician Statement: Pheochromocytoma The University of Pennsylvania's assortment of physician statements includes this Physician Data Query, provided in cooperation with the National Cancer Institute. Classification and staging information are reviewed. Visitors will also find sections addressing general treatment details as well as options recommended for localized, regional, metastatic, and recurrent disease.
http://cancer.med.upenn.edu/pdq_html/1/engl/102494.html

POLYCYSTIC OVARY SYNDROME (STEIN-LEVENTHAL SYNDROME)

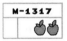

Merck Manual Home Edition: Polycystic Ovary Syndrome Intended for consumer viewing, this *Merck* reference discusses typical symptoms of polycystic ovary disease, clues to diagnosis, and a review of possible treatment options. http://www.merck.com/pubs/mmanual_home/sec22/236.htm

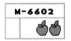

Vanderbilt Medical Center: Polycystic Ovary Syndrome Polycystic ovary syndrome is described in this clinical article, which discusses in detail this clinically heterogeneous syndrome. Incidence, symptoms, common clinical features, diagnosis, and treatment are summarized, and links are available to other topics, organized by body system.
http://www.mc.vanderbilt.edu/peds/pidl/adolesc/polcysov.htm

13.8 ENT DISORDERS

GENERAL RESOURCES

Karolinska Institutet: Otorhinolaryngologic Diseases Dedicated to otorhinolaryngologic diseases, this site offers a comprehensive directory of Web resources. The links are organized into broad categories such as ear diseases, laryngeal diseases, pharyngeal diseases, and nose diseases.
http://www.mic.ki.se/Diseases/c9.html

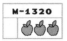

MEDLINEplus Health Information: Ear, Nose, and Throat More than 30 topics related to the ear, nose, and throat are featured on this Web page, including head and neck cancer, mouth and throat disorders, sinusitis, and tinnitus. Each topic offers additional information such as news, overviews, symptoms, treatment, and related organizations. Some topics have information specifically for children, women, seniors, and Spanish-speaking populations.
http://www.nlm.nih.gov/medlineplus/earnoseandthroat.html

EPIGLOTTITIS

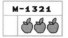

eMedicine: Epiglottitis, Adult Provided by an online textbook in emergency medicine, this site discusses the clinical presentation of epiglottitis in adults and offers several links to diagnostic differentials. Diagnostic workup procedure are outlined, and emergency care and antibiotic administration are reviewed. Visitors can view a full size or eMedicine Zoom View image consistent with epiglottitis.
http://www.eMedicine.com/emerg/topic169.htm

Virtual Children's Hospital: Acute Epiglottitis The ElectricAirway Library of University of Iowa Health Care offers this externally peer-reviewed site on acute epiglottitis, which examines the inflammation of the supraglottic structures and other disease characteristics. An online audio file, diagnosis based on history and observations, monitoring equipment, and a discussion of respiratory arrest are presented. The page contains an assortment of related, enlargeable images and a link to a summary diagram of epiglottitis protocol.
http://www.vh.org/Providers/Textbooks/ElectricAirway/Text/Epiglottitis.html

EPISTAXIS

eMedicine: Epistaxis Intended for physicians interested in epistaxis, this Web page addresses the causes, symptoms, diagnosis, and emergency room treatment of the condition.
http://www.emedicine.com/emerg/topic806.htm

Physician and Sports Medicine: Management of Epistaxis Drawn from the *Physician and Sportsmedicine,* this journal article provides a brief discussion on causes and treatment of epistaxis, as well as a look at several kinds of presenting cases and their appropriate diagnoses.
http://www.physsportsmed.com/issues/aug_96/davidson.htm

HOARSENESS

Practical ENT for Primary Care Physicians: Hoarseness Authored by David P. Goldstein of the University of Toronto, this site provides a review of

dysphonia, including hoarseness. The anatomy of the vocal apparatus, physiology of voice production, and a table describing the most common clinical entities associated with the symptom are provided. The author states organic and functional causes, emphasizing the importance of the symptom as a clue to both laryngeal pathology and systemic disease.
http://icarus.med.utoronto.ca/carr/manual/hoarse.html

University of Pittsburgh: Hoarseness: Common Causes   The University of Pittsburgh Voice Center provides information on hoarseness and its causes at this Web site, which offers a drop down menu and more information on their diagnostic lab, diagnostic services, and treatment. An image and video section illustrate common voice disorders, and the "Dos and Don'ts" section of the drop down menu provides special guidelines for singers.
http://www.upmc.edu/UPMCVoice/Hoarseness.htm

LABYRINTHITIS

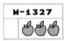

eMedicine: Labyrinthitis   Created to provide information on labyrinthitis, this physician-oriented site offers incidence, symptoms, causes, differential diagnosis, and treatment of the disease. A detailed section on drugs profiles, as well as a bibliography are provided.
http://www.eMedicine.com/EMERG/topic290.htm

MEDLINEplus Medical Encyclopedia: Labyrinthitis   Presented as a service of the National Library of Medicine, this page offers review of ear anatomy and information on causes, prevention, symptoms, and diagnosis of labyrinthitis. Treatment and prognosis are addressed, and a series of links to related information and definitions of terminology are supplied throughout the text.   http://www.nlm.nih.gov/medlineplus/ency/article/001054.htm

LARYNGEAL CANCER

CancerLinksUSA.com: Cancer of Larynx   Composed of general information, a regularly updated message board, links to treatment centers, fact sheets, and diagnostic pages, this physician-guided site offers interested viewers a broad selection of reputable information. Answers to frequently asked questions about the condition as well as descriptions of side effects and complications are provided.   http://cancerlinksusa.com/larynx/

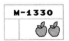

Voice Center: Cancer of the Larynx   An overview of cancer of the larynx is provided at this site by the Johns Hopkins Center for Laryngeal and Voice Disorders. Concise descriptions of symptoms, causes, and treatment, as well as images illustrating laryngeal tumors are found.
http://ww2.med.jhu.edu/voice/cancer.html

MASTOIDITIS

eMedicine: Mastoiditis Intended for physicians, this Web site provides information on mastoiditis. Incidence, causes, symptoms, differential connections within the eMedicine database, diagnosis, and emergency room treatment are discussed. A detailed discussion on pharmacologic intervention is also provided. http://www.eMedicine.com/emerg/topic306.htm

MEDLINEplus Medical Encyclopedia: Mastoiditis For consumers interested in mastoiditis, this site leads visitors to a brief overview of the condition, including symptoms, treatment, and prevention. For further information, images of mastoiditis and an illustration of the mastoid process are included. http://www.nlm.nih.gov/medlineplus/ency/article/001034.htm

MENIERE'S DISEASE

University of California San Diego (UCSD): Meniere's Disease Jeffrey P. Harris, M.D., Ph.D., has authored this site, addressing patient and professional questions about Meniere's disease. Characteristic findings of the condition and long-term consequences of untreated disease are explored, as well as several disease forms and their causes. Assessment and diagnostic testing, drug treatment, and details on rarely performed surgical procedures are presented, as a service of the Department of Head and Neck Surgery at the University of California San Diego.
http://www-surgery.ucsd.edu/ent/PatientInfo/info_md.html

Washington University: Meniere's Disease The University of Washington Otolaryngology Clinic offers information on Meniere's disease at this Web site, geared toward a professional audience. Symptoms, necessary evaluations and diagnosis, medical management, prognosis, and surgical interventions are discussed. Hyperlinks throughout the text provide more detailed information on related terminology.
http://depts.washington.edu/otoweb/meniere.html

NASAL POLYPS

eMedicine: Nasal Polyps, Nonsurgical Treatment Originally authored by Sanford M. Archer, M.D., this eMedicine article supplies information on the background and pathophysiology of nasal polyposis. Multiple factors known to play a role in polyp formation, figures on prevalence, and a review of the clinical assessment are offered. In addition to diagnostic differential links, content of the page includes bulleted summaries of laboratory studies, imaging studies, and medical care. Enlargeable, interactive images are offered, as well as a useful link to a surgical treatment guideline.
http://www.emedicine.com/ent/topic334.htm

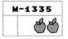

MEDLINEplus Medical Encyclopedia: Nasal Polyps Information on nasal polyps, such as causes, risk factors, symptoms, treatment, and prevention, can be accessed from this site. Hyperlinks are found within the text to further detail on terms used, and a diagram illustrating throat anatomy is provided.
http://www.nlm.nih.gov/medlineplus/ency/article/001641.htm

OBSTRUCTIVE SLEEP APNEA

American Family Physician: Obstructive Sleep Apnea Presented by the American Academy of Family Physicians, this article addresses common complaints associated with obstructive sleep apnea and methods of diagnosis. Review of polysomnography, home sleep studies, and treatment protocols are offered. Detailed, labeled illustrations of the normal and abnormal airway during sleep are displayed, and several images illustrate abnormalities contributing to the condition.
http://www.aafp.org/afp/991115ap/2279.html

University of Pennsylvania Health System: Sleep Apnea Diagnostic images of normal and apneic patients are displayed at this address, which provides an in-depth discussion about symptoms, diagnosis, and successful treatment.
http://www.uphs.upenn.edu/health/hi_files/topics/sleep/sleep_apnea/what_osahs.html

OTITIS EXTERNA

American Academy of Otolaryngology - Head and Neck Surgery, Inc.: Swimmer's Ear Consumer-oriented details on swimmer's ear are found at this fact sheet, which lists causes and stresses prevention. A print version of the article may be ordered through the site's online catalog link.
http://www.entnet.org/swimmers.html

Baylor College of Medicine: Otitis Externa Drawn from the Baylor College of Medicine Grand Rounds Archives, this page, intended for use by healthcare professionals, describes the clinical picture of otitis externa. Usually involved pathogens, malignant external otitis, and relevant laboratory studies are discussed. A case example and complete bibliography are included, as a service of the Bobby R. Alford Department of Otorhinolaryngology.
http://www.bcm.tmc.edu/oto/grand/101295.html

OTITIS MEDIA

eMedicine: Otitis Media Physicians will find a clinical discussion of otitis media at this site that includes incidence, symptoms, causes, differential diagno-

sis, and treatment. A discussion of European versus American treatment protocols of the condition is found.
http://www.emedicine.com/emerg/topic351.htm

 PDR's Getting Well Network: Ear Infection PDR.net's healthcare
information includes this page on otitis media, otherwise known as a common
ear infection. Links are found at the sidebar menu that address risk factors, detection, prevention, treatment, and related consumer information. An online
quiz tests one's knowledge of the condition.
http://www.pdr.net/gettingwell/otitismedia/

PHARYNGITIS, GENERAL

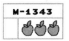 **eMedicine: Pharyngitis** A complete clinical guideline on the management
of all causes of pharyngitis is found at this online textbook chapter. Bacterial,
viral, and other causes; links to several differentials; laboratory workup and
other diagnostic information; and pharmacologic profiles for commonly prescribed antibiotics, corticosteroids, and antivirals are presented.
http://www.eMedicine.com/emerg/topic419.htm

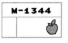 **Northwestern University: Sore Throat** The American Academy of
Otolaryngology offers this online booklet to educate the public about the causes
and cures of a sore throat. Self-treatment and advice on when to seek the help
of a physician are also provided.
http://www.cwru-ent.com/brochures/throataao.html

RHINITIS

 Canadian Medical Association: Assessing and Treating Rhinitis
Variations in effects on health of those affected by rhinitis are discussed at this
online guide, intended to unify practice of assessment and treatment of the
condition in Canada, the United States, and abroad. Anatomy and physiology
of the nasal passages, classifications and pathophysiology, key points in evaluation, diagnostic options, and optimal clinical approaches to management are
presented, as a service of the Canadian Rhinitis Symposium.
http://www.cma.ca/cpgs/rhinitis/

 McKinley Health Center: Allergic Rhinitis Providing a concise description of the causes, diagnosis, and treatment of allergic rhinitis, this site offers
interested viewers information on their condition and information on self-care
through prevention of allergen exposure.
http://www.mckinley.uiuc.edu/health-info/dis-cond/allergy/allergrh.html

Sinusitis, Acute and Chronic

 American Family Physician: Adult Rhinosinusitis: Diagnosis and Management Published by the American Academy of Family Physicians, this article addresses acute, recurrent, subacute, and chronic versions of adult rhinosinusitis, with a downloadable PDF version connection. Tables at the site outline signs and symptoms, disease classifications, and antibiotic therapy protocols. A schematic representation of the nasal cavity and diagnostic figures and images are included.
http://www.aafp.org/afp/20010101/69.html

 MEDLINEplus Health Information: Sinusitis Resources on sinusitis are provided at this site's links, including an overview of the condition, anatomy, clinical trials, diagnosis, research, treatment, and statistical information. Specific aspects of the condition and links to related organizations are provided.
http://www.nlm.nih.gov/medlineplus/sinusitis.html

Streptococcal Throat Infections

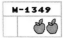 **American Heart Association (AHA): Treatment of Acute Streptococcal Pharyngitis and Prevention of Rheumatic Fever** The American Heart Association provides this statement for health professionals on treatment of acute streptococcal pharyngitis and prevention of rheumatic fever. A detailed discussion on diagnosis as well as primary and secondary treatment protocols are included.
http://www.americanheart.org/Scientific/statements/1995/109501.html

 eMedicine: Pediatrics, Pharyngitis A clinical discussion of group-A beta-hemolytic streptococcal pharyngitis is provided at this site. Information on causes, symptoms, differentials, diagnosis, and treatment in the emergency room are provided, as well as a detailed discussion of drugs used in treatment. A bibliography is included.
http://www.eMedicine.com/cgi-bin/foxweb.exe/showsection@d:/em/ga?book=emerg&topicid=395

Tinnitus

 American Tinnitus Association The American Tinnitus Association (ATA) site offers information on tinnitus, the *Tinnitus Today* journal, research and grant details, as well as related links at its home page. A products catalog, bibliography research service, and members-only sections are included.
(some features fee-based) http://www.ata.org/

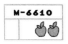 **Merck Manual of Diagnosis and Therapy: Tinnitus** Included as part of a *Merck Manual* searchable chapter, this page offers a discussion of subjective

tinnitus. Variations in patient experiences and information on possible related mechanisms are relayed at the site. Treatment, directed toward the underlying cause, is briefly reviewed.
http://www.merck.com/pubs/mmanual/section7/chapter82/82c.htm

VESTIBULAR DISORDERS, GENERAL

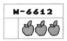

Merck Manual of Diagnosis and Therapy: Inner Ear   After accessing this page, visitors are provided with direct links to several subchapters of the online *Merck Manual*, including those on Meniere's disease, vestibular neuronitis, labyrinthitis, and acoustic neuroma. Symptoms, signs, diagnosis, and treatment are considered for each condition, and separate, main divisions of the publication are available, addressing hearing loss, vertigo, and hearing deficits in children. http://www.merck.com/pubs/mmanual/section7/chapter85/85a.htm

Virtual Hospital: Vertigo and Dizziness   Excerpted from the *University of Iowa Family Practice Handbook,* this site examines vertigo and dizziness. A concise description of the signs and symptoms of vertigo and dizziness, as well as a detailed discussion of the various vertigo syndromes are provided. A table at the site compares peripheral and central vertigo.
http://www.vh.org/Providers/ClinRef/FPHandbook/Chapter14/12-14.html

13.9   GASTROINTESTINAL/HEPATIC DISORDERS

GENERAL RESOURCES

Karolinska Institutet: Digestive System Diseases   This comprehensive site offers links for information on digestive system diseases. Gastrointestinal diseases, esophageal diseases, digestive system abnormalities, biliary tract diseases, pancreatic diseases, and liver diseases are featured. The sites are drawn primarily from universities and nonprofit organizations in the United States, Canada, the United Kingdom, and Australia.
http://www.mic.ki.se/Diseases/c6.html

MEDLINEplus Health Information: Digestive System   Topics related to the digestive system are featured on this Web page, including appendicitis, cirrhosis, colorectal cancer, diarrhea, and stomach disorders. Each topic offers a list of resources such as news, overviews, diagnosis, treatment, and research. There are also materials specific to children, women, and seniors. Some resources are available in Spanish.
http://www.nlm.nih.gov/medlineplus/digestivesystem.html

New York Online Access to Health (NOAH): Gastrointestinal Disorders   This consumer health resource offers links to information on gastrointes-

tinal disorders. The links are organized into topics such as the basics, care and treatment, conditions, and related information resources. Conditions covered include celiac disease, Crohn's disease, *E. coli* infections, food allergies and intolerances, peptic ulcer, and rectal polyps.
http://www.noah-health.org/english/illness/gastro/gastro.html

APPENDICITIS

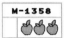

eMedicine: Appendicitis   A clinical perspective on acute appendicitis is offered at this physician-oriented site. Information on incidence, symptoms, causes, differential diagnostic procedures, and emergency room treatment options are provided. Special concerns for pregnant women and women of childbearing age, children, and geriatric patients are also addressed.
http://www.emedicine.com/emerg/topic41.htm

MEDLINEplus Health Information: Appendicitis   Appendicitis is featured at this address of the National Library of Medicine, which connects visitors to a condition explanation, a flow chart for assisted self-diagnosis, and an illustrated description of an appendectomy. Articles on recognizing appendicitis in children and a patient page, courtesy of the *Journal of the American Medical Association* (JAMA), are available.
http://www.nlm.nih.gov/medlineplus/appendicitis.html

CELIAC DISEASE

American Family Physician: Detecting Celiac Disease in Your Patients   Hosted by the American Academy of Family Physicians, this site features an online article on detecting this immune inflammatory response to gluten. A problem with underdiagnosis, new prevalence data, and its association with other autoimmune conditions are examined. Causes, symptoms, diagnosis, the value of antibody testing, and treatment of the condition are presented, along with an extensive list of references and a related patient guide.
http://www.aafp.org/afp/980301ap/pruessn.html

National Digestive Diseases Information Clearinghouse: Celiac Disease   Primarily for patients, this online fact sheet explains celiac disease, its causes, symptoms, diagnosis, and treatment. The gluten-free diet is highlighted, along with examples of appropriate foods.
http://www.niddk.nih.gov/health/digest/pubs/celiac/

CIRRHOSIS

Family Practice Notebook.com: Cirrhosis   Assorted topics in cirrhosis can be accessed from this Family Medicine Resource, as well as related topics

from the Pathology and Laboratory Medicine chapter. Each connection provides a summary of pathophysiology, symptoms and signs, and links to further information on related terminology.
http://www.fpnotebook.com/GICh2.htm

MEDLINEplus Health Information: Cirrhosis Resources offered at this site include an overview of cirrhosis, a link to clinical trials, diagnostic tests, causes, and documents on treatment. Under the "Specific Conditions" subsection, visitors can read about alcohol and the liver and cirrhosis-related liver conditions. http://www.nlm.nih.gov/medlineplus/cirrhosis.html

COLONIC POLYPS

Clinical Reference Systems: Polyps in the Colon (Colonic Polyps)
Presenting general information on occurrence, symptoms, and diagnosis, this fact sheet offers visitors a primer on what to expect at the office. Advice on taking care of oneself following surgical polyp removal, and colonic polyp prevention are emphasized.
http://www.realage.com/Connect/healthadvisor/adulthealth/crs/colonicp.htm

Society for Surgery of the Alimentary Tract: Management of Colonic Polyps and Adenomas The Society for Surgery of the Alimentary Tract provides information on diagnostic methods, polyp types, and management of patients undergoing colonoscopic treatment. Post-polypectomy surveillance, potential complications, and information regarding physician qualifications are presented.
http://www.ssat.com/guidelines/polyps.htm

CROHN'S DISEASE

Hospital Practice: Updating the Approach to Crohn's Disease
Authored by Stephen Hanauer of the University of Chicago, this article emphasizes identification of clinical and pathologic scenarios in Crohn's disease, as well as treatments and the advent of a new therapeutic option for refractory disease. A case presentation and management algorithm are presented.
http://www.hosppract.com/issues/1999/08/dmmhan.htm

MEDLINEplus Health Information: Crohn's Disease Provided by the National Library of Medicine, this site contains a comprehensive set of links for information on Crohn's disease. Basic facts, several clinical trials, coping tips, diagnostic procedures, and treatment options are featured. Separate categories of links for children, teenagers, and women with the disease are found.
http://www.nlm.nih.gov/medlineplus/crohnsdisease.html

DIARRHEAL DISEASES

 Division of Bacterial and Mycotic Diseases: Foodborne and Diarrheal Diseases Foodborne and diarrheal diseases are addressed in this subsection of the Centers for Disease Control and Prevention (CDC) Web site. By clicking on the links at the left side of the page, information on CDC's surveillance programs for disease outbreaks can be accessed. Statistics on food-related illness and frequently asked questions about foodborne disease and food irradiation are also featured.
http://www.cdc.gov/ncidod/dbmd/foodborn.htm

 Virtual Hospital: Acute Diarrhea Authored by Peter Toth, M.D., Ph.D., and externally peer-reviewed, this page examines causes, diagnosis, and treatment of acute diarrhea. A link to a related chapter on rehydration and fluid repletion is found.
http://www.vh.org/Providers/ClinRef/FPHandbook/Chapter04/01-4.html

DIVERTICULAR DISEASE

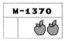 **National Digestive Diseases Information Clearinghouse: Diverticulosis and Diverticulitis** The causes, symptoms, diagnosis, and treatment of diverticulosis and diverticulitis are examined at this consumer-friendly brochure. The importance of a high-fiber diet is stressed.
http://www.niddk.nih.gov/health/digest/pubs/divert/divert.htm

 University of Florida: Diverticulitis: Is There any Science to the Pain? A slide presentation at this site, which may be enhanced with the use of RealAudio, offers information on the presentation of diverticulitis and evidence-based treatment and management approaches. Visitors can listed to the lecture while viewing notes that accompany the discussion. Chapters on terminology, diverticular bleeding, segmentation, and an algorithm for acute disease management are presented.
http://www.medinfo.ufl.edu/cme/grounds/mishra/

DYSPHAGIA

 Dysphagia Resource Center The Dysphagia Resource Center offers a comprehensive listing of links, organized by category, for swallowing and swallowing disorders. Categories include anatomy, case studies and pathologic images, diseases associated with dysphagia, Internet journals, organizations, and tutorials that include many related Web pages.
http://www.dysphagia.com/

 National Institute on Deafness and Other Communication Disorders (NIDCD): Dysphagia The National Institute on Deafness and Other Communication Disorders (NIDCD) site contains this page on dysphagia. Patients with dysphagia can learn about swallowing mechanisms, as well as causes, treatment, current research, and where to obtain additional information on the condition. http://www.nidcd.nih.gov/textonly/health/pubs_vsl/dysph.htm

ESOPHAGEAL MOTILITY DISORDERS, GENERAL

CliniWeb International: Esophageal Motility Disorders   Providing a variety of information, this site of Oregon Health Sciences University links visitors to PubMed query results related to various esophageal motility conditions. Also found are article and fact sheet connections from the Medical College of Wisconsin, Baylor College of Medicine, and other reputable health-related organizations and centers.
http://www.ohsu.edu/cliniweb/C6/C6.306.418.html

Society of Thoracic Surgeons: Achalasia and Esophageal Motility Disorders   The Society of Thoracic Surgeons maintains this site, which offers patient information on achalasia and esophageal motility disorders. Common questions and their answers are posted that explain symptoms, diagnosis, and treatment of the disorders.
http://www.sts.org/doc/4120

FATTY LIVER

Mayo Health: Fatty Liver   Fatty liver and the related disease, nonalcoholic steatohepatitis, are explained at this patient-oriented site. Causes, symptoms, treatment, and additional resources are offered. Illustrative photos accompany the text. http://www.mayohealth.org/home?id=MC00012

Merck Manual of Diagnosis and Therapy: Fatty Liver   Diffuse and focal fatty changes, pathogenesis, pathology, and symptoms and signs of fatty liver, and prognosis and treatment are discussed at this online *Merck* chapter.
http://www.merck.com/pubs/mmanual/section4/chapter39/39a.htm

GALLSTONES

American Family Physician: Gallstones   Presented by the American Academy of Family Physicians, this online article examines the management of gallstones and their complications. Risk factors, causes, diagnosis, and treatment are covered. There is also a link to a patient guide to gallstones and their treatment. http://www.aafp.org/afp/20000315/1673.html

National Digestive Diseases Information Clearinghouse: Gallstones This section of the National Institute of Diabetes and Digestive and Kidney Diseases (NIDDK) offers this fact sheet on the causes, risks, symptoms, and di-

agnosis of gallstones. Interested visitors are also provided with information on treatment modalities and facts regarding gallbladder removal.
http://www.niddk.nih.gov/health/digest/pubs/gallstns/gallstns.htm

GASTRITIS

 eMedicine: Gastritis and Peptic Ulcer Disease Primarily for physicians, this Web page describes gastritis and peptic ulcer disease. The causes, symptoms, diagnosis, and emergency intervention of the diseases are examined. Several links to differential diagnosis, medication profiles, and an image of the gross pathology of a gastric ulcer are provided.
http://www.eMedicine.com/emerg/topic820.htm

 Merck Manual of Diagnosis and Therapy: Gastritis This searchable publication examines the symptoms, diagnosis, and treatment for several kinds of gastritis, including acute and chronic erosive gastritis, nonerosive gastritis, and related syndromes. Prophylaxis and treatment as well as links to related chapters are found.
http://www.merck.com/pubs/mmanual/section3/chapter23/23b.htm

GASTROENTERITIS

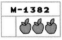 **eMedicine: Gastroenteritis** A comprehensive discussion of gastroenteritis is offered at this site, which includes the many causes, information on historical outbreaks, symptoms, diagnosis, differential links, treatment, follow-up, and prevention measures.
http://www.eMedicine.com/EMERG/topic213.htm

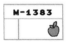 **National Center for Infectious Diseases: Viral Gastroenteritis** In a simple question and answer format, this site provides information on the most common patient concerns about viral gastroenteritis. Visitors will learn about the causes, symptoms, contagious nature, incidence, diagnosis, and treatment of the condition, provided as a service of the Centers for Disease Control and Prevention. http://www.cdc.gov/ncidod/dvrd/gastro.htm

GASTROESOPHAGEAL REFLUX DISEASE (GERD)

 American Family Physician: Gastroesophageal Reflux Disease: Diagnosis and Management Published by the American Academy of Family Physicians, this online article examines management and treatment options, including a thorough discussion of pharmacologic interventions. A connection to a related patient guide is offered.
http://www.aafp.org/afp/990301ap/1161.html

National Digestive Diseases Information Clearinghouse: Gastroesophageal Reflux Disease Gastroesophageal reflux disease is featured at this online brochure of the National Institute for Diabetes and Digestive and Kidney Diseases (NIDDK). The document explains the condition, the role of hiatal hernia, risk factors, symptoms, and treatment for the condition.
http://www.niddk.nih.gov/health/digest/pubs/heartbrn/heartbrn.htm

HEMORRHOIDS

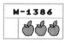

eMedicine: Hemorrhoids Created to provide information to physicians on hemorrhoids, this article addresses the causes, symptoms, diagnosis, and treatment of this common cause of hematochezia. Pathophysiology, clinical presentation, an image, and medication profiles are provided.
http://www.eMedicine.com/emerg/topic242.htm

MEDLINEplus Health Information: Hemorrhoids Resources at this site include an overview, images of the condition, and information on a surgical treatment procedure.
http://www.nlm.nih.gov/medlineplus/hemorrhoids.html

HEPATITIS

National Center for Infectious Diseases: Viral Hepatitis Links to information on hepatitis A, B, C, D, and non-A, non-B variants are provided at this index of the Centers for Disease Control and Prevention. An online training connection offers visitors clinical management details, as well as the opportunity to earn CME credit. http://www.cdc.gov/ncidod/diseases/hepatitis/index.htm

National Institute of Diabetes and Digestive and Kidney Diseases (NIDDK): Hepatitis Publications Patient publications on hepatitis A-E are featured at this site in both English and Spanish. Overviews of the three diseases, along with management of chronic hepatitis C and vaccination schedules for hepatitis A and B are offered. A treatment algorithm, formatted for download to a handheld computer, is available.
http://www.niddk.nih.gov/health/digest/pubs/hep/index.htm

HEPATOMA

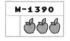

CancerNet: Liver Cancer In addition to introductory overviews of the disease, visitors will find a wide variety of articles on causes, diagnosis, treatment, and coping. Intended for both consumer and professional reference, the site supplies patient-oriented and clinical guidelines and offers links to information on clinical trials, complications, emotional concerns, and cancer literature.
http://cnetqc.nci.nih.gov/Cancer_Types/Liver_Cancer.shtml

Family Practice Notebook.com: Hepatocellular Carcinoma A concise outline of hepatoma is offered at this site that includes incidence, risk factors, symptoms, diagnosis, treatment, and prevention measures.
http://www.fpnotebook.com/GI49.htm

HERNIAS

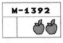

All About Inguinal Hernias: Symptoms and Causes Authored by Charles H. Booras, M.D., this page provides an illustration of the defect in the abdmoninal wall, in addition to a description of the condition, causes, symptoms, and surgical information.
http://www.jaxmed.com/articles/surgery/inguinalhernia.htm

Complete Book of Men's Health: Hernias Excerpted from *The Complete Book of Men's Health,* this site addresses femoral, indirect inguinal hernias, and umbilical hernias, with details on their causes, symptoms, and treatment. Illustrative diagrams complement the text.
http://www.lineone.net/mens_health/part2_014-2.html

INFLAMMATORY BOWEL DISEASE

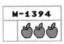

American Family Physician: Management of Inflammatory Bowel Disease The management of inflammatory bowel disease is examined at this online article, which additionally provides a related patient guide. Incidence, management algorithms, and a thorough discussion of medications are included. Coexisting problems and inciting factors are noted.
http://www.aafp.org/afp/980101ap/botoman.html

eMedicine: Inflammatory Bowel Disease William Shapiro, M.D., of the Scripps Clinic and Research Foundation describes inflammatory bowel disease and its causes, symptoms, diagnosis, differentials, and treatment at this site. Detailed sections of the article address follow-up and prognosis.
http://www.eMedicine.com/emerg/topic106.htm

INTESTINAL PARASITES

National Center for Infectious Diseases: Parasites of the Intestinal Tract Created by the Centers for Disease Control and Prevention to assist in the identification and diagnosis of parasitic diseases, this site offers a comprehensive A-to-Z listing of organisms with additional connections to further information. Causal agents, life cycle illustrations and information, clinical features, laboratory diagnosis, and geographic distribution are reviewed.
http://www.dpd.cdc.gov/dpdx/HTML/Frames/body_intest_listing.htm

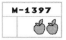

World Health Organization (WHO): Intestinal Parasites Infection by soil-transmitted helminths and additional organisms of significance are discussed at these pages of the World Health Organization. Links to relevant WHO documents, ongoing collaborations, and recent epidemiological data can be accessed. http://www.who.int/ctd/intpara/links.htm

IRRITABLE BOWEL SYNDROME

Irritable Bowel Syndrome Sites by individuals, as well as descriptions and connections to educational institutions, health centers, and associations and organizations with a focus on irritable bowel syndrome can be accessed from this Internet collection. Testing, clinical handbook pages, and book lists are offered. http://www.panix.com/~ibs/

National Digestive Diseases Information Clearinghouse: Irritable Bowel Syndrome A patient-friendly discussion of irritable bowel syndrome is provided at this site, which examines causes, symptoms, diagnosis, the effects of diet and stress, and treatment of the condition. http://www.niddk.nih.gov/health/digest/pubs/irrbowel/irrbowel.htm

ISCHEMIC COLITIS

MEDLINEplus Medical Encyclopedia: Ischemic Colitis A brief description of ischemic colitis is available from this site for those interested in learning more about the symptoms and treatment of the disease. Information on symptoms and diagnostic testing is also found. http://www.nlm.nih.gov/medlineplus/ency/article/000258.htm

Postgraduate Medicine: When to Suspect Ischemic Colitis The proper diagnosis of ischemic colitis is the focus of this online article originally published in *Postgraduate Medicine*. Symptoms, risk factors, diagnosis, differentials, and treatment methods are discussed. http://www.postgradmed.com/issues/1999/04_99/alapati.htm

MALABSORPTION, GENERAL

MEDLINEplus Medical Encyclopedia: Malabsorption Written for a consumer audience, offers explanations of malabsorption syndromes and lists several causes. Hypertext listed within the causes offers readers additional information on symptoms and treatment for the conditions that lead to malabsorption. http://www.nlm.nih.gov/medlineplus/ency/article/000299.htm

Merck Manual of Diagnosis and Therapy: Malabsorption For those interested in malabsorption syndromes, this site covers symptoms and diagnosis

of the condition. Links to subchapters on seven specific causes of malabsorption are provided. http://www.merck.com/pubs/mmanual/section3/chapter30/30a.htm

PANCREATITIS

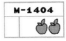

Merck Manual of Diagnosis and Therapy: Pancreatitis A general description of pancreatitis is featured at this site with links for a more thorough discussion of the acute and chronic forms. Symptoms, diagnosis, and treatment options are covered.
http://www.merck.com/pubs/mmanual/section3/chapter26/26a.htm

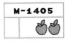

National Digestive Diseases Information Clearinghouse: Pancreatitis This online fact sheet explains the causes, symptoms, diagnosis, and treatment of both acute and chronic pancreatitis, courtesy of this division of the National Institute of Diabetes and Digestive and Kidney Diseases.
http://www.niddk.nih.gov/health/digest/pubs/pancreas/pancreas.htm

PEPTIC ULCERS

eMedicine: Gastritis and Peptic Ulcer Disease General information on the background, frequency, and physical presentation of gastritis and peptic ulcer disease is presented at this page, which offers access to an extensive collection of related problems to be considered in establishing a firm diagnosis. Outlines of information on medical care and profiles of commonly prescribed medications are offered.
http://www.emedicine.com/emerg/byname/gastritis_and_peptic_ulcer_disease.htm

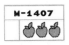

Merck Manual of Diagnosis and Therapy: Peptic Ulcer Disease Peptic ulcer disease is explained in clinical terms at this site, which emphasizes diagnosis and treatment of the condition. Related chapters and information on perforation, recurrence, and antibacterial therapy are presented.
http://www.merck.com/pubs/mmanual/section3/chapter23/23c.htm

ULCERATIVE COLITIS

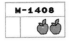

Merck Manual of Diagnosis and Therapy: Ulcerative Colitis Written for physicians, this site describes the symptoms, diagnosis, prognosis, and treatment options for ulcerative colitis.
http://www.merck.com/pubs/mmanual/section3/chapter31/31c.htm

National Digestive Diseases Information Clearinghouse: Ulcerative Colitis The purpose of this site is to explain, in a patient-friendly manner, the causes, symptoms, diagnosis, and treatment of ulcerative colitis. Both medication and surgery options are discussed along with current research findings,

courtesy of the National Institute of Diabetes and Digestive and Kidney Diseases (NIDDK).
http://www.niddk.nih.gov/health/digest/pubs/colitis/colitis.htm

13.10 GYNECOLOGIC DISORDERS AND TOPICS

GENERAL RESOURCES

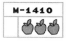

Healthfinder: Women's Health Approximately 400 Web sites related to women's health are listed on this Web page. The sites are organized into two broad categories: Web resources and organizations. Each site has a brief description and a search tool to find similar sites.
http://www.healthfinder.gov/scripts/SearchContext.asp?topic=920

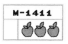

Karolinska Institutet: Female Genital Diseases and Pregnancy Complications Female genital diseases and pregnancy complications are featured in this comprehensive directory of links. Female genital conditions include sexually transmitted, vulvar, and vaginal diseases as well as genital neoplasms and salpingitis. Topics covered under pregnancy complications include dystocia, eclampsia, fetal distress, premature rupture of membranes, and ectopic pregnancy. http://www.mic.ki.se/Diseases/c13.html

MEDLINEplus Health Information: Women's Health Topics More than 75 topics related to women's health are featured on this Web site, including birth control, breast cancer, menopause, and sexually transmitted diseases. Each topic offers information such as news, overviews, symptoms, diagnosis, treatment, research, and related organizations. Some resources are available in Spanish.
http://www.nlm.nih.gov/medlineplus/womenshealth.html

AMENORRHEA

Hospital Practice: Analyzing Amenorrhea Authored by Glenn D. Braunstein of Cedars-Sinai Medical Center, this article provides three case presentations that include histories, test results, and diagnostic algorithms. A case commentary emphasizes specific disorders to be concerned about in anovulation and amenorrheic women.
http://www.hosppract.com/issues/1998/07/dmmbrau.htm

RxMed: Amenorrhea, Secondary A brief discussion of secondary amenorrhea is featured at this site. Patients will find information on causes, risk factors, diagnosis, and treatment of the condition.
http://www.rxmed.com/illnesses/amenorrhea,_secondary.html

Breast Cancer

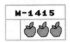

Doctor's Guide: Breast Cancer This Web site directs visitors to a comprehensive set of connections on breast cancer and related disorders. Medical news, general information, discussion groups, and additional sources of breast cancer information are found, including a statement from the National Cancer Institute. http://www.pslgroup.com/BREASTCANCER.HTM

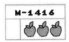

OncoLink: Breast Cancer General Information This section of the larger Oncolink site offers connections to comprehensive information about breast cancer, including discussions on screening, risk factors and prevention, treatment options, and related topics. Visitors can also find answers to frequently asked questions, news stories, support information centers, courtesy of the University of Pennsylvania.
http://cancer.med.upenn.edu/disease/breast

Cervical Cancer

CancerNet: Cervical Cancer The National Cancer Institute sponsors this comprehensive site on cervical cancer that includes access documents addressing the causes, prevention, treatment, clinical trials, and diagnosis of the disorder. A wide variety of patient guides covering physical and emotional effects of cervical cancer are available in a section on coping with disease.
http://www.cancernet.nci.nih.gov/Cancer_Types/Cervical_Cancer.shtml

MEDLINEplus Health Information: Cervical Cancer Information links on cervical cancer, excerpted from a variety of sources, are displayed at this comprehensive resource of the National Library of Medicine. Primarily patient-oriented, hyperlinks take consumers to information on clinical trials, detection and symptoms, prevention, treatment, and the latest news on cervical cancer.
http://www.nlm.nih.gov/medlineplus/cervicalcancer.html

Contraception

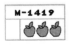

JAMA Contraception Information Center Sponsored by the American Medical Association (AMA), information on contraception is presented at this physician-oriented site. Recent articles, clinical guidelines, patient education material, and a list of related resources are provided from the *Journal of The American Medical Association*.
http://www.ama-assn.org/special/contra/contra.htm

MEDLINEplus Health Information: Birth Control/Contraception A variety of resources regarding contraception are found at this site, including links to patient fact sheets on specific methods, clinical trials, and statistics.

Special sections are dedicated to men and teenagers respectively, and some brochures are available in Spanish.
http://www.nlm.nih.gov/medlineplus/birthcontrolcontraception.html

DYSFUNCTIONAL BLEEDING

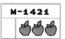

eMedicine: Dysfunctional Uterine Bleeding Serving as a clinical tutorial on dysfunctional uterine bleeding, this Web site provides information on the causes, symptoms, diagnosis, and treatment of the condition. A lengthy listing of links to diagnostic differentials is provided for convenient comparisons, and emergency care and an introduction to pharmacologic therapy are found.
http://www.eMedicine.com/EMERG/topic155.htm

MEDLINEplus Medical Encyclopedia: Dysfunctional Uterine Bleeding Visitors to this site will find information on dysfunctional uterine bleeding. A brief overview of the disorder can be accessed, and a discussion of symptoms and treatment are provided. Hyperlinks throughout the text provide further explanation of related terminology.
http://www.nlm.nih.gov/medlineplus/ency/article/000903.htm

ECTOPIC PREGNANCY

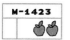

About.com: Pregnancy/Birth: Ectopic Pregnancy Ectopic pregnancy is described at this site, including causes, such as pelvic inflammatory disease, infertility, and previous abdominal surgery. Symptoms, diagnosis, treatments, and related topics are covered.
http://pregnancy.about.com/health/pregnancy/library/weekly/aa120197.htm

eMedicine: Ectopic Pregnancy Dedicated to ectopic pregnancy this site discusses causes, incidence, clinical presentation, and management of the condition. Diagnostic tests, several differential links, imaging study details, and eMedicine full size and interactive zoom view ultrasound images are available.
http://www.eMedicine.com/emerg/topic478.htm

ENDOMETRIAL CANCER

National Cancer Institute (NCI): Endometrial Cancer Healthcare professionals will find resources on endometrial cancer at this site, such as risk factors, patterns of metastasis, indicators of prognosis, cellular classification, and staging. An overview of treatment options is also available.
http://cancernet.nci.nih.gov/cancer_Types/endometrial_(uterine)_cancer.shtml

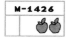

ViaHealth: Endometrial Cancer Endometrial cancer is described at this site, including risk factors, symptoms, causes, prevention, diagnosis, and treatment of the disease. Users can access other women's health resources from this page. http://www.viahealth.org/disease/gynecologicalhealth/endometr.htm

ENDOMETRIOSIS

National Institute of Child Health and Human Development (NICHD): Facts About Endometriosis   Authored by researchers of the institute, this site offers patients information about endometriosis, including an overview of the condition, symptoms, diagnosis, and treatment options. Visitors are also provided with information about other organizations that can provide answers to questions regarding endometriosis.
http://www.nichd.nih.gov/publications/pubs/endomet.htm

OBGYN.net: Endometriosis Pavilion   Offering clinical resources and sponsored by Innerdyne, Inc., this page of OBGYN.net provides connections to articles about endometriosis, hints to surviving chronic pain, news in laparoscopic surgery, and links to Hot Topics in the OBGYN.net Endometriosis Pavilion Forum. http://www.obgyn.net/endo/endo.asp

FIBROCYSTIC BREAST DISEASE

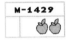

American Cancer Society: Fibrocystic Breasts: A Non-Disease
Information on fibrocystic breasts is presented at this site, sponsored by Fort Wayne Radiology. Causes of fibrocystic breast changes, details on actual lumps versus fibrocystic changes, and breast self-examination details are presented.
http://www.fwradiology.com/fibrobrst.htm

WebMDHealth: Fibrocystic Breast Disease   Intended for patients, this site features fibrocystic breast changes and their causes, symptoms, and associated diagnostic tests. Diagrams of breast anatomy are provided.
http://my.webmd.com/content/asset/adam_disease_mammary_dysplasia

HIRSUTISM

Endocrine Society: Endocrinology and Hirsutism   Examining this important issue in endocrinology, this online fact sheet explains hirsutism, incidence, and those most often affected. An explanation of when to see a specialist and the role of the endocrinologist are presented.
http://216.205.53.178/endo/pubrelations/patientInfo/hirsutism.htm

Postgraduate Medicine: Hirsutism in Women   Drawn from an issue of *Postgraduate Medicine*, this site features an article on hirsutism in women and effective long-term therapy. The article explains the causes of hirsutism, diagnostic evaluation, and long-term treatment options.
http://www.postgradmed.com/issues/2000/06_00/bergfeld.htm

HORMONE REPLACEMENT THERAPY (HRT)

Menopause and Hormone Replacement Therapy   Authored by EJ Mayeaux, Jr., M.D., of the Louisiana State University Medical Center, this online article provides physicians with information on the benefits and risks of prescribing hormone replacement therapy. The article also addresses dosage, administration, and alternative therapies.
http://lib-sh.lsumc.edu/fammed/grounds/menopaus.html

National Institute on Aging (NIA): Hormone Replacement Therapy Created by the National Institute on Aging, this Web page presents a patient fact sheet on hormone replacement therapy. The site addresses both the advantages and disadvantages of hormone replacement therapy and offers a list of related resources.
http://www.aoa.dhhs.gov/aoa/pages/agepages/hormone.html

INFERTILITY

Infertility Resources   Infertility resources are accessible through this Internet Health Resources Web site. Access to news, service providers, infertility clinics, male reproductive services, and sperm banks, as well as links to educational materials, organizations, and research programs are provided.
http://www.ihr.com/infertility/

RESOLVE: The National Infertility Association   The home page of RESOLVE, the National Infertility Association, offers consumers fact sheets, publications, advocacy information, and a list of related resources. Members can also access a physician and clinic referral service.
(some features fee-based) http://www.resolve.org/

MENOPAUSE

MEDLINEplus Health Information: Menopause   Visitors will find a large selection of information at this site on menopause. Overviews of menopause, clinical trials, research, and treatment information are available through site links. Of particular interest is the relationship between menopause and other medical conditions accessible from the "Specific Conditions/Aspects" section.
http://www.nlm.nih.gov/medlineplus/menopause.html

North American Menopause Society   For those interested in menopause, this site provides access to professional education, consensus opinions, and scientific meeting details. Information and abstracts from the professional journal, *Menopause;* consumer-related documents and events; and additional Internet resource listings are found at this page of the leading scientific organization in menopause education.   http://www.menopause.org/

OVARIAN DISORDERS

MEDLINEplus Health Information: Ovarian Cysts A comprehensive directory of sites related to ovarian cysts is found at this reference of the National Library of Medicine, including information on clinical trials, links to pages on diagnosis and symptoms, specific conditions, and an atlas of the female body.
http://www.nlm.nih.gov/medlineplus/ovariancysts.html

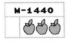

Ovarian Disorders Clinical Resources Clinical resources for ovarian disorders are presented at this site, with links to directories of information for both ovarian cysts and ovarian neoplasms. Comprehensive sets of links are available, with information on diagnostic procedures, clinical guidelines, clinical trials, and pathology.
http://www.slis.ua.edu/cdlp/WebDLCore/clinical/gynecology/ovariandisorders/

PELVIC INFLAMMATORY DISEASE (PID)

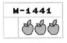

eMedicine: Pelvic Inflammatory Disease Clinical and physical presentation, causes, and links to diagnostic differentials are all contained at this eMedicine article. Diagnostic workups, therapeutic goals and drug profiles, and details on prevention and complications are offered.
http://www.eMedicine.com/emerg/topic410.htm

National Institute of Allergy and Infectious Diseases (NIAID): Pelvic Inflammatory Disease Possible causes of pelvic inflammatory disease, along with symptoms, risk factors, diagnostic measures, treatment, and preventative measures, are explored at this online fact sheet. Provided as a service of NIAID, the page also offers a brief discussion of related research.
http://www.niaid.nih.gov/factsheets/stdpid.htm

VAGINITIS

Common Simple Emergencies: Vaginitis Excerpted from *Common Simple Emergencies,* this electronic publication offers a short clinical discussion of vaginitis. Patient presentation, diagnostic procedures, and appropriate treatment are described.
http://www.clark.net/pub/electra/cse0803.html

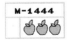

National Vaginitis Association The home page of the National Vaginitis Association offers healthcare professionals access to the latest news on vaginal and reproductive health, along with detailed reports on recent research developments. Patients can learn more about vaginal health by reading the *Women's Guide* and the FAQ sections.
http://www.vaginalinfections.com/00f03.html

13.11 INFECTIOUS DISEASES

GENERAL RESOURCES

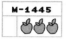

Centers for Disease Control and Prevention (CDC): Alphabetical Disease Directory A comprehensive list of infectious diseases and related disorders resources from the CDC is available at this address. Each listing links to a fact sheet on the topic. Information on selected CDC prevention programs is also available.
http://www.cdc.gov/ncidod/diseases/index.htm

Johns Hopkins Infectious Diseases A specialty page from Johns Hopkins University is available at this address, which posts medical education materials, case rounds, and news in the field of infectious disease. A variety of additional disease resources and guides are found, including the Johns Hopkins University AIDS Service, Epidemiology and Infection Control, and Web sites specific to hepatitis, tuberculosis, and antibiotic treatment.
http://hopkins-id.edu/

MEDLINEplus Health Information: Infectious Disease Topics Dedicated to infectious disease, this site offers resources for a variety of topics such as AIDS, bacterial infections, chickenpox, the common cold, and fungal infections. Each topic offers information such as the latest news, overviews, clinical trials, research, specific aspects of the disease, treatment, and related organizations. http://www.nlm.nih.gov/medlineplus/infections.html

New York State Department of Health: Communicable Disease Fact Sheets Weekly influenza activity updates and fact sheets on more than 70 communicable diseases common to both the United States and tropical areas are provided by the New York State Department of Health at this site. Fact sheets on vaccine-preventable diseases are also available.
http://www.health.state.ny.us/nysdoh/consumer/commun.htm

AMEBIASIS

London School of Hygiene and Tropical Medicine: The Entamoeba Homepage This informative resource provides materials on Entamoeba species and amebiasis, including background, the phylogeny of Entamoeba, journal links, and a directory of researchers. Laboratory resources for diagnosis as well as treatment details are provided.
http://www.lshtm.ac.uk/mp/bcu/enta/homef.htm

National Center for Infectious Diseases: Amebiasis Topics discussed at this article of the Centers for Disease Control and Prevention include the causal agent of the disease, geographic distribution, clinical features, laboratory

diagnosis, and treatment. A description of the organism's life cycle is accompanied by a detailed illustration.
http://www.dpd.cdc.gov/DPDx/HTML/Amebiasis.htm

BOTULISM

Center for Food Safety and Applied Nutrition: Clostridium botulinum   Containing valuable information on botulism, this site of the U.S. Food and Drug Administration (FDA) features background on the organism causing botulism, infant botulism, and wound botulism; nature of the disease; diagnosis; and details on selected outbreaks.
http://vm.cfsan.fda.gov/~mow/chap2.html

eMedicine: Botulism   Nine sections of information are contained at this eMedicine resource, addressing disease classification, pathophysiology, and morbidity and mortality of food-borne disease. The clinical presentation of botulism is outlined, and links to differentials are offered. Emergency care and a profile of antitoxin therapy are found.
http://www.eMedicine.com/emerg/topic64.htm

CANDIDIASIS

Division of Bacterial and Mycotic Diseases: Candidiasis   A page containing technical information about candidiasis infection is found at this site, including clinical features, etiologic agent, incidence, sequelae, risk groups, and surveillance. The general information link takes visitors to three separate pages on oropharyngeal, invasive, and genital candidiasis, and a reference listing is provided.
http://www.cdc.gov/ncidod/dbmd/diseaseinfo/candidiasis_t.htm

MEDLINEplus Health Information: Candidiasis   Links to resources on cadidiasis are featured at this site, including an overview, information on specific kinds of infection, and treatment options. The latest news, research, and connections to fact sheets regarding infection in children are offered.
http://www.nlm.nih.gov/medlineplus/candidiasis.html

CAT SCRATCH DISEASE

eMedicine: Cat Scratch Disease   The physical presentation and causes of cat scratch disease are addressed at this eMedicine article, which also provides review of the diagnostic workup and pharmacologic therapy. Links to several differentials within the eMedicine database are included.
http://www.eMedicine.com/MED/topic304.htm

Vanderbilt Medical Center: Cat Scratch Disease   Directed toward medical professionals, this site features clinical manifestations, treatment, and discussion of the etiologic agent. Recent studies on systemic manifestations are reviewed, and references are provided.
http://www.mc.vanderbilt.edu/peds/pidl/infect/catscrat.htm

E. COLI INFECTION

Division of Bacterial and Mycotic Diseases: Escherichia coli   A clinical description of *E. coli* is featured at this site, with a discussion of symptoms, etiology, incidence, transmission, and clinical challenges. Intended for a consumer audience, the general information link connects visitors to a list of FAQs concerning diagnosis, treatment, and prevention. PDF files regarding surveillance, related links, references, and articles drawn from the *Morbidity and Mortality Weekly Report* are also provided.
http://www.cdc.gov/ncidod/dbmd/diseaseinfo/escherichiacoli_t.htm

MEDLINEplus Health Information: E. Coli Infections   The latest news, fact sheets, and research update connections are provided at this site from the National Library of Medicine. MEDLINEplus provides a comprehensive resource for information on *E. coli,* and visitors will find an assortment of accessible material on transmission, prevention, and related links.
http://www.nlm.nih.gov/medlineplus/ecoliinfections.html

ENCEPHALITIS

eMedicine: Encephalitis   A general description of encephalitis, as well as other article sections devoted to pathophysiology, demographic details, and clinical and physical presentation are found at this eMedicine reference. Causes are discussed, and several differential links to similar articles within this online textbook are offered.
http://www.eMedicine.com/EMERG/topic163.htm

MEDLINEplus Health Information: Encephalitis   For those interested in encephalitis, this site features an overview, clinical trials, diagnosis, information on the several types of encephalitis, and connections to statistical information.
http://www.nlm.nih.gov/medlineplus/encephalitis.html

FOOD POISONING

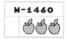

Centers for Disease Control and Prevention (CDC): Foodborne Illnesses   Information on more than 25 foodborne illnesses and topics are available from this site, which offers links to FAQs about each disease, clinical information connections, and additional, related articles, links, and reference listings. http://www.cdc.gov/health/foodill.htm

MEDLINEplus Health Information: Food Contamination/Poisoning
Food poisoning is the focus of this site, which contains links to consumer advice, food safety information, clinical trials, and prevention measures. A variety of connections to specific conditions and information on protecting children are also provided.
http://www.nlm.nih.gov/medlineplus/foodcontaminationpoisoning.html

GASTROENTERITIS, GENERAL

eMedicine: Gastroenteritis   Authored by Arthur Diskin, M.D., of Mount Sinai Medical Center, this eMedicine article addresses the pathophysiology, clinical presentation, and epidemiologic factors associated with gastroenteritis. Examination guidelines, causes, and differential diagnoses are presented, as well as laboratory workup information and treatment.
http://www.eMedicine.com/EMERG/topic213.htm

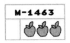

Merck Manual of Diagnosis and Therapy: Gastroenteritis, General
Complete coverage of the etiology and epidemiology, pathophysiology, symptoms, and general principles of treatment for gastroenteritis are found at this *Merck* reference page. Connections to further information on a variety of organisms, viral gastroenteritis, travelers' diarrhea, and additional specific conditions are found.
http://www.merck.com/pubs/mmanual/section3/chapter28/28a.htm

GIARDIASIS

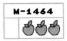

eMedicine: Giardiasis   Examining giardiasis, this site provides physicians with information on incidence, causes, symptoms, differentials, diagnostic workup, and emergency room treatment. Descriptions of appropriate medications and follow-up care are also provided.
http://www.eMedicine.com/emerg/topic215.htm

Virtual Hospital: Giardiasis   As part of the University of Iowa Health Care network, this public health fact sheet intended for patients describes the symptoms, diagnosis, treatment and prevention of giardiasis.
http://www.vh.org/Patients/IHB/IntMed/Infectious/Giardiasis.html

HEPATITIS

National Center for Infectious Diseases: Viral Hepatitis   Information on hepatitis A, B, C, delta virus, and hepatitis E is available from this single location. By visiting any particular part of this resource center, visitors are af-

forded access to documents and links on all varieties of hepatitis, including fact sheets, answers to frequently asked questions, clinical information, and surveillance reports.
http://www.cdc.gov/ncidod/diseases/hepatitis/

National Institute of Diabetes and Digestive and Kidney Diseases (NIDDK): Hepatitis Patient publications on hepatitis A, B, and C are featured at this site in both English and Spanish. Overviews of the three diseases along with management of chronic hepatitis C and vaccinations for hepatitis A and B are offered.
http://www.niddk.nih.gov/health/digest/pubs/hep/index.htm

HISTOPLASMOSIS

Division of Bacterial and Mycotic Diseases: Histoplasmosis Histoplasmosis resources are available from the Centers for Disease Control and Prevention at this address. Information for healthcare professionals includes a clinical fact sheet and links to related articles and resources. Answers to frequently asked questions about the disease are also included.
http://www.cdc.gov/ncidod/dbmd/diseaseinfo/histoplasmosis_g.htm

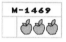

Indiana University: Histoplasmosis Reference Laboratory Indiana University's Histoplasmosis Reference Laboratory offers an information guide that describes transmission, risk factors, symptoms, treatment, drugs, and prevention. Diagnostic testing details, an FAQ document, references, and selected, downloadable lectures on therapy and management are provided.
http://www.iupui.edu/~histodgn

INFECTIOUS MONONUCLEOSIS (EPSTEIN-BARR VIRUS)

MEDLINEplus Health Information: Infectious Mononucleosis Visitors to this site will find a variety of links to information on infectious mononucleosis. A general description of the disease along with discussions of the illness in children and teenagers are found.
http://www.nlm.nih.gov/medlineplus/infectiousmononucleosis.html

National Center for Infectious Diseases: Epstein-Barr Virus and Infectious Mononucleosis The Centers for Disease Control and Prevention have provided this clinical fact sheet on Epstein-Barr Virus. The document describes incidence, symptoms, and diagnostic tests along with their interpretation. http://www.cdc.gov/ncidod/diseases/ebv.htm

INFLUENZA

Centers for Disease Control and Prevention (CDC): Influenza Prevention and Control Various types of the influenza virus are profiled at this CDC site, as well as the influenza vaccine and antiviral drugs available to treat the disease. Updates on influenza surveillance efforts and information for international travelers are also found at the site.
http://www.cdc.gov/ncidod/diseases/flu/fluvirus.htm

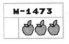

National Foundation for Infectious Diseases: Influenza This online presentation provides access to facts, statistics, tables, and surveillance reports on the highly contagious influenza virus. Symptoms, complications, vaccines, specific structure information, and diagnostic laboratory tests are covered.
http://www.nfid.org/library/influenza/index.html

LEGIONNAIRES' DISEASE

Division of Bacterial and Mycotic Diseases: Legionellosis: Legionnaire's Disease (LD) and Pontiac Fever A clinical description of Legionnaires' disease and its symptoms, etiology, incidence, transmission, and clinical challenges are presented at this site, courtesy of the Centers for Disease Control and Prevention. Visitors can also access answers to several frequently asked questions or jump to related *Morbidity and Mortality Weekly Reports.*
http://www.cdc.gov/ncidod/dbmd/diseaseinfo/legionellosis_t.htm

Legionnaires' Disease This Veterans Administration Medical Center site on Legionnaires' disease features professional resources, such as links to recent publications, laboratory testing services, and a listing of experts in the field. Summaries and full-text of recent, peer-reviewed literature are offered.
http://www.legionella.org

LYME DISEASE

Centers for Disease Control and Prevention (CDC): Lyme Disease Dedicated to providing information on Lyme disease infection, this site of the Division of Vector-Borne Infectious Diseases offers an introduction to Lyme disease, including details on disease transmission and disease risk. Additional pages available from the site menu address diagnosis, epidemiology, prevention, control, and vaccine recommendations. Answers to commonly asked questions and a complete reference list are offered.
http://www.cdc.gov/ncidod/dvbid/lyme/index.htm

University of Connecticut: Lyme Disease Education Information at the site is divided into general Lyme disease information, instructional materials for teachers, and research related to Lyme disease. Each page contains several connections to a variety of Internet resources on Lyme disease, including a Power Point slide presentation, online brochures, popular literature, and professional organizations. http://www.ucc.uconn.edu/~wwwlyme/index.html

MEASLES

eMedicine: Measles (Rubeola) This article offers a detailed, clinical discussion of measles, including pathophysiology, appropriate laboratory diagnostics, differential diagnosis, and treatment protocols. The measles vaccine is also described, including drug category, preparation, and vaccine schedule.
http://www.eMedicine.com/DERM/topic259.htm

National Foundation for Infectious Diseases: Facts About Measles for Adults Examining measles and the Measles, Mumps, Rubella (MMR) vaccine, this site offers a general description of measles including routes of infection, symptoms, prevention, and vaccine safety. Many useful facts about measles, including incidence and related statistics, are available.
http://www.nfid.org/factsheets/measlesadult.html

MENINGITIS

eMedicine: Meningitis A general description of meningitis, factors influencing its development, and incidence of several disease variations are presented at this eMedicine reference. Information on distinguishing among acute, subacute, and chronic varieties and pathogen identification is found, along with history, clinical presentation, and differential Web links.
http://www.eMedicine.com/emerg/topic309.htm

MEDLINEplus Health Information: Meningitis A variety of connections to information on meningitis is provided at this site including an overview, clinical trials, diagnosis, and prevention fact sheets from several reputable government and private organizations. Readers will find a discussion of the disease in college students and of disease variations.
http://www.nlm.nih.gov/medlineplus/meningitis.html

MYCOPLASMAL INFECTIONS, GENERAL

Medical Microbiology: Mycoplasmas This chapter of an online textbook, authored by Shmuel Razin, presents general concepts in mycoplasmal infection; structure, classification, and antigenic types; pathogenesis; and diagnostic details. An electron micrographic image, schematic presentations, and taxonomy and properties are provided.
http://gsbs.utmb.edu/microbook/ch037.htm

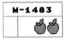 **Pathogenesis and Treatment of Mycoplasmal Infections** Originally published in the *Antimicrobial Infectious Disease Newsletter,* this online article addresses the pathogenesis and treatment of mycoplasmal infections. Also examined, is the link between these infections and unexplained chronic illnesses.
http://www.immed.org/publications/fatigue_illness/pub1.html

Mycotic Diseases (Fungal)

 Doctor Fungus This medical mycology site offers disease descriptions and images, histopathology, and an online procedure manual. Links for patients, further education, and downloadable software are offered.
http://www.doctorfungus.org/aboutdrf/index.htm

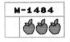 **Merck Manual of Diagnosis and Therapy: Systemic Fungal Diseases** A discussion of systemic fungal infections is presented at this *Merck* page, with diagnostic and general therapeutic principles and antifungal treatments addressed. Additional sub-topic connections provide in-depth coverage of more than 10 fungal opportunists. Additionally, related chapters on dermatohpytoses and fungal infections involving the genitourinary and pulmonary system are available from this address.
http://www.merck.com/pubs/mmanual/section13/chapter158/158a.htm

Osteomyelitis

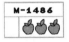 **eMedicine: Osteomyelitis** Osteomyelitis is the focus of this physician-oriented site. The discussion includes incidence, symptoms, causes, differential diagnosis, and emergency room treatment. Medication profiles and follow-up management are presented.
http://www.eMedicine.com/emerg/topic349.htm

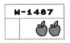 **MEDLINEplus Medical Encyclopedia: Osteomyelitis** Patients with osteomyelitis will find an overview of the condition, along with links to symptoms, diagnostic tests, and treatment options at a page of this National Library of Medicine database. Powered by adam.com, this reference also includes schematic representations of bone infection and diagnostic tests.
http://www.nlm.nih.gov/medlineplus/ency/article/000437.htm

Parasitic Infections

 Division of Parasitic Diseases: Professional Information Healthcare professionals will find a variety of resources on parasitic infection at this site, including an alphabetical listing of parasite connections and information, laboratory assistance for diagnosis of parasites, and guidelines for issuing immunobiologics and drugs. A page accessible from the site is dedicated to preventing infections during travel, courtesy of the Centers for Disease Control and Prevention. http://www.cdc.gov/ncidod/dpd/professional/default.htm

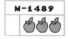

Karolinska Institutet: Parasitic Diseases A comprehensive listing of links related to parasitic disease is featured at this site. The connections are intended for a variety of audiences, with pathologic images, diagnostic procedures, and information on parasites from around the world. Lectures, textbook chapters, and an assortment of disease-specific fact sheets are here.
http://www.mic.ki.se/Diseases/c3.html

PERTUSSIS (WHOOPING COUGH)

Division of Bacterial and Mycotic Diseases: Pertussis Pertussis is featured at this site of the Centers for Disease Control and Prevention, with information on clinical features, etiologic agent, incidence, complications, transmission, and clinical challenges. Current opportunities for research in pertussis are also suggested, and additional articles, links, and references are provided.
http://www.cdc.gov/ncidod/dbmd/diseaseinfo/pertussis_t.htm

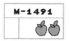

MEDLINEplus Medical Encyclopedia: Pertussis Visitors to this consumer-oriented site, will find information on pertussis and its causes, symptoms, diagnostic tests, treatment, and prevention measures.
http://www.nlm.nih.gov/medlineplus/ency/article/001561.htm

PHARYNGITIS

Kansas University Medical Center: Common Problems of the Throat A slide presentation offers visitors information on several etiologies of a sore throat, details on differential decision-making, and clinical management of viral, strep, and other disorders associated with pharyngitis.
http://www2.kumc.edu/instruction/nursing/nrsg814/ppthroat/

Merck Manual of Diagnosis and Therapy: Pharyngitis In addition to an overview of inflammation of the pharynx, this *Merck* site provides several links to related conditions, including peritonsillar abscess and tonsillitis.
http://www.merck.com/pubs/mmanual/section7/chapter87/87c.htm

PINWORMS

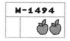

Division of Parasitic Diseases: Pinworm Infection Supported by the Centers for Disease Control and Prevention, this site offers professionals links to laboratory assistance in the identification of pinworms and a host of related articles. Patients will find a fact sheet and an article on infection prevention in the child care setting.
http://www.cdc.gov/ncidod/dpd/parasites/pinworm/default.htm

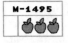 **eMedicine: Pinworms (Enterobiasis Vermicularis)** This Continuing Medical Education article offers background, pathophysiology, and demographic information related to pinworm infection. Clinical details, links to information on differential diagnoses, laboratory diagnostics, complete management, and medication information are available.
http://www.eMedicine.com/EMERG/topic424.htm

PNEUMONIA

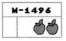 **American Lung Association (ALA): Pneumonia** Sections on causes of pneumonia; bacterial, viral, and mycoplasmal pathogens; other types of pneumonia; and intervention are presented at this online brochure of the ALA. Information on prevention of viral and pneumonococcal varieties and access to related sites are offered.
http://www.lungusa.org/diseases/lungpneumoni.html

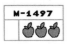 **eMedicine: Pneumonia, Bacterial** Authored by James Stephen, MD, this eMedicine topic addresses bacterial infection of the lungs, with pathophysiology, clinical presentation, pathogenic details, differential links, and complete diagnostic workup information offered.
http://www.eMedicine.com/EMERG/topic465.htm

RICKETTSIAL INFECTIONS

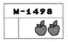 **American Society for Rickettsiology** The American Society for Rickettsiology fosters the exchange of information among scientists engaged in research on rickettsiae and rickettsial diseases. The site contains online newsletters, a member directory, and links to related sites.
http://www.cas.umt.edu/rickettsiology/

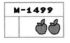 **Merck Manual Home Edition: Rickettsial Infections** This site provides a brief tutorial on rickettsial infection. Symptoms, diagnosis, and treatment are addressed, with particular attention to Rocky Mountain spotted fever and murine typhus. http://www.merck.com/pubs/mmanual_home/sec17/183.htm

SALMONELLA INFECTIONS

 Center for Food Safety and Applied Nutrition: Salmonella The U.S. Food and Drug Administration's (FDA) Center for Food Safety and Applied Nutrition provides this site on Salmonella. Background on the organism causing salmonella poisoning, nature of acute infection, diagnosis, and selected outbreak information are featured.
http://vm.cfsan.fda.gov/~mow/chap1.html

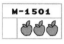

MicroBioNet: Salmonella Profile   Offering a broad overview of Salmonella species, this site also provides information on classification, biochemistry, genetics, serology, virulence factors, pathogens, laboratory identification, and vaccines.
http://www.sciencenet.com.au/frames/profiles/negative/families/enteroba/profile2.htm

Sepsis

Merck Manual of Diagnosis and Therapy: Bacteremia and Septic Shock   General information on sepsis is reviewed at this site of the authoritative *Merck* reference. Additional topic links address bacteremia and septic shock, and connections to related *Merck* chapters are available.
http://www.merck.com/pubs/mmanual/section13/chapter156/156a.htm

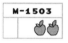

Virtual Hospital: University of Iowa Family Practice Handbook, 3rd Edition: Infectious Disease: Sepsis   A clinical outline of sepsis is the focus of this site, which includes a definition, causes, epidemiology, symptoms, diagnosis, and treatment options.
http://www.vh.org/Providers/ClinRef/FPHandbook/Chapter18/02-18.html

Streptococcal Infections, General

Boston University: Streptococcal Infections   Resources on streptococcal infections at this site include a description of possible infections, routes of infection, risk groups, symptoms, diagnosis, and treatment.
http://www.bu.edu/cohis/infxns/bacteria/strep.htm

University of Texas Medical Branch: Streptococcus   Intended for healthcare professionals, this site on Streptococcus covers clinical manifestations, bacterial structure, classification and antigenic types, pathogenesis, host defenses, epidemiology, diagnosis, and control. Also included are morphological illustrations, tables of medically important pathogens, and vaccination discussion. http://gsbs.utmb.edu/microbook/ch013.htm

Tetanus

Centers for Disease Control and Prevention (CDC): Tetanus   Available in PDF format, this document includes chapters on clinical features, tetanus complications, and medical and wound management. Immunogenicity and vaccine efficacy are fully addressed, as well as vaccine schedule and adverse reactions. http://www.cdc.gov/nip/publications/pink/tetanus.pdf

New York State Department of Health: Tetanus (Lockjaw)   A summary of tetanus is offered at this site, including a description of the causative organism and disease, symptoms, treatment, and details of the tetanus vaccine.
http://www.health.state.ny.us/nysdoh/consumer/tetanus.htm

TOXIC SHOCK SYNDROME

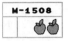 **Centers for Disease Control and Prevention (CDC): Toxic Shock Syndrome** The Division of Bacterial and Mycotic Diseases of the CDC offers this technical fact sheet on toxic shock syndrome, which describes clinical features, transmission, national surveillance, and challenges. A list of related references can be accessed.
http://www.cdc.gov/ncidod/dbmd/diseaseinfo/toxicshock_t.htm

 eMedicine: Toxic Shock Syndrome Toxic shock syndrome is examined at this site, which, in addition to background on the infection, provides information on pathophysiology, causes, workup, treatment, and follow-up management. Several differentials within the eMedicine database are accessible, as well as links to related, indexed literature.
http://www.eMedicine.com/emerg/topic600.htm

TOXOPLASMOSIS

 Division of Parasitic Diseases: Toxoplasmosis This section of the Centers for Disease Control and Prevention offers a collection of resources related to toxoplasmosis for both professional and consumer visitors. A fact sheet on the condition; a document examining life cycle, geographic distribution, and clinical features; and related *Morbidity and Mortality Weekly Report* documents are found. http://www.cdc.gov/ncidod/dpd/parasites/toxoplasmosis/default.htm

 University of Kentucky Lexington: Toxoplasmosis A comprehensive listing of links on toxoplasmosis is offered at this site. Information includes several fact sheets, the disease in humans, and protecting against the disease during pregnancy. http://www.uky.edu/Agriculture/FoodScience/FSC632/fsc632toxop.html

TUBERCULOSIS

 Division of Healthcare Quality Promotion: Tuberculosis This section of the Centers for Disease Control and Prevention examines tuberculosis, with a variety of educational materials accessible from the site. Visitors will discover fact sheets, prevention and control guidelines, documents addressing respiratory protection, and standards for diagnosis and treatment.
http://www.cdc.gov/ncidod/hip/guide/tuber.htm

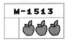 **Johns Hopkins Center for Tuberculosis Research** In addition to regularly updated news, this site of Johns Hopkins Medical Institutions offers information on treatment of latent disease, drug information, a question and answer forum designed for healthcare professionals, and details on epidemiology and the natural history of tuberculosis infection.
http://www.hopkins-tb.org/

VARICELLA-ZOSTER

 Centers for Disease Control and Prevention (CDC): Varicella-Zoster Virus A comprehensive introduction to the varicella-zoster virus (VZV) is found at this address, provided by the National Center for Infectious Diseases. Devoted to chickenpox, shingles, and postherpetic neuralgia (PHN), the material provides quick facts, references, and statistics, as well as varicella-zoster vaccine information.
http://www.cdc.gov/ncidod/srp/varicella.htm

 Varicella Zoster Virus (VZV) Research Foundation (RF) Dedicated to research and education on VZV infection, this organization offers patient and physician pages about VZV, addressing chickenpox, shingles, and post-herpetic neuralgia (PHN). The site contains information on research, question and answer pages, and the online *VZVRF Focus* newsletter.
http://www.vzvfoundation.org

VIRAL INFECTIONS, GENERAL

 Karolinska Institutet: Virus Diseases Viral illnesses are the focus of this large Internet link collection, which connects visitors to fact sheets, textbook pages, virology databases, and comprehensive information on a variety of viral infectious diseases. Site selections include pages of reputable research centers, educational institutions, and governmental and private, disease-oriented organizations. http://www.mic.ki.se/Diseases/c2.html

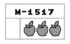 **Merck Manual of Diagnosis and Therapy: Viral Diseases** General information on viruses, including diagnosis, prophylaxis, and treatment, is contained at this page of the noteworthy, online *Merck* publication. Links are available to related topics include respiratory, herpesvirus, central nervous system viral disease, and arbovirus and arenavirus illness.
http://www.merck.com/pubs/mmanual/section13/chapter162/162a.htm

13.12 NEUROLOGICAL DISORDERS

GENERAL RESOURCES

 Karolinska Institutet: Nervous System Diseases Created to provide information about nervous system diseases, this site offers a directory of links for autonomic nervous system diseases, central nervous system diseases, cranial nerve diseases, demyelinating diseases, nervous system malformations, neurologic manifestations, and neuromuscular diseases.
http://www.mic.ki.se/Diseases/c10.html

Merck Manual of Diagnosis and Therapy: Neurological Disorders
Drawn from the *Merck Manual of Diagnosis and Therapy,* this site features section 14 on neurologic disorders. Chapters in the section cover pain, headache, coma, dementia, central nervous system infections, spinal cord disorders, and muscular disorders. Each chapter offers clinical information on the diseases, such as the causes, symptoms, diagnosis, and treatment.
http://www.merck.com/pubs/mmanual/section14/sec14.htm

New York Online Access to Health (NOAH): Neurological Problems
A comprehensive directory of links related to neurological and neuromuscular disorders is featured on this Web site. Disorders covered include amyotrophic lateral sclerosis (Lou Gehrig's disease), carpal tunnel syndrome, cerebral palsy, multiple sclerosis, and Tay Sachs syndrome. In addition, there are links for information on children and neurology, procedures used with neurological disorders, and general neurology information.
http://www.noah-health.org/english/illness/neuro/neuropg.html

ALZHEIMER'S DISEASE

Alzheimer Web A directory of current Alzheimer's disease research endeavors, links to research laboratories, current literature via PubMed, and a listing of FAQs are included at this Web site. An up-to-date listing of cholinesterase inhibitors and other Alzheimer's drugs and a colorful depiction of the cholinergic pathways affected in the Alzheimer's brain can be viewed.
http://home.mira.net/~dhs/ad3.html

MEDLINEplus Health Information: Alzheimer's Disease Alzheimer's resources from a variety of governmental and reputable private organizations are collected at this page of listings, selected as a service of the National Library of Medicine. The latest news, fact sheets from the National Institute of Aging and the National Institute of Neurological Disorders and Stroke, clinical trial details, and a variety of other links to research, journals, and statistics are offered. http://www.nlm.nih.gov/medlineplus/alzheimersdisease.html

BELL'S PALSY

Bell's Palsy Resource Center The Bell's Palsy Resource Center provides a comprehensive list of online resources devoted to Bell's palsy. Hundreds of links are categorized by headings that include general information sites, treatment and clinical studies, surgical procedures, and foundations and medical centers.
http://www.findinfo.com/bellspalsy.htm

eMedicine: Bell Palsy This informative site examines the management of Bell palsy, including pathophysiology, incidence, clinical and physical findings, differential diagnoses, treatment, follow-up, complications, prognosis, and recommended patient education.
http://www.eMedicine.com/emerg/topic56.htm

CEREBRAL PALSY

American Academy for Cerebral Palsy and Developmental Medicine
The Web site of the academy offers online research opportunities with a connection to an electronic library catalog, appropriate for both healthcare professionals and patients. The "Posters" page allows physicians to present ideas online via the academy's forum.
http://www.aacpdm.org

United Cerebral Palsy The latest information regarding cerebral palsy is contained at the United Cerebral Palsy (UCP) Web site. Articles, press releases, and the UCP Research and Educational Foundation's research are highlighted. Assistive technology resources are found, including an online course in funding assistive technology.
http://www.ucp.org

DEMENTIA, GENERAL

Internet Mental Health: Dementia In addition to both American and European descriptions of dementia, visitors can access expert consensus guidelines for management of Alzheimer's disease, agitation, and other dementias of late life. Information for caregivers, important research, and electronic booklets on memory and other relevant subjects are available.
http://www.mentalhealth.com/dis/p20-or05.html

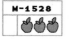

MEDLINEplus Health Information: Dementia This Web site, courtesy of the National Library of Medicine, offers general overviews on dementia, a listing of CenterWatch clinical trials concerning dementia and memory loss, management and research documents, and an additional section with links to specific conditions associated with dementia.
http://www.nlm.nih.gov/medlineplus/dementia.html

ENCEPHALITIS

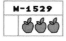

MEDLINEplus Health Information: Encephalitis For those interested in encephalitis, this site features an overview, clinical trials, diagnosis, fact sheets addressing several types of encephalitis, and statistics.
http://www.nlm.nih.gov/medlineplus/encephalitis.html

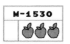

Postgraduate Medicine: Encephalitis Identification of the specific cause of encephalitis is the focus of this online symposium. Key clinical features, diagnostic possibilities, and a comprehensive approach to evaluation are all offered at this in-depth discussion for general practitioners.
http://www.postgradmed.com/issues/1998/03_98/guti.htm

EPILEPSY

Doctor's Guide: Epilepsy Information and Resources Patients, family, and friends of those diagnosed with epilepsy will find current information and resources, including press releases on current therapeutics, epilepsy newsgroups and Web forums, and links to organizations dedicated to treatment, research, and patient support at this page. http://www.pslgroup.com/EPILEPSY.HTM

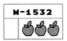

Postgraduate Medicine: Epilepsy Management Professionals are presented with an online symposium article at this page, which offers coverage of issues related to the complete management of epilepsy. Appropriate pharmacologic therapy, determination of prognosis, and examination of several additional issues surrounding medical and surgical management are found.
http://www.postgradmed.com/issues/1997/07_97/sperling.htm

GUILLAIN-BARRE SYNDROME

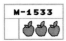

Guillain-Barre Syndrome Fact Sheet A description of Guillain-Barre syndrome is concisely presented at this online brochure, courtesy of the National Institute of Neurological Disorders and Stroke. Visitors will find a listing of potential triggers of the syndrome, as well as information on diagnosis and procedures. http://www.ninds.nih.gov/health_and_medical/disorders/gbs.htm

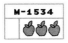

Guillain-Barre Syndrome Foundation International Guillain-Barre syndrome is summarized at this Web site along with information on diagnosis and treatment. A brochure entitled "A Handbook for Caregivers" is available upon request, and the GBS message boards provide opportunities for information exchange with an online chapter of the Foundation.
http://www.webmast.com/gbs

HEADACHE: MIGRAINE, CLUSTER, TENSION

Neuroland: Headache Index Online review articles addressing the management of headache are accessible from this collection of Neuroland resources. Visitors will additionally find coverage of special topics in diagnosis and treatment and several references for further reading.
http://neuroland.com/ha/index.htm

Upstate Medical University: Headache Cybertext This online tutorial is devoted to headache diagnosis and management. The diagnosis, classification, and treatment of common headaches encountered in office practice, including migraine, tension-type headache, analgesic and ergotamine abuse headaches, cluster headaches, and chronic post-traumatic headaches are discussed. More than 100 headache and migraine references are listed.
http://www.upstate.edu/neurology/haas/

HEMORRHAGIC SYNDROMES, GENERAL

eMedicine: Subarachnoid Hemorrhage Examining subarachnoid hemorrhage, this Web site offers a description of the symptoms, causes, differentials, diagnostic tests, emergency room treatment, and appropriate medications for the condition.
http://www.eMedicine.com/emerg/topic559.htm

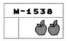

Merck Manual of Diagnosis and Therapy: Hemorrhagic Syndromes
This electronic *Merck* focuses on the symptoms, diagnosis, and treatment for both intracerebral hemorrhage and subarachnoid hemorrhage.
http://www.merck.com/pubs/mmanual/section14/chapter174/174c.htm

MENINGITIS

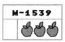

Division of Bacterial and Mycotic Diseases: Meningococcal Disease
This division of the Centers for Disease Control and Prevention offers answers to frequently asked questions, clinical information for practitioners, and additional articles of the *Morbidity and Mortality Weekly Report*. Links to management recommendations and guidelines for travelers are found.
http://www.cdc.gov/ncidod/dbmd/diseaseinfo/meningococcal_g.htm

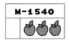

MEDLINEplus Health Information: Meningitis Information on meningitis is accessible from this site, including an overview, clinical trials, diagnosis, and prevention pages. A discussion of the disease in college students and pages of disease variations are offered.
http://www.nlm.nih.gov/medlineplus/meningitis.html

MOVEMENT DISORDERS, GENERAL

MEDLINEplus Health Information: Movement Disorders Links to an overview of movement disorders and to fact sheets on several specific diseases are offered at this National Library of Medicine link collection. In addition, connections to information on clinical trials, diagnostic tests, and treatment are provided. http://www.nlm.nih.gov/medlineplus/movementdisorders.html

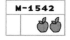

Neurologychannel: Movement Disorders Summaries of several types of movement disorders are offered at this online brochure, which provides overviews of symptoms, diagnosis, and treatment for tremors, dystonias, tics, and Huntington's chorea, in addition to Parkinson's disease information.
http://neurologychannel.com/movementdisorders/

MULTIPLE SCLEROSIS

MEDLINEplus Health Information: Multiple Sclerosis The National Library of Medicine offers links to an assortment of online fact sheets and brochures related to various aspects of multiple sclerosis (MS). The latest news in MS treatment, information from private organizations and governmental divisions, and research and statistical details are accessible.
http://www.nlm.nih.gov/medlineplus/multiplesclerosis.html

University of Utah: Multiple Sclerosis Designed to serve as an introduction to multiple sclerosis for practitioners-in-training, this online tutorial presents a clinical overview; lectures specific to etiology, laboratory findings, differential diagnosis, and treatment options; several videos characterizing signs and symptoms; and an accompanying, educational image index.
http://www-medlib.med.utah.edu/kw/ms/

MYASTHENIA GRAVIS

Myasthenia Gravis Links An index to myasthenia gravis Web sites is found at this comprehensive online collection. General disease information, current treatment, research, and support pages for patients are offered, as well as organizational listings and an active LISTSERV of over 600 myasthenia gravis patients. http://pages.prodigy.net/stanley.way/myasthenia

Yale University: Myasthenia Gravis Information on myasthenia gravis is presented at this Web site, as a service of the Yale Neuromuscular Program. Clinical features and presentation are described, and special attention to pathophysiology is found. Pharmacological management of the disease is outlined, and related links are provided.
http://pandora.med.yale.edu/neurol/CNeurophysiol/MG.html

NARCOLEPSY

National Institute of Neurological Disorders and Stroke (NINDS): NINDS Narcolepsy Information Page This disabling neurological disorder of sleep regulation is concisely described at this NINDS Web link. The four classic symptoms of the condition are presented and the use of various pharmacological therapies for symptom reduction is discussed. Information on prognosis and current research efforts is also provided.
http://www.ninds.nih.gov/health_and_medical/disorders/narcolep_doc.htm

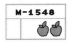

Stanford School of Medicine: Center for Narcolepsy The Stanford Center for Narcolepsy is a world leader in the treatment and research of narcolepsy. The site provides information on the epidemiology, symptoms, diagnosis,

and socioeconomic impact of narcolepsy, in addition to research updates, related links, publications, and video files of cataplectic attacks.
http://www-med.stanford.edu/school/Psychiatry/narcolepsy

NEUROMUSCULAR DISEASES, GENERAL

Muscular Dystrophy Association (MDA): Neuromuscular Diseases
Part of the larger Muscular Dystrophy Association Web site, this address provides access to information on 40 diseases in the MDA program, with each connection providing basic disease characteristics, usual age of onset, progression and inheritance type, and listings of related materials.
http://www.mdausa.org/disease

Washington University School of Medicine: Neuromuscular Disease Center Providing comprehensive access to all aspects of neuromuscular disease, this portal guides visitors to professionally-oriented information on symptoms, diagnosis, and disease management. An index and search engine are available to assist users in navigating this large database of information. Syndromes may be searched alphabetically, and education in basic concepts in neuromuscular disease is offered.
http://www.neuro.wustl.edu/neuromuscular/

PARKINSON'S DISEASE

Doctor's Guide: Parkinson's Disease Information and Resources
Current information on Parkinson's disease may be found at this site, including medications, nonpharmacological management, and surgical interventions; a Parkinson's glossary; and information on young-onset Parkinson's disease. Also included are three discussion groups and links to related Parkinson's disease associations. http://www.pslgroup.com/Parkinson.htm#TOPMENU

National Parkinson Foundation The National Parkinson Foundation (NPF) site offers information on Parkinson's disease, including an online library and educational information for both patients and healthcare professionals. In addition, details on research grants, NPF-funded research centers, and clinical trials are provided.
http://www.parkinson.org

RESTLESS LEGS SYNDROME

National Institute of Neurological Disorders and Stroke (NINDS): Restless Legs Syndrome Information Page Answers to commonly asked questions regarding restless legs syndrome are presented at this online informa-

tion sheet, courtesy of NINDS. Pharmacological treatment options and sleep-onset insomnia are explained.
http://www.ninds.nih.gov/health_and_medical/disorders/restless_doc.htm

Postgraduate Medicine: How to Help People with Restless Legs (RLS) Syndrome This article presented at this *Postgraduate Medicine* site describes diagnostic criteria for restless legs syndrome, secondary and often curable causes of RLS, and current treatment options. Information also includes pharmacologic and nonpharmacological management as well as a list of references. http://www.postgradmed.com/issues/1999/03_99/evidente.htm

SLEEP DISORDERS, GENERAL

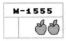

American Academy of Sleep Medicine This site's professional section offers access to position papers, links to related sites, and additional professional education resources, including pages from the journal, *Sleep.* The public portion of the site provides explanations of sleep disorders, information on where to go for diagnosis and treatment, and related resource listings.
http://www.asda.org

National Center on Sleep Disorders Research The National Center on Sleep Disorders Research, a division of the National Institutes of Health, offers healthcare professionals information on research funding, publications, and related Internet links at its site. A separate portion of the site is dedicated to patient education. http://www.nhlbi.nih.gov/about/ncsdr/

SPINAL CORD INJURY

National Spinal Cord Injury Association The National Spinal Cord Injury Association Web page offers a national resource directory, online pamphlets and fact sheets, a newsletter, and access to several streaming video case presentations. http://www.spinalcord.org

Spinal Cord Injury Resource Center Providing information on the anatomy, physiology, and complications resulting from spinal cord trauma, this site links visitors to basic questions and answers, forums for community discussion, information on rehabilitation, and a collection of current news excerpts.
http://www.spinalinjury.net/

STROKE

Acute Stroke Toolbox Created by the Brain Attack Coalition, this site offers tools for healthcare professionals working to develop systems for rapid diagnosis and treatment of acute stroke. Management guidelines, the Stroke Coding Guide of the American Academy of Neurology, and the Stroke Preven-

tion Guidelines of the National Stroke Association are available. Patient education materials are also provided.
http://www.stroke-site.org

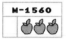 **Internet Stroke Center** The Internet Stroke Center site provides healthcare professionals with current research findings and connections to consensus statements, pharmacologic profiles, diagnostic procedures, images, teaching links, and brain anatomy. General stroke information for patients is also available. http://www.strokecenter.org

SUBDURAL HEMATOMA

 eMedicine: Subdural Hematoma A clinical discussion of subdural hematoma is featured at this eMedicine article, including causes, symptoms, differentials, diagnostic tools, and emergency treatment. Recommendations for follow-up and potential complications are also provided.
http://www.eMedicine.com/EMERG/topic560.htm

 Lycos Health with WebMD: Acute (Subacute) Subdural Hematoma
A definition; causes, incidence, and risk factors; and links to a related illustration, symptoms, and treatment information are provided at this encyclopedic entry of the adam.com database.
http://webmd.lycos.com/content/asset/adam_disease_acute-suba_subdural_hematoma

TRANSIENT ISCHEMIC ATTACK (TIA)

 eMedicine: Transient Ischemic Attack Information for healthcare professionals is presented at this eMedicine document, which addresses the causes, symptoms, diagnosis, differentials, and emergency management of transient ischemic attack. Medication profiles, discharge criteria, follow-up, and prognosis are reviewed.
http://www.eMedicine.com/EMERG/topic604.htm

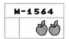 **National Institute of Neurological Disorders and Stroke (NINDS): Transient Ischemic Attack** Visitors to this site will find a concise fact sheet examining the symptoms, treatment, and prognosis of transient ischemic attack. Current research of this division of the National Institutes of Health is discussed, and related links are provided.
http://www.ninds.nih.gov/health_and_medical/disorders/tia_doc.htm

13.13 NUTRITIONAL DISORDERS

GENERAL RESOURCES

Karolinska Institutet: Nutritional and Metabolic Diseases This comprehensive directory of links features nutritional and metabolic diseases. Nutrional conditions covered include obesity, starvation, and anemia. For metabolic diseases, there are resources on topics such as acid-base imbalance, mitochondrial disorders, and inborn errors of metabolism.
http://www.mic.ki.se/Diseases/c18.html

MEDLINEplus Health Information: Food, Nutrition, and Metabolism Topics A broad array of topics related to food, nutrition, and metabolism is featured on this site, including eating disorders, diabetes, food safety, and hypoglycemia. Under each topic, there are links to news, overviews, symptoms, diagnosis, and treatment. Many sections contain information specifically for women, children, and seniors. Some of the resources are available in Spanish.
http://www.nlm.nih.gov/medlineplus/foodnutritionandmetabolism.html

MALNUTRITION

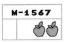

MEDLINEplus Medical Encyclopedia: Malnutrition In addition to causes, incidence, and risk factors associated with malnutrition, summaries of a variety of related topics are accessible from this National Library of Medicine Web site. Links to related information on eating disorders and kwashiorkor can be located, courtesy of adam.com.
http://www.nlm.nih.gov/medlineplus/ency/article/000404.htm

Merck Manual of Diagnosis and Therapy: Malnutrition With related tables and figures accessible, this site address malnutrition from both undernutrition and overnutrition. Information on malnutrition in pregnant women, patients with chronic disease, vegetarians, and alcoholics is presented. Chapters on protein-energy malnutrition, carnitine deficiency, and essential fatty acid deficiency are reviewed, with each topic offering information on detection and management. http://www.merck.com/pubs/mmanual/section1/chapter2/2a.htm

OBESITY

American Family Physician: Management of Obesity After reading this monograph, physicians should be familiar with the epidemiology, identification, evaluation, and management of obesity. Behavioral and lifestyle strategies and pharmacologic agents and their indications are reviewed. Visitors will also gain access to a variety of useful patient education resources.
http://www.aafp.org/afp/monograph/199902/

HealthAtoZ: Obesity Condition Forum for the Consumer and Medical Health Professional. Examining obesity, this comprehensive site offers information on the criteria, causes, health consequences, and treatment of the condition. Additional Internet links are provided to related resources.
http://www.healthatoz.com/atoz/Obesity/OBindex.asp

VITAMIN AND MINERAL DEFICIENCY AND TOXICITY

Medic-Planet Vitamin-deficiency Diseases Vitamin deficiencies are summarized in easy-to-understand terms at this site. Each vitamin, bodily requirements and functions, food sources of the vitamin, and its diseases of deficiency are explained.
http://www.medic-planet.com/MP_article/internal_reference/Vitamin-deficiency_diseases

Merck Manual of Diagnosis and Therapy: Vitamin Deficiency, Dependency, and Toxicity Comprehensive information on vitamin deficiencies is accessible from this site, courtesy of the authoritative *Merck* reference. Each connection offers review of the etiology, symptoms and signs, and laboratory findings and diagnosis. Prophylaxis and treatment of deficiency are included, as well as information on conditions of toxicity.
http://www.merck.com/pubs/mmanual/section1/chapter3/3a.htm

13.14 OCCUPATIONAL AND ENVIRONMENTAL DISEASE

GENERAL RESOURCES

American Environmental Health Foundation: Medical Articles on Environmental Health More than 35 full-text medical articles related to environmental aspects of health and disease are provided on this site. The articles cover topics such as chemical sensitivity, environmentally triggered disorders, pesticides and brain function changes, and formaldehyde sensitivity.
http://www.aehf.com/articles/MedArtl.htm

Centers for Disease Control and Prevention (CDC): Safety and Health Topics Provided by the National Institute for Occupational Safety and Health, this site offers an A-to-Z listing of safety and health topics, covering everything from asbestos to stress. Each topic has a listing of links to fact sheets, articles, databases, and related Internet resources.
http://www.cdc.gov/niosh/toplst.html

CHEMICAL SENSITIVITIES

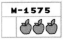

National Academy Press: Multiple Chemical Sensitivities Offered in an educational, online version, the publication at this page includes everything from key concepts associated with chemical sensitization to information on diagnostic markers. Individual chapters can be accessed directly from this online book, which is available for printing in PDF format.
http://www.nap.edu/books/0309047366/html/

Occupational Safety and Health Administration (OSHA): Multiple Chemical Sensitivities A fact sheet discusses recognition of multiple chemical sensitivities, and a report is available from the site, courtesy of the Interagency Workgroup on Multiple Chemical Sensitivity. More detailed information on particular hazardous and toxic substances suspected as part of the disorder and other educational material can be accessed at this divisional site of the U.S. Department of Labor. http://www.osha-slc.gov/SLTC/multiplechemicalsensitivities/

HIGH-ALTITUDE SICKNESS

High Altitude Medicine Guide Health issues affecting travelers to mountainous regions are addressed at this comprehensive Web site. Information, provided by Thomas E. Deitz, M.D., offers a fact sheet on altitude illness, case reports, and a complete physician's guide to clinical diagnosis and management of acute mountain sickness and high altitude cerebral and pulmonary edema. http://www.high-altitude-medicine.com/

Priory Lodge Education, Ltd.: Common High Altitude Medical Problems Altitude-related medical problems are discussed at this page, which offers a particular emphasis on recognition of symptoms and appropriate management. The basis of medical problems, information on acute mountain sickness, and a self-assessment table are found. Also included is information on high altitude cerebral edema and often overlooked eye problems at altitude.
http://www.priory.com/anaes/altitude.htm

MOTION SICKNESS

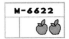

Canada Communicable Disease Report: Statement on Motion Sickness From the Health Protection Branch of Canada's Laboratory Centre for Disease Control, this document addresses the etiology of motion sickness, as well as symptom development and time course. Incidence, depending on individual susceptibility and surrounding factors; differential diagnosis; and methodologies used in the assessment of proper management are discussed. Several supportive measures are outlined at the page, including restriction of both visual activity and motion stimulus.
http://www.hc-sc.gc.ca/hpb/lcdc/publicat/ccdr/96vol22/dr2213ea.html

Don't type in long URLs – add the site number to the eMedguides URL: www.eMedguides.com/**G-1234**.

Medical College of Wisconsin: Motion Sickness   Offering a guide to prevention and treatment, this fact sheet reviews symptoms of motion sickness and strategies to lessen the effects. Effective over-the-counter and prescription medications are introduced at the page, authored by Gary P. Barnas, M.D.
http://healthlink.mcw.edu/article/907367055.html

OCCUPATIONAL LUNG DISEASE

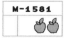

American Lung Association (ALA): Occupational Lung Disease   A brochure addressing occupational lung disease is found at this subsite of the ALA. Fast facts about a variety of occupationally-related disorders are introduced and address lung cancer, asbestosis, silicosis, occupational asthma, and hypersensitivity pneumonitis. Related links are accessible.
http://www.lungusa.org/diseases/occupational_factsheet.html

Dynamics of Disease: Environmental and Occupational Lung Diseases   Authored by Gary R. Epler, M.D., this primer on environmental and occupational lung disease offers several methods for disease classification, criteria for diagnosis, and pulmonary evaluation guidelines. In addition to asbestos lung, visitors will find coverage of silicosis, inert metal pneumoconiosis, metal effects, and lung disease of toxic fume exposure. Accompanied by illustrative tables, this site addresses selected occupations, occupational lung cancer, and additional, related topics.
http://www.epler.com/occu1.html

PESTICIDE POISONING

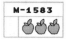

Texas A & M University: Physician's Guide to Pesticide Poisoning   Researched and authored by Douglass E. Stevenson, this reference book for physicians offers a quick guide to management of pesticide poisoning cases. Intended as reference material, the site provides easily accessible information on symptoms and directs professionals to reputable sources of additional information.   http://www-aes.tamu.edu/doug/med/pgpp.htm

University of Nebraska: Signs and Symptoms of Pesticide Poisoning   In addition to routes of exposure and recognition of signs and symptoms of poisoning, this handy guide offers details specific to several commonly used pesticides, including action to take, references, and emergency contact information.
http://www.ianr.unl.edu/pubs/pesticides/ec2505.htm

SICK BUILDING SYNDROME

Environmed Research Inc.: Indoor Environments: Chemicals   Health problems associated with indoor air pollution are outlined at this document,

prepared by Tom Fairley and Stephen Gislason, M.D. Sick buildings and environmentally-related illness, review of a study by the Environment Protection Agency, common chemical contaminants, and sources are discussed.
http://www.nutramed.com/environment/handbook.htm

Environmental Protection Agency (EPA): Sick Building Syndrome (SBS) The United States Environmental Protection Agency introduces "sick building syndrome" at this brochure and details indicators of the condition, cited causes or contributing factors, and information on surveys of indoor air quality. Solutions, important elements of education, and a connection to the Indoor Air Quality Information Clearinghouse are provided by the division.
http://www.epa.gov/iaq/pubs/sbs.html

13.15 ORTHOPEDICS/SPORTS MEDICINE

GENERAL RESOURCES

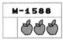

About.com: Orthopedics Resources related to orthopedics are offered on this site, covering topics such as fractures and dislocations, sprains and strains, sports medicine, hip surgery, knee surgery, and alternative treatments. Additional topics covered include physical therapy, arthritis, anatomy, amputations, orthopedic journals, and orthopedic news. Each topic has several more subtopics with hyperlinks to information on other Web pages.
http://orthopedics.about.com/health/orthopedics/mlibrary.htm

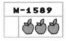

Karolinska Institutet: Musculoskeletal Diseases More than 100 links related to musculoskeletal diseases are provided on this site. In addition to general information on musculoskeletal diseases, there is information on specific diseases and conditions such as foot deformities, bone diseases, musculoskeletal abnormalities, and rheumatic diseases.
http://www.mic.ki.se/Diseases/c5.html

MEDLINEplus Health Information: Bones, Joints, and Muscles Topics Information on a variety of bone, joint, and muscle topics is provided on this Web page, including bone diseases, cartilage disorders, chronic fatigue syndrome, and fractures. Each topic offers links to further information on symptoms, diagnosis, treatment, clinical trials, and related organizations. Some resources are available in Spanish.
http://www.nlm.nih.gov/medlineplus/bonesjointsandmuscles.html

BACK PAIN

Agency for Healthcare Research and Quality (AHRQ): Acute Low Back Problems in Adults A clinical practice guideline is provided at this

site, which can be searched by diagnosis, sign, symptom, or other phrase or keyword. Initial assessment methods, clinical care, and special studies and diagnostic considerations of low back pain are addressed. Attachments include algorithms, pain assessment instruments, and patient discussion handouts.
http://text.nlm.nih.gov/ftrs/pick?dbName=lbpc&
ftrsK=45732&cp=1&t=897020630&collect=ahcpr

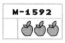 **MEDLINEplus Health Information: Back Pain**　A collection of resources, provided as a service of the National Library of Medicine, includes information from the National Institutes of Health on back pain, general overviews on understanding acute low-back problems, clinical trial information, and a self-care flowchart, courtesy of the American Academy of Family Physicians.
http://www.nlm.nih.gov/medlineplus/backpain.html

CARPAL TUNNEL SYNDROME

 MEDLINEplus Health Information: Carpal Tunnel Syndrome　Visitors can access a variety of educational material at this page, including information on diagnosis, an online atlas image, prevention and screening information, and documents related to treatment of carpal tunnel syndrome. A statistical fact sheet is offered, courtesy of the American Academy of Orthopaedic Surgeons, as well as a Spanish-language publication.
http://www.nlm.nih.gov/medlineplus/carpaltunnelsyndrome.html

 Patient's Guide to Carpal Tunnel Syndrome　Available for printing, downloading, and distribution, this colorful, online material offers pages on the anatomy, diagnosis, and treatment of carpal tunnel syndrome. Authored by Randale C. Sechrest, M.D., the site provides hyperlinks that lead visitors to further definition, close-up anatomical illustrations, and a separate document on endocscopic treatment.
http://www.medicalmultimediagroup.com/pated/ctd/cts/cts.html

CONCUSSIONS

 American Family Physician: Assessment and Management of Concussion in Sports　Presented by the American Academy of Family Physicians, this site offers a complete practice management guide, with a compilation of concussion guidelines, a table outlining symptoms, evaluation details, and details on evaluation of the patient with loss of consciousness. Post-concussion syndrome is addressed, and a related patient information handout is provided.
http://www.aafp.org/afp/990901ap/887.html

 National Center for Injury Prevention and Control: Facts About Concussion and Brain Injury　Sponsored by the Centers for Disease Control and Prevention, this electronic material offers facts about brain injury and is available in Adobe Acrobat format. By clicking on the appropriate link, visitors

will gain access to information on danger signs, symptoms, tips for healing, and help for those affected and their caregivers.
http://www.cdc.gov/ncipc/tbi/default.htm

DISK DISORDERS

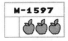

eMedicine: Lumbar (Intervertebral) Disk Disorders This ten-part eMedicine reference examines the pathophysiology, clinical presentation, and causes of lumbar disk disease. Visitors will find several links to diagnostic differentials within the eMedicine database and will also discover information on laboratory workup, imaging studies, and complete treatment information.
http://www.eMedicine.com/emerg/topic303.htm

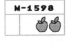

Sciatica.org Answers to frequently asked questions about sciatica, anterior and posterior body views highlighting possible causes of pain, and a discussion of the diagnosis and treatment of *piriformis syndrome* are included at this Internet location.
http://www.sciatica.org/

ELBOW INJURIES AND DISORDERS

MEDLINEplus Health Information: Elbow Injuries and Disorders Documents accessible from this collection address several specific conditions, including arthritis of the elbow, elbow bursitis, dislocation, and lateral epicondylitis. Treatment, links to related organizations, and a statistical fact sheet, provided as a service of the National Institute for Occupational Safety and Health, are provided.
http://www.nlm.nih.gov/medlineplus/elbowinjuriesanddisorders.html

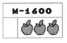

Physician and Sports Medicine: Assessment and Treatment Guidelines for Elbow Injuries This professional reference offers coverage of both acute elbow injuries and overuse disorders, with anatomy and biomechanics of the elbow examined. Patient history, mechanism of injury, differential, and treatment are reviewed, offering a complete guide for primary care.
http://www.physsportsmed.com/issues/may_96/nirschl.htm

FOOT/ANKLE INJURIES AND DISORDERS

eMedicine: Ankle Sprain Background information on ankle injury, functional anatomy, and history and physical injury presentation are reviewed at this eMedicine site. Full size images and eMedicine Zoom Views are available, in addition to several links to differential articles within the eMedicine online database.
http://www.eMedicine.com/sports/topic6.htm

Don't type in long URLs – add the site number to the eMedguides URL: www.eMedguides.com/**G-1234**.

MEDLINEplus Health Information: Foot/Ankle Injuries and Disorders In addition to the latest news on causes of ankle injuries, visitors to this site will find a compilation of links to articles, brochures, and specific discussions of various ankle injuries. Treatment information is provided by a variety of reputable, private organizations.
http://www.nlm.nih.gov/medlineplus/footankleinjuriesanddisorders.html

FRACTURES

 HealthCyclopedia: Fractures Health portals available from this page address the basics of fracture diagnosis and treatment, and a Web directory provides a comprehensive listing of links to information about broken bones and resources that address fracture types and treatment modalities.
http://www.healthcyclopedia.com/fractures.html

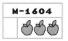 **MEDLINEplus Health Information: Fractures** Provided by the National Library of Medicine, this compilation of sites includes Reuters news releases, general overviews on bone fractures, bone imaging information, and fact sheets addressing specific aspects of fractures. Care of casts and splints, healing information from the Food and Drug Administration, and information about fractures in the elderly are offered.
http://www.nlm.nih.gov/medlineplus/fractures.html

HAND/WRIST/ARM INJURIES AND DISORDERS

 MEDLINEplus Health Information: Hand/Wrist/Arm Injuries and Disorders Created by the U.S. National Library of Medicine, this collection offers material on symptoms, diagnosis, prevention, and rehabilitation related to common injuries of the hand, wrist, and arm. Documents accessible include those from governmental and reputable, private organizations.
http://www.nlm.nih.gov/medlineplus/handwristarminjuriesanddisorders.html

 Merck Manual of Diagnosis and Therapy: Common Hand Disorders This section of the online *Merck Manual of Diagnosis and Therapy* offers access to six chapters of the publication, including guides to hand deformities, neurovascular syndromes, trauma, infection, and tendon problems of the hand. Descriptions of each condition, characteristic findings, and treatment strategies are presented. http://www.merck.com/pubs/mmanual/section5/chapter61/61a.htm

KNEE INJURIES AND DISORDERS

 MEDLINEplus Health Information: Knee Injuries and Disorders In addition to Reuters news releases regarding knee injuries, this collection of links offers a variety of diagnosis and treatment information. Specific aspects of knee

injuries are addressed at several Web brochures and fact sheets, provided by preeminent organizations in the field.

http://www.nlm.nih.gov/medlineplus/kneeinjuriesanddisorders.html

Physician and Sports Medicine: Acute Knee Injuries   At this comprehensive online article, visitors are introduced to the sideline evaluation of knee injuries, with answers to assessment questions and procedures likely to reveal significant injuries reviewed. Mechanisms of injury and a guide to the physical examination are included.

http://www.physsportsmed.com/issues/1999/10_01_99/laprade.htm

Leg Injuries and Disorders

About.com: Sports Medicine: Common Leg Injuries   Detailed descriptions of leg injuries and their treatments are accessible from this assortment of sites, including information on chronic leg pain, shin splints, and treatment of quadricep pulls. Related resources, information from other guides, and external Web links are available.

http://sportsmedicine.about.com/health/sportsmedicine/cs/leg_injuries/

MEDLINEplus Health Information: Leg Injuries and Disorders   With guides to diagnosis, symptoms, rehabilitation, and specific injuries of the leg, this compilation of links, offered by the National Library of Medicine, provides both consumers and professional viewers an organized resource for several orthopaedic conditions.

http://www.nlm.nih.gov/medlineplus/leginjuriesanddisorders.html

Rotator Cuff Injuries and Disorders

eMedicine: Rotator Cuff Injuries   In addition to review of anatomic structure and function, readers will find information on the clinical presentation, diagnostic workup, and management of shoulder injuries. Diagnostic differential links are accessible, and Medline reference links are available.

http://www.eMedicine.com/emerg/topic512.htm

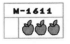

Patient's Guide to Rotator Cuff Tear   This page provides a tutorial on rotator cuff injuries, addressing shoulder anatomy, causes of rotator cuff tears, symptoms, and diagnosis. Provided by the Medical Multimedia Group, conservative treatment options, surgical alternatives, and rehabilitation are available, with links found to labeled illustrations of related terms and phrases.

http://www.medicalmultimediagroup.com/pated/shoulder_problems/cufftear.html

Sprains and Strains, General

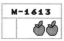

About.com: Orthopedics: Sprains and Strains Caring for and rehabilitation from sprains and strains are the focus of this collection of sites. A sprains- and-strains section of answers to frequently asked questions and information on both upper and lower extremity sprains and strains are presented, as well as resources for treating these common conditions.
http://orthopedics.about.com/health/orthopedics/cs/sprainsstrains/

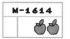

eMedicine: Sprains and Strains This emergency medicine and family healthcare guide offers information on causes, signs and symptoms, and basic care for common strains and sprains. Recognizing the need for hospital care, physician care, diagnosis, treatment, and prevention are emphasized.
http://www.eMedicine.com/aaem/topic410.htm

Tendonitis

American College of Rheumatology (ACR): Tendinitis/Bursitis Provided by the authoritative organization in rheumatology, this fact sheet on tendinitis and bursitis highlights the causes, health impact, diagnosis, and treatment of these two conditions. The American College of Rheumatology's membership directory and the Arthritis Foundation Web site links are offered.
http://www.rheumatology.org/patients/factsheet/tendin.html

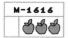

eMedicine: Tendonitis This article from eMedicine.com provides background information, history and physical presentation, causes, and an extensive list of differential links for tendonitis. Outlines of imaging studies, emergency department care, complications, and prognosis are included. Principles of patient education and medical and legal pitfalls are introduced.
http://www.emedicine.com/emerg/topic570.htm

Whiplash and Cervical Spine Disorders

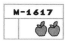

American Association of Neurological Surgeons: The Primary Care Physician's Guide to Cervical Spine Disorders As its name implies, this guideline offers general information and signs signifying potentially serious conditions of the cervical neck and spine. Initial treatment and assessment and summaries of common disorders of the cervical spine are presented, including whiplash, cervical disc herniation, and osteoarthritis/degenerative disc disease. A variety of corrective, surgical techniques are discussed.
http://www.spineuniverse.com/1p/aans/091900_cerv_primarycare.html

Hospital Practice: Management of Neck Pain: Primary Care This *Hospital Practice* article, authored by David G. Bornstein of George Washington University, offers review of biomechanical stress and its role in causing neck pain. Nonoperative treatment, further information for management of chronic or radicular pain, and coverage of systemic illness and spinal compression are presented. http://www.hosppract.com/issues/1998/10/boren.htm

13.16 PSYCHIATRIC/BEHAVIORAL DISORDERS

GENERAL RESOURCES

Internet Mental Health   Internet Mental Health offers fact sheets on more than 50 of the most common mental disorders. Information includes descriptions, diagnoses, treatments, current research, and links to online brochures offering additional information on the disorders. Disorders are listed both alphabetically and categorically for easy reference.
http://www.mentalhealth.com/fr20.html

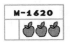

Medical College of Wisconsin: Health Link: Neurological Disorders
An A-to-Z listing of neurological disorder descriptions and links to related articles are presented at the Medical College of Wisconsin Physicians and Clinics Web site. Disease description information is provided by the National Institute of Neurological Disorders and Stroke subdivision of the National Institutes of Health. http://www.healthlink.mcw.edu/neurological-disorders

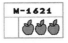

Merck Manual of Diagnosis and Therapy: Psychiatric Disorders   This chapter of the online *Merck Manual of Diagnosis and Therapy* presents 12 psychiatric disorder chapters, from anxiety disorders to schizophrenia and related diseases. Each section offers general information about the disorder classification, as well as relevant etiological, diagnostic, and therapeutic considerations.
http://www.merck.com/pubs/mmanual/section15/sec15.htm

National Institute of Mental Health (NIMH): Public Resources   This National Institute of Mental Health site for the public offers links to pages devoted to information on major mental disorders, including anxiety disorders, learning disorders, bipolar disorder, obsessive-compulsive disorder, depression, panic disorder, attention deficit hyperactivity disorder, phobias, autism, post-traumatic stress disorder, generalized anxiety disorder, and schizophrenia. Information on medications, other mental disorders, and clinical trials is also available. http://www.nimh.nih.gov/publicat/index.cfm

ABUSIVE SYNDROMES

Center for Mental Health Resources: Abuse   This site provides a variety of abuse-related links such as the National Clearinghouse on Child Abuse and Neglect Information and Survivor Connections. Resources for abuse survivors, such as details on forming a self-help group and communicating with other victims of abuse, are provided.

http://www.mentalhealth.org/links/abuse.htm

University of Pennsylvania: Useful Victimology Links Supported by the University of Pennsylvania School of Nursing, this site contains resources on the study of victims, including numerous links to organizations, articles, Web sites, documents, and support organizations. The resources are divided into forensic resources, rape and child abuse, government and university resources, and domestic violence connections.

http://www.nursing.upenn.edu/Victimology

ALCOHOLISM/SUBSTANCE ABUSE

Mental Health Net: Substance Abuse and Alcoholism Web resources for drug and alcohol abuse, nicotine addiction, and related categories are found at this comprehensive listing of described and rated Internet sites. Recovery, treatment, and support links, and articles and publications from Harvard Medical School and the Mental Health Net are part of this collection.

http://mentalhelp.net/guide/substnce.htm

Substance Abuse and Mental Health Services Administration The public information connection of this pubic health federal agency includes a facility treatment locator, substance abuse statistics, and access to Prevention Online, a database of information related to alcohol and drug education. Drug-specific topics, information related to a variety of patient populations, research briefs, and expert panel Webcasts are found.

http://www.samhsa.gov/public/public.html

ANXIETY DISORDERS

Anxiety Network International The Anxiety Network home page provides support and therapy information for three of the most commonly diagnosed anxiety disorders: social anxiety, panic/agoraphobia, and generalized anxiety disorder. Over 100 individual articles and the Anxiety Network bookstore provide a broad base of information, with some individual publication ratings provided.

http://www.anxietynetwork.com

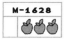

National Institute of Mental Health (NIMH): Anxiety Disorders Education Program The site of the Anxiety Disorders Education Program offers healthcare professionals educational resources, such as a list of books and videos and hyperlinks to online articles through the library section. Patient fact sheets on anxiety disorders are provided with connections to videos of personal recovery stories.

http://www.nimh.nih.gov/anxiety/anxiety/whatis/objectiv.htm

BIPOLAR DISORDER

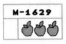

MEDLINEplus Health Information: Bipolar Disorder   Resources on bipolar disorder at this site include an overview, research information, publications in Spanish, law and policy-related material, news sites, organizations, information for teenagers, and treatment details.
http://medlineplus.nlm.nih.gov/medlineplus/bipolardisorder.html

Psycom.net: Bipolar Disorder   This site provides links to many resources on bipolar disorder, offering news of research advances, general information for patients, answers to frequently asked questions, and support resources. Professionals will also find practice guidelines, consensus statements, and links to sites focused on diagnosis and treatment issues.
http://www.psycom.net/depression.central.bipolar.html

DEPRESSION

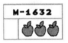

Internet Mental Health: Major Depressive Disorder   Visitors to this site will find an assortment of consumer and professionally-related resources on major depressive disorder, including an online diagnostic tool, articles on treatment from the U.S. Surgeon General, management algorithms, and several treatment guidelines and patient booklets. Additional accessible publications address causation, epidemiology, and treatment resources.
http://www.mentalhealth.com/dis/p20-md01.html

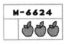

National Institute of Mental Health (NIMH): Depression   This division of the National Institutes of Health (NIH) focuses exclusively on clinical depression at this site. An online brochure, available in PDF format, provides a description of major depression and its variants, as well as information on possible causes, diagnosis, and treatment options available. Additional links at the site connect visitors to an assortment of fact sheets and disease summaries, addressing bipolar disorder, depression in children, depression in older adults, and related topics. Clinical trial information, prevention and treatment guidelines, landmark study reviews, and a connection to the National Library of Medicine's MEDLINEplus site collection of resources on depression are offered.
http://www.nimh.nih.gov/publicat/depressionmenu.cfm

EATING DISORDERS

Academy for Eating Disorders   In addition to a fact sheet addressing anorexia nervosa, bulimia, binge eating, and eating disorders not otherwise specified, this site provides a professional forum for the promotion of effective treatment and care of patients. Archived newsletters, related links and support networks, conference listings, and practice parameters for professional members are offered. (some features fee-based) http://www.aedweb.org

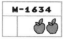

American Anorexia Bulimia Association, Inc.   Dedicated to the prevention and treatment of eating disorders, this association site offers general information about eating disorders geared toward sufferers, family and friends, and professionals. Details regarding risk factors for the development of eating disorders and recommendations for further reading are found.
http://www.aabainc.org/home.html

OBSESSIVE-COMPULSIVE DISORDER (OCD)

Expert Consensus Guidelines: Obsessive-Compulsive Disorder
Information for consumers on obsessive-compulsive disorder, such as symptoms, heritability, treatment, and support information are reviewed at this comprehensive article. Related reading materials and organizations are listed.
http://www.psychguides.com/oche.html

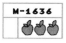

Obsessive-Compulsive Disorder (OCD) Resource Center   The OCD Resource Center provides patients with information on the condition, including symptoms, diagnosis, treatment, and getting help. A physician-only section of the site is provided, and material just for kids explains the condition in an easy-to-understand manner. Links to related sites are provided.
(free registration) http://www.ocdresource.com/

PANIC DISORDERS

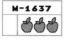

Healing Panic   Divided into self-help, healing, and treatment aids sections, this site offers basic, yet comprehensive, information on all aspects of panic disorders and their treatment. Informative links to diagnosis, treatment, and causes of these disorders as well as referral links and a bibliography are included.
http://www.eadd.com/~berta/

National Institute of Mental Health (NIMH): Panic Disorder Consensus Statement   The NIMH, a division of the National Institutes of Health, offers this review of the incidence, causes, assessment, clinical signs, and current treatment practices for panic disorders. Consequences of treatment, future research questions, and recommendations regarding assessment, treatment identification, and education are provided.
http://www.nimh.nih.gov/anxiety/resource/constate.htm

PERSONALITY DISORDERS

Mental Health Infosource: Personality Disorders   Answers to both consumer and professional questions are available in archive from this page and address the origin of personality disorders, definitions, and comparisons of

various disorders. Articles excerpted from the *Psychiatric Times,* conference listings by topic, and an index of related sites at Internet Mental Health are found.
http://www.mhsource.com/disorders/person.html

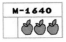

Mental Health Net: All About Personality Disorders   Offering a comprehensive portal dedicated solely to personality disorders, this page offers basic information and descriptions of ten different personality disorder categories. Aims of treatment, additional online resources, organization referral, and online support networks are compiled at this single location.
http://personalitydisorders.mentalhelp.net/

PHOBIAS

MEDLINEplus Health Information: Phobias   Resources on phobias found at this site include an overview and specific information on anxiety disorders, social phobia, and fighting phobias. In addition, visitors are offered links to information on clinical trials, social phobia treatment, a Spanish fact sheet, and related organizations.
http://www.nlm.nih.gov/medlineplus/phobias.html

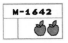

Phobia List   This site contains an alphabetized list of phobias, both common and rare. Included are links to information on phobia nomenclature, categories, treatment of phobias, and links to sites for information and support with respect to phobic disorders.
http://phobialist.com/

SCHIZOPHRENIA

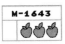

Internet Mental Health: Schizophrenia   Attention to schizophrenia includes American and European disease descriptions, documents provided by the U.S. Surgeon General, an online diagnostic tool, and related Web communities. Treatment guidelines can be accessed, as well as external links to management algorithms.
http://www.mentalhealth.com/dis/p20-ps01.html

Schizophrenia.com   Providing an online support and education center, this site includes discussion and chat areas; information on causes, diagnosis, and treatment of schizophrenia; and in-depth articles geared toward patient, student, and professional audiences. Each link offers general reading and related Internet connections.
http://www.schizophrenia.com/

SOCIAL ANXIETY DISORDER

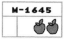

Anxiety Network International: Social Anxiety Home Page   Several discussions on social anxiety are accessible from this educational site, including information on its common misdiagnosis and distinctions between social anxiety and panic disorder. Additional links include personal accounts of the condition, case studies, and information on publications and audio material.
http://www.anxietynetwork.com/sphome.html

Social Anxiety Disorder   A short definition of social anxiety disorder is presented at this site, courtesy of the Midwest Center for Stress and Anxiety. Links provide answers to FAQs, symptoms, causes, treatment, recovery, and details on seeking help for the condition. A patient education booklet and video are available to physicians.
http://degnanco.com/anxiety/main.html

SUICIDE

American Foundation for Suicide Prevention   Professional resources at this page include monthly CME articles, research initiatives of the organization, and reprints of the quarterly *Lifesaver* newsletter.
http://www.afsp.org

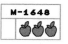

Psycom.net: Suicide and Suicide Prevention   Suicide prevention, awareness, and support resources are offered at this Psycom.net collection. In addition to hotline links, warning signs, and suicidal behaviors, these connections also examine statistics regarding suicide, coexisting depression, biological markers associated with increased risk, and suicide prevention programs.
http://www.psycom.net/depression.central.suicide.html

13.17 RESPIRATORY AND PULMONARY DISORDERS

GENERAL RESOURCES

American Lung Association (ALA): Lung Diseases A-to-Z   More than 100 topical disease resources are found in this directory from the American Lung Association. Resources provide information on specific diseases, smoking, infectious diseases, the environment and air quality, exercise, and minority health. http://www.lungusa.org/diseases/A-Z.html

Karolinska Institutet: Respiratory Tract Diseases   A directory of more than 100 links related to respiratory tract diseases is featured at this site. General information, tracheal diseases, pleural diseases, bronchial diseases, respiratory tract infections, respiration disorders, and lung diseases are among the topics included, with a variety of fact sheets and clinical information available for each. http://micf.mic.ki.se/Diseases/c8.html

Merck Manual of Diagnosis and Therapy: Pulmonary Disorders The online *Merck Manual of Diagnosis and Therapy* offers this comprehensive directory of pulmonary topics available through the publication. Visitors can access specific sections devoted to pulmonary function testing, special procedures, respiratory failure, adult respiratory distress syndrome, chronic obstructive airway disorders, acute bronchitis, bronchiectasis, pulmonary embolism, pneumonia, lung abscess, pleural disorders, tumors of the lung, and other related topics. Each section typically offers a discussion of the etiology and pathology, symptoms and signs, diagnosis, and prognosis and treatment associated with each disease group, including links to more specific subtopics.
http://www.merck.com/pubs/mmanual/section6/sec6.htm

New York Online Access to Health (NOAH): Respiratory Disorders Links provided by NOAH offer general information about respiratory disorders, childhood respiratory disorders, and diagnosis and prevention details. Visitors will also find links to resources on specific conditions, including asthma, bronchitis, bronchiolitis, chronic obstructive pulmonary disease (COPD), emphysema, lung cancer, pertussis, pneumonia, pulmonary fibrosis, sarcoidosis, sinusitis, sore throat, streptococcal infections, and tuberculosis. Resources on care and treatment, drug therapies, living with COPD, lung transplantation, and therapeutic alternatives are also available. Other resources, including links to national hospital rankings, clinical trials, magazine articles, and professional organizations, are also listed.
http://www.noah-health.org/english/illness/respiratory/resp.html

ADULT RESPIRATORY DISTRESS SYNDROME

American Lung Association (ALA): Adult (Acute) Respiratory Distress Syndrome (ARDS) This online fact sheets offers information on incidence, common precursors to the condition, and a concise statement on requirements of management. Related links, such as the ARDS Support Center are available directly from the site.
http://www.lungusa.org/diseases/ards_factsheet.html

Merck Manual of Diagnosis and Therapy: Adult Respiratory Distress Syndrome The etiology; pathophysiology; and symptoms, signs, and diagnosis for this type of respiratory failure are reviewed at this page of the online *Merck* reference. Management principles and information on mechanical ventilation are provided, in addition to related chapters within this online publication. http://www.merck.com/pubs/mmanual/section6/chapter67/67a.htm

ASBESTOS-RELATED DISEASE

MEDLINEplus Health Information: Asbestos/Asbestosis A collection of resources on asbestos and asbestos-related disease is gathered at this page, maintained by the National Library of Medicine. General disease overviews from government and private research organizations are featured, and an article addressing asbestos in the home is offered by the Environmental Protection Agency. Additional links to related organizations are included.
http://www.nlm.nih.gov/medlineplus/asbestosasbestosis.html

Mt. Sinai Medical Library: Asbestos Lung Disease Authored by a physician with experience in diagnosing asbestosis and additional asbestos-related lung disease, this primer answers commonly asked questions and provides several Web links and medical references. A document focusing on the physician's perspective in diagnosis is accessible.
http://www.mtsinai.org/pulmonary/Asbestos/asbestos-questions.htm

ASTHMA

American Lung Association (ALA): Asthma Information Index In its mission to prevent lung disease and promote lung health, the ALA has created this comprehensive page dedicated solely to asthma education and management. Reports from asthma research centers, fact sheets on asthma medications and therapies, and an asthma management guideline from the National Heart, Lung, and Blood Institute are a small selection of the available material at this site. http://www.lungusa.org/asthma/

Global Initiative for Asthma Offered in collaboration with the National Heart, Lung, and Blood Institute and the World Health Organization, goals of the Global Initiative for Asthma (GINA) effort are outlined at this site, with an assortment of GINA documents and resources readily available. Visitors have access to a directory of patient organizations, quick reference and practical guides for asthma management, and an online patient manual.
http://www.ginasthma.com/

ATELECTASIS

Adam.com: Atelectasis Providing information on symptoms, treatment, and prevention, this encyclopedia entry contains an organized summary of information on the common occurrence of atelectasis. Review of causes, incidence, and risk factors is found, as well as access to related images and illustrations. http://pcs.adam.com/ency/article/000065.htm

Merck Manual of Diagnosis and Therapy: Atelectasis Sponsored by an educational leader in medical information, this Web site provides readers with a

general review of both acute and chronic atelectasis. Causes, related chapters within the online *Merck* reference, symptoms and signs, and diagnostic details are included.
http://www.merck.com/pubs/mmanual/section6/chapter71/71a.htm

BRONCHITIS

American Family Physician: Acute Bronchitis Offering both a professionally-oriented article and a patient information handout, this site of the American Academy of Family Physicians provides visitors with a comprehensive look at the epidemiology, diagnosis, and treatment of acute bronchitis. Tables at the site detail differential diagnosis, antibiotic trials, and bronchodilator efficacy. http://www.aafp.org/afp/980315ap/hueston.html

American Family Physician: Chronic Bronchitis: Primary Care Management Characterization of the clinical diagnosis of bronchitis is found in this comprehensive article, sponsored by the American Academy of Family Physicians. Healthcare professionals and other interested readers will find discussions of organism microbiology, diagnostic testing, and an overall management algorithm provided. A related patient information handout is conveniently accessible from the site.
http://www.aafp.org/afp/980515ap/heath.html

CHRONIC OBSTRUCTIVE PULMONARY DISEASE (COPD)

MEDLINEplus Health Information: COPD (Chronic Obstructive Pulmonary Disease) The latest news on treatment and management guidelines for COPD, general disease overviews, and an assortment of additional links related to diagnosis and disease management are accessible from this page of the National Library of Medicine. With over 40 links in all, the site provides a comprehensive variety for both consumers and healthcare professionals alike.
http://www.nlm.nih.gov/medlineplus/copdchronicobstructivepulmonarydisease.html

WebMDHealth: Drug and Nonsurgical Treatments for Chronic Obstructive Lung Disease Intended to serve as a complete review of therapies, this document addresses the use of a variety of bronchodilators, corticosteroids, and both continuous and noncontinuous oxygen delivery. Delivery systems, administration devices, and treatment of complications are also examined. Visitors to the site will find a review of surgical procedures and breathing exercises, including pursed-lip breathing and spirometry.
http://my.webmd.com/content/dmk/dmk_article_53213

EMPHYSEMA

American Lung Association (ALA): Emphysema The serious nature of emphysema, its causes, its development, and both treatment and prevention information are reviewed at this online brochure of the preeminent lung disease prevention organization. Related links on the web, such as the National Heart, Lung, and Blood Institute, are available.
http://www.lungusa.org/diseases/lungemphysem.html

National Emphysema Foundation Striving to improve the quality of life for those with chronic lung disease, the home page of the National Emphysema Foundation offers an interactive tutorial on pulmonary health and function, exercises for physical reconditioning of the lungs, articles on pulmonary diseases, and feature articles. A Gateway to Related Health Links is found.
http://www.emphysemafoundation.org/

INTERSTITIAL LUNG DISEASE, GENERAL

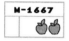

American Lung Association (ALA): Facts About Pulmonary Fibrosis and Interstitial Lung Disease Facts about interstitial lung disease, including common features, known causes, symptoms, diagnosis, and treatment, are offered at this online brochure. Related links accessible from the site include a medical fact sheet from the Mayo Clinic and definitions of terms.
http://www.lungusa.org/diseases/pulmfibrosis.html

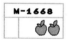

Temple University: Interstitial Lung Disease Universal clinical manifestations of interstitial lung disease are outlined at this document, which also emphasizes the impact of these diseases on pulmonary function, respiration, and gas exchange. Disease classifications, physiologic alterations, and pathogenesis are examined, as is a general approach to the patient.
http://blue.temple.edu/~pathphys/pulmonary/interstitial_lung_disease.html

PNEUMONIA

American Lung Association (ALA): Pneumonia Several types of pneumonia are outlined at this comprehensive brochure, provided as a service of the ALA. Bacterial conditions, viral pathogens, mycoplasma pneumonia, and other types are reviewed. Treatment, prevention and steps to take if one has symptoms are all addressed at this consumer-oriented information sheet.
http://www.lungusa.org/diseases/lungpneumoni.html

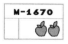

Yahoo! Health: Pneumonia A definition of pneumonia is provided on this site, along with its causes, incidence, and risk factors. A list of several different types of pneumonia is presented, with hyperlinks to additional information for each type. Prevention measures, symptoms, and diagnostic tests are described. A

hyperlink at the bottom of the site leads to information on treatment, prognosis, and complications.
http://health.yahoo.com/health/diseases_and_conditions/disease_feed_data/pneumonia

PULMONARY EMBOLISM

Boston University: Pulmonary Embolism Discussion of the fatal nature of pulmonary embolism, links to information on a variety of causes, and summaries of symptoms, diagnosis, and treatment are offered at this site of the Community Outreach Health Information System.
http://web.bu.edu/cohis/cardvasc/vessel/vein/pe.htm

eMedicine: Pulmonary Embolism An in-depth review of pulmonary embolism includes pathophysiology, demographic information, history and physical presentation, and a listing of differential links. Causes, complete laboratory and imaging, and other tests that may demonstrate the presence of pulmonary embolism are included at this comprehensive continuing education resource. http://www.eMedicine.com/emerg/topic490.htm

SLEEP DISORDERED BREATHING (SDB)/SLEEP APNEA

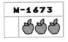

American Sleep Apnea Association Information for both healthcare professionals and consumers is available at this site of the American Sleep Apnea Association. An assortment of online publications on sleep apnea evaluation and management are found, as well as an "Ask the Doctor" forum and the opportunity to order or view an online version of the organization's General Information Packet.
http://www.sleepapnea.org/

National Heart, Lung, and Blood Institute (NHLBI): Facts About Sleep Apnea As a service of the institute, visitors are offered access to a four-page brochure that discusses the serious nature of sleep apnea and its treatment. ASCII and PDF formats are available, and printed copies can be ordered online, by telephone, fax, or e-mail.
http://www.nhlbi.nih.gov/health/public/sleep/sleepapn.htm

SMOKING/CESSATION

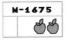

About.com: Smoking Cessation Resources for smokers and those thinking of kicking the habit are available at this collection, including online news and discussions, a how-to guide for the first smoke-free week, and sites that review smoking cessation aids.
http://quitsmoking.about.com/health/quitsmoking/mbody.htm

Physician's Guide to the Internet: Help Your Patients Stop Smoking
Derived from *American Medical News*, this resource provides several clinical guides, intended to help physicians assist their patients in smoking cessation. A quick reference guide from the Agency for Healthcare Research and Quality, recommendations on the use of nicotine gum, an executive summary on smoking cessation interventions, and a patient information handout are included.
http://www.physiciansguide.com/smoke1.html

TUBERCULOSIS

American Lung Association (ALA): Tuberculosis (TB) Symptoms of tuberculosis and information on disease development are reviewed at this consumer-friendly brochure of the ALA. Treatment, multi-drug resistance, and related TB topics are reviewed. In addition, visitors can go directly to the World Health Organization's tuberculosis Web site or the Centers for Disease Control's Division of Tuberculosis Elimination.
http://www.lungusa.org/diseases/lungtb.html

World Health Organization (WHO): Tuberculosis Strategy and Operations After outlining organization goals and objectives, this site invites visitors to learn more about tuberculosis (TB) control, prevention, and treatment with a series of online material. A tuberculosis fact sheet, the Global TB Control WHO Report, and online catalogues of WHO TB documents, books and reports, and references by subject are provided.
http://www.who.int/gtb/

UPPER RESPIRATORY TRACT INFECTIONS, GENERAL

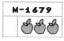

American Lung Association (ALA): Guidelines for the Prevention and Treatment of Influenza and the Common Cold Cold and influenza symptoms, prevention, and treatment are all included at this electronic reference of the ALA. Groups at increased risk for influenza-related complications, vaccination, and links to specific information addressing symptom relief are offered.
http://www.lungusa.org/diseases/c&fguide/lungcolds_flu.html

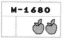

Virtual Hospital: Viral Upper Respiratory Tract Infections The online *Family Practice Handbook* of the University of Iowa outlines the common cold, influenza, and bronchitis infections at this reference page. Externally peer-reviewed, the document includes clinical presentation, management, and complications. http://www.vh.org/Providers/ClinRef/FPHandbook/Chapter03/08-3.html

13.18 RHEUMATOLOGIC DISORDERS

GENERAL RESOURCES

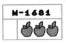

About.com: Arthritis and Related Diseases A directory of links related to rheumatologic disorders is provided on this site. The links are organized into categories such as general arthritis information, ankylosing spondylitis, fibromyalgia, gout, juvenile rheumatoid arthritis, Lyme disease, osteoporosis, and rheumatoid arthritis.
http://arthritis.about.com/health/arthritis/cs/indexdiseases/index.htm

Johns Hopkins Arthritis The Johns Hopkins Arthritis site includes a variety of professional resources in the field of rheumatology, including a lecture series in clinical rheumatology, meeting highlights from professinal meetings, RealPlayer netcasts of rheumatic disease pathophysiolgy lectures, and CME opportunities. This site also provides the latest news in arthritis treatment and research, listings of ongoing clinical trials, case rounds, additional disease management tools, and an "Ask the Expert" forum.
http://www.hopkins-arthritis.org/

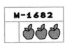

New York Online Access to Health (NOAH): Arthritis and Rheumatic Disease This consumer health resource offers more than 50 links to information on arthritis and rheumatic diseases. The links are organized under headings such as the basics of arthritis, diagnosis, types of disease, management, coping, and medications. There is also information on specific concerns such as arthritis and African-Americans, arthritis and children, and rheumatoid disease and pregnancy. http://www.noah-health.org/english/illness/arthritis/arthritis.html

ARTHRITIS, GENERAL

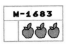

MEDLINEplus Health Information: Arthritis This collection of links, provided by the National Library of Medicine, offers information on topics such as clinical trials, diagnosis/symptoms, disease management, rehabilitation, specific conditions, treatments, news, and organizations. In addition, general overview sites and details on disease in specific patient populations are found.
http://www.nlm.nih.gov/medlineplus/arthritis.html

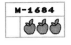

Weill Medical College of Cornell University: Arthritis This chapter of *Joint* describes rheumatic conditions, mechanisms of disease, arthritis types, and arthritis as a manifestation of systemic disease in a thorough and comprehensive format. Morphologic changes associated with a variety of arthritis types are viewable at several accessible images. Information on synovial fluid analysis, arthritic conditions of unknown etiology, degenerative forms of disease, metabolic arthritis, and arthritis types resulting from trauma are discussed.
http://edcenter.med.cornell.edu/CUMC_PathNotes/Skeletal/Joint_02.html

---

Don't type in long URLs – add the site number to the eMedguides URL: www.eMedguides.com/**G-1234**.

CHRONIC FATIGUE SYNDROME

About.com: Chronic Fatigue Syndrome/Fibromyalgia Resources related to chronic fatigue syndrome/fibromyalgia are provided on this site, including advocacy information, alternative medicine, news, coping strategies, medications, and organizations. There is also information on finding a doctor, personal stories, research, and support groups.
http://chronicfatigue.about.com/health/chronicfatigue/mlibrary.htm

Centers for Disease Control and Prevention (CDC): Chronic Fatigue Syndrome Detailed information on Chronic Fatigue Syndrome (CFS) is available at this CDC-sponsored Web site. The site explains why and how the definition of CFS was recently revised; offers guidelines for the evaluation and study of CFS; discusses the demographics of this disorder, its possible causes, and how it is diagnosed; and provides an overview of the strategy and objectives of the CDC's program for CFS research.
http://www.cdc.gov/ncidod/diseases/cfs/index.htm

MEDLINEplus Health Information: Chronic Fatigue Syndrome MEDLINEplus provides links to numerous sources for both clinical and patient education about chronic fatigue syndrome. Links fall into the categories of general/overviews, clinical trials, disease management, directories of patient resources, and related organizations.
http://www.nlm.nih.gov/medlineplus/chronicfatiguesyndrome.html

FIBROMYALGIA

MEDLINEplus Health Information: Fibromyalgia This resource from MEDLINEplus provides numerous links to information about fibromyalgia for both patients and healthcare professionals. Two articles from the National Institutes of Health provide an overview of fibromyalgia. Other links included at this site are categorized as general/overviews, clinical trials, coping, disease management, research, treatment, and specific conditions/aspects of the disorder. http://www.nlm.nih.gov/medlineplus/fibromyalgia.html

Merck Manual of Diagnosis and Therapy: Fibromyalgia This site features information on the etiology, symptoms, diagnosis, and treatment of a group of nonarticular disorders, collectively known as fibromyalgia. Primary fibromyalgia syndrome is discussed, and information on myofascial pain syndrome, a closely related disorder, is available through a site link.
http://www.merck.com/pubs/mmanual/section5/chapter59/59e.htm

Gout

American Family Physician: Gout and Hyperuricemia   A fully-referenced clinical discussion of gout and hyperuricemia is available at this Web site from the American Academy of Family Physicians (AAFP). The article discusses the four clinical phases of gout, clinical features, diagnosis, and treatment at each of these stages and is supported by figures and tables.
http://www.aafp.org/afp/990215ap/925.html

MEDLINEplus Health Information: Gout and Pseudogout   More than a dozen gout resources are indexed here and include overviews, clinical trials, disease management sites, directories, organizations, and sites that cover specific aspects of the condition. Sources of information include the Arthritis Foundation, the American Academy of Family Physicians, and the American College of Rheumatology.
http://www.nlm.nih.gov/medlineplus/goutandpseudogout.html

Lyme Disease

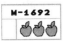

American College of Physicians-American Society of Internal Medicine Online: Initiative on Lyme Disease   Part of a three-year project by the American College of Physicians to educate doctors on the evaluation and treatment of Lyme disease, this site offers a case report form, a probability calculator, a case study quiz, and a patient's guide to Lyme disease. Additionally, related organization links are found, including the American Lyme Disease Foundation and the Infectious Disease Society of America.
http://www.acponline.org/lyme/

Centers for Disease Control and Prevention (CDC): Lyme Disease Home Page   Part of the Division of Vector-Borne Infectious Diseases, this site provides a variety of information on Lyme disease transmission and infection. The introduction emphasizes risks and is accompanied by a map illustrating approximate distribution of predicted Lyme disease risk in the United States. Additional pages of the site provide details on diagnosis, epidemiology, and prevention and control. http://www.cdc.gov/ncidod/dvbid/lyme/index.htm

Myofascial Pain, General

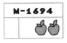

Arthritis Foundation: Myofascial Pain   A consumer-oriented overview of myofascial pain, including its symptoms, causes, and treatment options, is found at this Web site, provided by the Arthritis Foundation. A list of resources and suggestions is provided, including links to *Arthritis Today Magazine,* the *Arthritis Today Drug Guide,* and other sources of information on medical treatments and self-care.
http://www.arthritis.org/conditions/DiseaseCenter/myofascial_pain.asp

Family Village: Myofascial Pain Syndrome Information and resources regarding myofascial pain syndrome are available at this site from Family Village, a global community of disability-related resources. This site provides links to organizations dedicated to pain management, sites offering more information about myofascial pain syndrome, and online discussion groups.
http://www.familyvillage.wisc.edu/lib_mps.htm

OSTEOARTHRITIS

Merck Manual of Diagnosis and Therapy: Osteoarthritis A definition and classification of osteoarthritis are found at this online reference. Additional information is offered concerning pathophysiology, symptoms and signs, diagnosis, prognosis, and treatment.
http://www.merck.com/pubs/mmanual/section5/chapter52/52a.htm

National Institute of Arthritis and Musculoskeletal and Skin Diseases (NIAMS): Osteoarthritis This publication of the National Institutes of Health includes information on signs, diagnosis, and treatment, with tips on self-management programs and information on current research included. Descriptions of diagnostic tools, genetic studies, and comprehensive treatment strategies are provided.
http://www.niams.nih.gov/hi/topics/athritis/oahandout.htm

RAYNAUD'S PHENOMENON

National Institute of Arthritis and Musculoskeletal and Skin Diseases (NIAMS): Questions and Answers About Raynaud's Phenomenon Raynaud's phenomenon is the subject of this article, courtesy of the National Institutes of Health. The article describes the disorder, its classifications, and diagnostic criteria. Treatment options for Raynaud's phenomenon and several non-drug interventions are presented.
http://www.niams.nih.gov/hi/topics/raynaud/ar125fs.htm

Virtual Hospital: Raynaud's Phenomenon This Virtual Hospital site outlines primary and secondary Raynaud's phenomenon, along with diagnosis and treatment of the condition.
http://www.vh.org/Providers/ClinRef/FPHandbook/Chapter06/08-6.html

RHEUMATOID ARTHRITIS

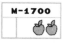

American College of Rheumatology (ACR): Rheumatoid Arthritis Health impact information is provided at this fact sheet, along with information on the cause, diagnosis, and treatment of rheumatoid arthritis. A short discussion of the rheumatologist's role in treatment and management of the condition is provided, and a link to criteria for the classification of acute disease is found. http://www.rheumatology.org/patients/factsheet/ra.html

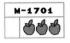

Merck Manual of Diagnosis and Therapy: Rheumatoid Arthritis This chapter in the *Merck Manual of Diagnosis and Therapy* addresses the etiology, pathology, symptoms and signs, laboratory findings, and diagnosis of rheumatoid arthritis. Several treatment and drug programs are outlined. http://www.merck.com/pubs/mmanual/section5/chapter50/50a.htm

SYSTEMIC LUPUS ERYTHEMATOSUS

Merck Manual of Diagnosis and Therapy: Systemic Lupus Erythematosus At this site of the searchable *Merck Manual of Diagnosis and Therapy* pathology, symptoms, and signs are described, along with laboratory findings, diagnosis, and prognosis. Treatment options, including suppressive therapy and general medical management, are discussed for mild or remittent and severe disease. http://www.merck.com/pubs/mmanual/section5/chapter50/50e.htm

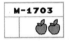

Virtual Hospital: Systemic Lupus Erythematosus A clinical summary of systemic lupus erythematosus is offered at this site, with an overview of the disorder, 11 diagnostic criteria, descriptions of nine clinical features, laboratory findings, and treatment options reviewed. Reference to preventative care and specific medications is included. http://www.vh.org/Providers/ClinRef/FPHandbook/Chapter06/09-6.html

SYSTEMIC/VASCULITIC RHEUMATIC DISEASE, GENERAL

American Family Physician: An Approach to Diagnosis and Initial Management of Systemic Vasculitis The American Academy of Family Physicians (AAFP) presents this fully-referenced clinical review of the diagnosis and treatment of systemic vasculitis. The article discusses the classification of vasculitis and details the clinical features, diagnostic workup, differential diagnosis, treatment, and prognosis of this group of diseases. http://www.aafp.org/afp/991001ap/1421.html

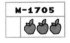

Merck Manual of Diagnosis and Therapy: Vasculitis The pathology and classifications of vasculitis are concisely reviewed at this site of *The Merck Manual of Diagnosis and Therapy*. Chapters on numerous vasculitic disorders are accessible from the topical listing of links. http://www.merck.com/pubs/mmanual/section5/chapter50/50k.htm

13.19 SEXUALLY TRANSMITTED DISEASES AND HIV/AIDS

GENERAL RESOURCES

HIVInSite: HIV/AIDS Information Dedicated to HIV/AIDS, this page offers a broad array of information related to the disease, including advice, community resources, medicine, policy, information for specific populations, and prevention. The medicine section is the largest and covers topics such as alternative medicine, blood safety, conferences, CME, infections, nutrition, patient fact sheets, and tuberculosis. Information for specific regions of the world and for settings such as healthcare settings, military, prisons, and rural communities is also featured.
http://hivinsite.ucsf.edu/InSite.jsp?page=Links

LookSmart: Sexually Transmitted Diseases A directory of resources related to sexually transmitted diseases is provided on this site. Topics include balanitis, chlamydia, genital herpes, gonorrhea, hepatitis B, HIV/AIDS, scabies, syphilis, and trichomoniasis.
http://www.looksmart.com/eus317837/eus317920/eus53948/eus54706/eus71099/r?l&

New York Online Access to Health (NOAH): Sexually Transmitted Diseases Visitors to this site will find more than 60 links related to sexually transmitted diseases. The links cover the basics of STDs, prevention, statistics, testing, and treatment. Specific diseases covered include AIDS/HIV, chlamydia, gonorrhea, herpes, and syphillis.
http://www.noah-health.org/english/illness/stds/stds.html

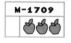

Sexually Transmitted Diseases Compiled by the Department of Obstetrics and Gynecology of Geneva University Hospital, this site offers links to information on sexually transmitted diseases. The links are organized under topics such as general information, diagnosis, and treatment. Specific conditions covered include chancroid, granuloma inguinale, mycoplasmas, pelvic inflammatory disease, and scabies.
http://matweb.hcuge.ch/matweb/endo/cours_4e_MREG/Infectious_diseases_STDs.htm

CHLAMYDIA

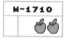

National Institute of Allergy and Infectious Diseases (NIAID): Chlamydial Infection Provided by the National Institutes of Health, this site contains a consumer brochure on chlamydial infection. An overview of the condition along with its symptoms, diagnostic tests, and treatment are found, as well as complications resulting from lack of prompt intervention.
http://www.niaid.nih.gov/factsheets/stdclam.htm

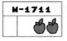

University of Wisconsin, Madison: Chlamydia Trachomatis Describing the most prevalent sexually transmitted disease in the U.S., this document offers a history and biological background, information on virulence factors, details about transmission and symptoms, and various modes of detection. Treatment and both personal and community-based prevention strategies are discussed. http://www.bact.wisc.edu/Bact330/lecturechlamydia

GENITAL HERPES

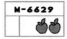

Association for Genito-Urinary Medicine: National Guideline for the Management of Genital Herpes Created by the Clinical Effectiveness Group of the Association for Genito-Urinary Medicine and the Medical Society for the Study of Venereal Diseases, this guideline describes disease features and viral detection of herpes lesions, with a table at the site reviewing the sensitivity, specificity, advantages, and disadvantages of several testing methods. Management with antiviral therapy, suppressive therapy, supportive measures, and counseling is introduced, and information on treatment in pregnant and immunocompromised individuals is provided. http://www.agum.org.uk/CEG/S24_herpes.html

National Institute of Allergy and Infectious Diseases (NIAID): Genital Herpes Examining genital herpes, this site offers patients an overview of the condition, with information on both *herpes simplex virus,* types one and two examined. Information on transmission, symptoms, and a discussion of outbreaks are provided, and diagnostic tests and treatment options are explained. The dangers of herpes infection in pregnant women are also examined, with tips on prevention, hotlines for counseling, and resources for further information provided. http://www.niaid.nih.gov/factsheets/stdherp.htm

GONORRHEA

Journal of the American Medical Association (JAMA): Gonococcal Infections Among Adolescents and Adults Treatment guidelines for gonococcal infections in adolescents and adults are featured at this Web page, which includes recommended regimens for uncomplicated gonococcal infections and alternative interventions. Information on follow-up, patient education regarding sex partners, and special considerations are addressed, such as allergy, pregnancy, HIV infection, and complications of gonococcal infections. http://www.ama-assn.org/special/std/treatmnt/guide/stdg3451.htm

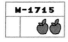

National Institute of Allergy and Infectious Diseases (NIAID): Gonorrhea A fact sheet on gonorrhea reviews general information about the disease and offers information on incidence and transmission. Descriptions of symptoms, diagnostic tests, and treatment are found, and disease complications

are addressed. Visitors will find protocols of prevention and descriptions of current research endeavors.
http://www.niaid.nih.gov/factsheets/stdgon.htm

HIV/AIDS

JAMA HIV/AIDS Information Center Produced by the *Journal of the American Medical Association,* this site serves as a comprehensive resource for HIV/AIDS information. Professionals will find news and special reports, training programs, clinical literature, and some full text articles. Clinical trials, treatment updates, drug information, and policy issues are presented. Patients can find educational materials and support group information, as well as a comprehensive list of reviewed Internet sites related to HIV/AIDS.
http://www.ama-assn.org/special/hiv/

Johns Hopkins AIDS Service The Johns Hopkins AIDS Service Web page offers a wealth of resources for both healthcare professionals and patients. Under the publications section, visitors can access the bimonthly *Hopkins HIV Report;* the full text of a clinical handbook on HIV/AIDS; and the *Moore News Quarterly,* an online consumer newsletter. Case studies, conference proceedings and multimedia presentation (audio and video clips) archives, information on clinical trials, and managed care details are offered. Separate discussion forums are available for professionals and patients, and a comprehensive list of related Internet resources is provided.
http://www.hopkins-aids.edu/

HUMAN PAPILLOMAVIRUS AND GENITAL WARTS

eMedicine: Warts, Genital Background information on genital warts and a comprehensive clinical guide to diagnosis and management are offered at this eMedicine resource. Drug profiles of keratolytics and interferons are featured, and full size and eMedicine interactive Zoom View images are available.
http://www.eMedicine.com/EMERG/topic640.htm

National Institute of Allergy and Infectious Diseases (NIAID): Human Papillomavirus and Genital Warts A patient's guide to human papillomavirus and genital warts is offered at this Web site, which explores aspects of genital warts and its transmission. Diagnostic tests, treatment, and potential complications are explained, with tips for prevention and resources for further information provided.
http://www.niaid.nih.gov/factsheets/stdhpv.htm

SYPHILIS

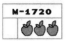

American Family Physician: Resolving the Common Clinical Dilemmas of Syphilis Providing both a professional guideline and a related patient information handout, this site of the American Academy of Family Physicians offers viewers an overview of common presentations at various disease stages. Details on serologic study interpretation, recommendations for diagnosis, and special concerns about the diagnosis and treatment of the disease in AIDS patients are presented. http://www.aafp.org/afp/990415ap/2233.html

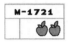

National Institute of Allergy and Infectious Diseases (NIAID): Syphilis An overview of syphilis and its transmission is provided, along with symptoms of primary syphilis, secondary syphilis, and neurosyphilis. Diagnostic tests, treatment, and the effects of syphilis in pregnant women are described. Tips for prevention are outlined, as well as future research needs.
http://www.niaid.nih.gov/factsheets/stdsyph.htm

TRICHOMONIASIS

Merck Manual of Diagnosis and Therapy: Trichomoniasis Drawn from the *Merck Manual of Diagnosis and Therapy*, a clinical tutorial on trichomoniasis is offered at this Web page. The site covers the etiology, symptoms in women and men, diagnosis, and treatment.
http://www.merck.com/pubs/mmanual/section13/chapter164/164e.htm

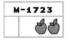

Urologychannel: Sexually Transmitted Diseases (STDs): Trichomoniasis Trichomoniasis is the focus of this patient fact sheet, which includes an overview of the condition, as well as information on its transmission, causes, symptoms, and diagnostic tests. Treatment with metronidazole is described, and recommendations for prevention are introduced.
http://www.urologychannel.com/std/trichomoniasis.shtml

13.20 UROLOGY DISORDERS AND TOPICS

GENERAL RESOURCES

CliniWeb International: Kidney Diseases Provided as a service of Oregon Health Sciences University, this collection of sites offers visitors easy access to disorder overviews, including Web sites from the University of Utah Webpath, OncoLink, Vanderbilt University, and the Medical College of Wisconsin. Some pages offer pathologic images and descriptions, while others provide clinical case discussions. Preformatted PubMed query links to disorder research reviews and article abstracts on therapy and diagnosis are provided.
http://www.ohsu.edu/cliniweb/C12/C12.777.419.html

Johns Hopkins Medical Institutions: Brady Urological Institute

Representing excellence in research and care in the field of urology, the Brady Urological Institute site offers information on normal function and anatomy, as well as overviews of urological condition symptoms, examination, and treatment. Additional features of the site include patient information resources, major research discoveries and details, innovative surgical techniques, and educational programs of the division.

http://prostate.urol.jhu.edu/

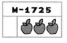

National Institute of Diabetes and Digestive and Kidney Diseases (NIDDK): Urologic Diseases

As part of the NIH Web site, this information resource provides current brochures and statistics on a variety of urologic conditions. Current subjects include bladder control, impotence, prostatitis, and urinary tract infections. A section of Spanish-language articles is included, and a bibliographical search engine for kidney and urological diseases is provided. Professionals may order bulk quantities of certain titles.

http://www.niddk.nih.gov/health/urolog/urolog.htm

Open Directory Project: Urologic Diseases

Access to information on close to 30 categories of conditions and diseases in urology is provided from this Web page. Brief condition-oriented articles, personal pages about specific diseases, and writings that focus on assessment, diagnosis, and therapeutic intervention are included.

http://dmoz.org/Health/Conditions_and_Diseases/Urological_Disorders/

ACUTE TUBULAR NECROSIS

MEDLINEplus Medical Encyclopedia: Acute Tubular Necrosis

This site offers information on acute tubular necrosis, which explains causes, risk factors, symptoms, diagnostic tests, and treatment options.

http://www.nlm.nih.gov/medlineplus/ency/article/000512.htm

OutlineMed: Acute Tubular Necrosis

Examining acute tubular necrosis, this Web page features short descriptions of the pathophysiology, etiology, symptoms, and treatment of the disease. Related outlines on renal tubular function, vascular pathophysiology, and acute renal failure are accessible.

http://www.outlinemed.com/demo/nephrol/8854.htm

BENIGN PROSTATIC HYPERPLASIA (BPH)

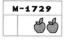

Merck Manual of Diagnosis and Therapy: Benign Prostatic Hyperplasia

Drawn from the authoritative *Merck* reference, this site offers a clinical tutorial on benign prostatic hyperplasia. The condition is defined, along with its incidence, theories on possible etiology, symptoms, diagnosis, and medical and surgical treatment options.

http://www.merck.com/pubs/mmanual/section17/chapter218/218a.htm

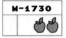

National Institute of Diabetes and Digestive and Kidney Diseases (NIDDK): Benign Prostatic Hyperplasia A patient's guide to benign prostatic hyperplasia (BPH) is featured at this Web page, maintained by the National Institutes of Health. The guide describes the prostate gland and BPH, theories on why BPH occurs, and a description of symptoms. Common diagnostic tests are explained, as well as drug, other nonsurgical, and surgical treatment options.
http://www.niddk.nih.gov/health/urolog/pubs/prostate/index.htm

BLADDER CANCER

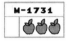

Bladder Cancer WebCafe This site provides information on bladder cancer and offers links to information on biomarkers, investigations, chemoprevention, gene therapy, superficial bladder cancer, and alternative treatment. An e-mail discussion list, extensive information for the newly diagnosed, and a list of references are offered.
http://blcwebcafe.org/default.asp

OncoLink: Bladder Cancer Provided as a service of the University of Pennsylvania Cancer Center, this OncoLink site offers visitors links to a bladder cancer support and information group, as well as the opportunity to subscribe to a professional Urology Network. OncoLink documents on bladder cancer evaluation, diagnosis, and management are accessible.
http://cancer.med.upenn.edu/disease/bladder/index.html

EPIDIDYMITIS

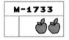

Adam.com: Epididymitis A concise definition of epididymitis and information related to the cause and incidence of the condition are reviewed at this Adam.com site. An illustration of the male reproductive system is accessible, and hyperlinks at each page offer connections to further details on symptoms, treatment, and prevention.
http://pcs.adam.com/ency/article/001279.htm

eMedicine: Epididymitis This site addresses the pathophysiology and incidence in the general population, as well as information on symptoms, causes, diagnostic work-up, and emergency intervention for epididymitis. A table of commonly prescribed antibiotics is found, along with recommendations for further inpatient and outpatient care.
http://www.eMedicine.com/emerg/topic166.htm

ERECTILE DYSFUNCTION

Digital Urology Journal: Erectile Dysfunction Underlying conditions associated with erectile dysfunction are reviewed at this page, with discussions of the physician's role in diagnosis, the diagnostic evaluation, and patient interview. Risk factors associated with organic erectile dysfunction and uncommon yet correctable causes are identified.
http://www.duj.com/erectile.html

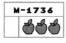

Urologychannel: Erectile Dysfunction Erectile dysfunction, often referred to as impotence, is explained at this online patient guide. The site examines levels of erectile dysfunction and provides links to information on causes, symptoms, diagnosis, and conventional and alternative treatment options.
http://www.urologychannel.com/erectiledysfunction/index.shtml

GLOMERULAR DISEASES, GENERAL

Merck Manual of Diagnosis and Therapy: Glomerular Diseases Summarizing glomerulonephropathies, this overview provides links to discussions of the causes, etiology, incidence, and classification of nephritic and nephrotic syndromes. Visitors will find tables illustrating pathogenesis, information on treatment and prognosis, and access to related chapters within this online *Merck* reference.
http://www.merck.com/pubs/mmanual/section17/chapter224/224a.htm

National Kidney and Urologic Diseases Information Clearinghouse: Glomerular Diseases Geared toward consumers, this site discusses glomerular diseases and their interference with kidney function. Disease causes, diagnosis, and related information on renal failure are provided, as well as a glossary of terms and key points to remember.
http://www.niddk.nih.gov/health/kidney/pubs/glomer/glomer.htm

HYDROCELE

eMedicine: Hydrocele Directed toward practitioners, an introduction to hydrocele is featured at this Web page, authored by physicians of the University of California Irvine Medical Center. Discussion of adult hydroceles, clinical presentation, differential links, diagnosis, and management are reviewed.
http://www.eMedicine.com/emerg/topic256.htm

MEDLINEplus Medical Encyclopedia: Hydrocele An overview, symptoms, and treatment options for hydrocele are featured on this Web page. Causes, incidence, and risk factors are addressed, as a service of the National Library of Medicine.
http://www.nlm.nih.gov/medlineplus/ency/article/000518.htm

Infertility, Male Factor

M-1741

Postgraduate Medicine: Shattering the Myths About Male Infertility
Postgraduate Medicine offers this online CME opportunity, which reviews the current state of knowledge regarding male infertility factors and frequency. The article focuses primarily on significant male factors, the importance of patient education, and diagnosis and treatment of easily correctable factors.
http://www.postgradmed.com/issues/2000/02_00/sandlow.htm

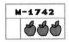
M-1742

Urologychannel: Male Infertility This Urology Forum contains a wealth of information on male infertility assessment, diagnosis, and treatment, directed at a variety of audiences. Pages on anatomy and physiology, risk factors, and therapeutic options make the site a comprehensive, online learning tool.
http://www.urologychannel.com/Maleinfertility/index.shtml

Interstitial Cystitis

M-1743

Interstitial Cystitis Association Healthcare providers and patients will find a variety of information on interstitial cystitis at this disease-oriented home page, including feature articles, the organization's quarterly publication, *Physician Perspectives,* fact sheets, treatment options, an "Ask the Expert" forum, and audio presentations that offer online multimedia educational opportunities.
http://www.ichelp.org/

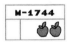
M-1744

Urologychannel: Interstitial Cystitis Those with interstitial cystitis can learn more about the incidence, risk factors, symptoms, diagnosis, and treatment of the condition at this informative, electronic brochure. A listing of several conditions that may mimic its symptoms is offered.
http://www.urologychannel.com/interstitialcystitis/index.shtml

Kidney Stones/Urinary Tract Stones

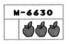
M-6630

eMedicine: Urolithiasis This eMedicine site reviews background information on the common occurrence of kidney stones and includes access to enlargeable images of renal calculi and a ureteral stone. Various theories of pathophysiology of urinary tract stone disease, as well as common patient complaints, are reviewed. In addition to recommendations for the patient evaluation, a large number of differential links can be accessed from the site, which also examines the significance and use of several laboratory and imaging studies. Issues regarding emergency department care, postsurgical follow-up, ongoing medical therapy, and complications of urinary tract stone disease are considered. http://www.emedicine.com/MED/topic1600.htm

M-1746

Urologychannel: Kidney Stones An introduction to kidney stones is presented at this Urology Forum site and includes a definition of the condition,

causes of stone formation, and details on stone type variation. Answers to questions about who develops kidney stones and recurrence details are provided.
http://www.urologychannel.com/kidneystones/index.shtml

NEPHROTIC SYNDROME

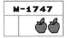

National Kidney and Urologic Diseases Information Clearinghouse: Nephrotic Syndrome in Adults Provided as a service of the National Kidney and Urologic Diseases Information Clearinghouse, this fact sheet offers an overview of nephrotic syndrome as it occurs with many diseases. Treatment, focused on identification of the underlying cause, is reviewed, and resources for further information are listed.
http://www.niddk.nih.gov/health/kidney/summary/nephsynd/nephsynd.htm

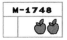

RenalNet Renal Pathology Tutorial: The Nephrotic Syndrome Examining the nephrotic syndrome, this Web page provides healthcare professionals with a clinical discussion of the condition. Hyperlinks within the text illustrate the histologic features of the disease. Links are also provided to other glomerular diseases.
http://www.gamewood.net/rnet/renalpath/ch3.htm

POLYCYSTIC KIDNEYS

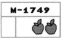

National Kidney and Urologic Diseases Information Clearinghouse: Polycystic Kidney Disease Sponsored by the National Kidney and Urologic Diseases Information Clearinghouse, this informative fact sheet offers visitors information on autosomal dominant, autosomal recessive, and acquired cystic kidney disease. A section devoted to the search for the precise genetic connection is provided.
http://www.niddk.nih.gov/health/kidney/pubs/polycyst/polycyst.htm

Polycystic Kidney Research Foundation Disease news, current research, and a members-only newsletter are all available at this site's links. Information about annual conferences and links to other resources are provided. By accessing the "What's New" connection, visitor will find the latest political action information and the "Hot List" of Web resources.
http://www.pkdcure.org/

PROSTATE CANCER

CancerNet: Prostate Cancer Directed toward healthcare professionals, the National Cancer Institute's Physician Data Query on prostate cancer is featured at this site. An overview of prostate cancer is offered, along with cellular classi-

fication, stage information, treatment options, and complications due to surgery, radiation, and hormone therapy.
http://cancernet.nci.nih.gov/cgi-bin/srchcgi.exe?DBID=pdq&TYPE=
search&UID=208+01229&ZFILE=professional&SFMT=pdq_treatment/1/0/0

 MEDLINEplus Health Information: Prostate Cancer Drawn from a variety of sources, this Web site offers information on prostate cancer including clinical trials, symptoms, and treatment connections. Of interest to patients and physicians are links to recent research from the Mayo Clinic as well as the latest news articles. Some patient publications are available in Spanish.
http://www.nlm.nih.gov/medlineplus/prostatecancer.html

PROSTATITIS

 American Family Physician: Treatment of Prostatitis Recommendations for treatment of prostatitis are offered at this comprehensive management article of the American Academy of Family Physicians. Diagnostic tests and correct classification of the condition are emphasized, along with respective treatment protocols. A related patient guide to prostatitis is available at a convenient site connection.
http://www.aafp.org/afp/20000515/3015.html

 Prostatitis Foundation Both consumer and healthcare professionals will find an assortment of resources on prostate-related disease at the home page of the Prostatitis Foundation. Links to scientific publications and books, conference proceedings, information on the causes of prostatitis, methods of treatment, and patient testimonials are offered. http://prostatitis.org/aboutpf.html

PYELONEPHRITIS

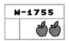 **Adam.com: Pyelonephritis** Intended for a variety of audiences, this Web page focuses on pyelonephritis and provides a definition, types, causes, and incidence descriptions. Links to additional information on symptoms, diagnostic tests, treatment, and prevention tips can be accessed.
http://pcs.adam.com/ency/article/000522.htm

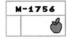 **National Center for Emergency Medicine Informatics: Pyelonephritis** Drawn from *Common Simple Emergencies,* this site provides a case description and concise information on how to treat a patient with pyelonephritis.
http://www.ncemi.org/cse/cse0702.htm

RENAL CELL CARCINOMA

 National Cancer Institute (NCI): Renal Cell Cancer The National Cancer Institute provides a comprehensive patient information statement on re-

nal cell cancer at this site. An overview, explanation of stages, a detailed discussion of treatment options, and brief coverage of recurrent renal cell carcinoma are presented. Resources for further information are provided.
http://www.graylab.ac.uk/cancernet/201070.html

OncoLink: Kidney Cancer Created by the University of Pennsylvania Cancer Center, this site features consumer and professional resources related to kidney cancer. More than 50 sites are accessible, along with general resources related to cancer, symptom management, and psychosocial support.
http://www.oncolink.upenn.edu/disease/kidney/

Renal Failure, Acute

American Family Physician: Acute Renal Failure Published by the American Academy of Family Physicians, this cover article offers visitors a comprehensive discussion of disease etiology, a systematic approach to diagnosis, management considerations, and possible cases for prevention.
http://www.aafp.org/afp/20000401/2077.html

Merck Manual of Diagnosis and Therapy: Acute Renal Failure Primarily for healthcare professionals, this site examines prerenal, postrenal, and renal types. The pathophysiology and symptoms of each subtype are described, with detailed information on diagnostic tests, findings, treatment options, and prognosis presented.
http://www.merck.com/pubs/mmanual/section17/chapter222/222b.htm

Testicular Cancer

MEDLINEplus Health Information: Testicular Cancer Geared toward a consumer audience, this site provides a number of sources for general information on testicular cancer, symptoms, and treatment. Several articles on early detection and a self-care flowchart are also available through hyperlinks.
http://www.nlm.nih.gov/medlineplus/testicularcancer.html

OncoLink: Testicular Cancer For those interested in testicular cancer, this site offers a listing of resources, including journal abstracts and information from the National Cancer Institute. Links to information on germ cell tumors, screening and prevention details, and general information on cancer, symptom management, and support are provided.
http://oncolink.upenn.edu/disease/testicular/

Urethritis

eMedicine: Urethritis, Male Offering a clinical discussion of urethritis in men, eMedicine provides discussion of the pathophysiology, symptoms, causes,

and links to differentials. Information on diagnostic workup and detailed information on several antibiotics are offered, along with discussions of follow-up and potential complications.
http://www.eMedicine.com/emerg/topic623.htm

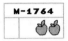

MEDLINEplus Medical Encyclopedia: Urethritis This National Library of Medicine site offers consumer-oriented information on urethritis. Causes, risk factors, symptoms, and diagnostic testing details are provided, along with treatment, potential complications, and prevention tips.
http://www.nlm.nih.gov/medlineplus/ency/article/000439.htm

URINARY INCONTINENCE

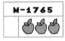

Agency for Healthcare Research and Quality (AHRQ): Urinary Incontinence in Adults This clinical practice guideline is provides an overview of the condition, as well as information on causes, evaluation, and treatment. Recommended treatments include pelvic muscle rehabilitation and behavioral, pharmacologic, and surgical therapies, as well as a discussion of treatments for the chronically incontinent. The need for public education is emphasized, and references are provided. http://www.ahcpr.gov/news/press/overview.htm

MEDLINEplus Health Information: Urinary Incontinence Links on anatomy and physiology, general overviews, clinical trial details, and disease management pages are all accessible from this collection of Internet sites, courtesy of the National Library of Medicine. Both consumer and professional viewers will find an assortment of useful prevention and management resources at this collection, sponsored by government divisions and reputable private organizations. http://www.nlm.nih.gov/medlineplus/urinaryincontinence.html

URINARY RETENTION

National Center for Emergency Medicine Informatics: Urinary Retention The presentation of urinary retention and concise management information are presented at this online portion of *Common Simple Emergencies*. Causes and urethral catheterization are outlined.
http://www.ncemi.org/cse/cse0709.htm

Urinary Retention Pages accessible from this site describe this common clinical problem, with causes, clinical assessment, investigations, and management options summarized.
http://medmic02.wnmeds.ac.nz/groups/rmo/urinary_retention/retention_toc.html

URINARY TRACT INFECTION

American Family Physician: Urinary Tract Infections in Adults A full-text article, courtesy of the American Academy of Family Physicians, is presented at this page, which includes diagnostic approach and treatment discussion. Acute uncomplicated cystitis in young women, recurrent cystitis, acute uncomplicated pyelonephritis, complicated urinary tract infection (UTI), UTI-related infection, infection in men, and asymptomatic bacteriuria are addressed. A link to a related patient handout on urinary tract infections is provided.
http://www.aafp.org/afp/990301ap/1225.html

Merck Manual of Diagnosis and Therapy: Urinary Tract Infections
This professional resource introduces visitors to the etiology and pathogenesis of a variety of bacterial urinary tract infections, including urethritis, cystitis, prostatitis, and acute pyelonephritis. Symptoms and signs, diagnostic details, and prevention are emphasized, with links offered to related *Merck* chapters.
http://www.merck.com/pubs/mmanual/section17/chapter227/227a.htm

VASECTOMY

American Family Physician: Vasectomy Techniques Presented by the American Academy of Family Physicians, this article describes vasectomy techniques and practices. A vasectomy procedure checklist, sections on the preoperative evaluation, patient preparation details, and anesthesia requirements are discussed. This well-illustrated site includes an accessible patient information handout, provided by the authors of this article.
http://www.aafp.org/afp/990700ap/137.html

Urologychannel: Vasectomy This informational brochure, maintained by the Urologychannel, offers sections on basic physiology of the procedure, tips on preparation, discussions of how it is performed, and what to expect postoperatively. Possible complications and details on vasectomy reversal are provided. http://www.urologychannel.com/Vasectomy/index.shtml

GENERAL MEDICAL
WEB RESOURCES

14

REFERENCE INFORMATION
AND NEWS SOURCES

14.1 GENERAL MEDICAL SUPERSITES

Visitors interested in medical supersites may also find similar information under the medical search engine section.

American Medical Association (AMA) The AMA develops and promotes standards in medical practice, research, and education; acts as advocate on behalf of patients and physicians; and provides discourse on matters important to public health in America. General information is available at the site about the organization; journals and newsletters; policy, advocacy, activities, and ethics; education; and accreditation services. AMA news and consumer health information are also found at the site. Resources for physicians include membership details; information on the AMA's current procedural terminology (CPT) information services, the resource-based relative value scale (RBVS), and electronic medical systems; information on the AMA Alliance (a national organization of physicians' spouses); descriptions of additional AMA products and services; a discussion of legal issues for physicians; and information on AMA's global activities. Information for consumers includes medical news; detailed information on a wide range of conditions; family health resources for children, adolescents, men, and women; interactive health calculators; healthy recipes; and general safety tips. Specific pages are devoted to comprehensive resources related to HIV/AIDS, asthma, migraines, and women's health.
http://www.ama-assn.org

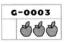

BioSites BioSites is a comprehensive catalog of selected Internet resources in the medical and biomedical sciences. The sites were selected as part of a project by staff members of Resource Libraries within the Pacific Southwest Region of the National Network of Libraries of Medicine. Sites are organized by medical topic or specialty field, and users can also search the site by keyword. Featured Web sites are listed by title; details are provided within each hyperlink.
http://www.library.ucsf.edu/biosites

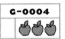

Doctor's Guide The Doctor's Guide to the Internet, provided by PSL Consulting Group, Inc., contains a professional edition for healthcare professionals and a section directed at patients. Information of medical and professional interest includes medical news and alerts, new drugs or indications, medical conferences, the Congress Resource Center, a medical bookstore, and Internet medical resources. Patient resources are organized by specific diseases or condition. Users can search the World Wide Web through Excite, InfoSeek, McKinley, and Alta Vista search engines or can search the Doctor's Guide medical news and conference database.

(free registration) http://www.docguide.com

Emory University: MedWeb Maintained by the library staff of Emory University, MedWeb offers more than 100 subjects encompassing a comprehensive catalog of thousands of biomedical and health-related sites. Visitors can perform a keyword search or browse through categories such as biological and physical sciences, clinical practice, consumer health, diseases and conditions, drugs, healthcare, institutions, mental health, publications, and specialties. A subject index is available to browse the entire catalog.

http://www.medweb.emory.edu/Medweb/

Galaxy: Medicine Intended primarily for consumer reference, Galaxy Health provides topic-specific search engines in over 30 health-related areas. Categories include diseases, fitness, mental health, weight loss, and dentistry. Each topic contains links to online articles, discussion groups, periodicals, and organizations. http://health.galaxy.com

Hardin MD: Meta Directory Hosted by the Hardin Library for the Health Sciences at the University of Iowa, this site features a meta-directory of Internet health sites. More than 40 subjects are listed in the directory such as AIDS, cancer, dermatology, neurology, pregnancy, and pediatrics. The directory contains thousands of sites. By clicking on a subject, visitors will find lists of Internet sites compiled from other Web pages. Each list is ranked according to depth of content. In addition to the meta-directory, links are provided to an array of news sources, medical libraries, free journals online, and consumer-oriented sites. http://www.lib.uiowa.edu/hardin/md/

Health On the Net (HON) Foundation The Health On the Net Foundation site offers an engine that searches the Internet as well as the foundation's database for medical sites, hospitals, and support communities. HON also provides a dossier with in-depth information on topics such as mother and child, allergy, vision and eye care, smoking cessation, hepatitis B, rare diseases, and aging. A media gallery contains a database of medical images and videos from various sources. The site also features articles from a daily news archive, a conference locator, and surveys of health trends. Users can select a target group, such as healthcare providers, medical professionals, or patients and other individuals, to receive more tailored search results. http://www.hon.ch

HealthWeb With support from a National Library of Medicine grant, this collaborative effort of over 20 health sciences libraries offers a meta-directory of health-related, noncommercial Web sites. The sites are categorized into approximately 70 different subject areas such as AIDS, anatomy, dermatology, hematology, and toxicology. Within each subject, sites are further classified by clinical resources, academic institutes, statistics, conferences, consumer health resources, online publications, and organizations. For each site listed, there is a brief description of its contents.

http://healthweb.org/index.cfm

Karolinska Institutet: Diseases, Disorders and Related Topics
Karolinska Institutet, a medical university, offers ample resources for both professionals and the general public at this collection. Covering every major field of medicine, the site provides a database of fact sheets and Web sites on individual diseases, pathology databases, clinical guidelines, research, and anatomy and other medical tutorials. Databases for biological sciences, bioethics, medical images, and medical news are also available, as well as "Ask the Doctor" and second-opinion services. Visitors can locate information via an alphabetical list of diseases or through more than 20 directories in a particular field of medicine. Other resources of the Karolinska Institutet include MEDLINE access, electronic journals, and a Medical Subject Headings (MeSH) tree tool for finding references and links to other resources.

http://micf.mic.ki.se/Diseases

Martindale's Health Science Guide: Virtual Medical Center The Virtual Medical Center claims to have more than 61,500 teaching files, 129,800 medical cases, 1,155 courses/textbooks, 1,580 tutorials, 4,100 databases, and thousands of movies. The information is listed in categories on the home page such as biomechanics, cancer, immunology, microbiology, sports medicine, and toxicology. Separate sections contain information on public health, environmental health, and travel warnings. The site also provides resources such as a physician finder, clinical trials, CME, medical codes, laboratory diagnostics, blood-related information, hospitals worldwide, medical auctions, and medical dictionaries in eight languages.

http://www.sci.lib.uci.edu/~martindale/Medical.html

MedExplorer Created by a Canadian paramedic, MedExplorer provides a database of Web sites covering a wide array of health topics for health professionals and the public. Links to an enormous number of sites, along with brief descriptions of site contents, are categorized into nearly 30 health-related topics such as allied health, alternative medicine, education, employment, government, laboratory, medical imaging, research, and specialty medicine. There are also discussion forums, an employment center, and health news headlines. Health centers of resources for women, men, children, and seniors are also included, as well as a nutrition database, an online health exam, access to MEDLINE, and more than 250 health newsgroups.

http://www.medexplorer.com/

Medical Matrix Medical Matrix offers a list of directories categorized into specialties, diseases, clinical practice resources, literature, education, healthcare and professional resources, medical computing, Internet and technology, and marketplace resources containing classifieds and employment opportunities. Additional features include a site search engine; access to MEDLINE, clinical searches, and links to symposia on the Web; medical textbook resources; patient education materials; CME information; news; and online journals. Free registration is necessary to access the site.

(free registration) http://www.medmatrix.org

Medicine Online   Offering a broad range of medical information, this site contains resources of interest to both physicians and patients. The reference section features a medical dictionary, fact sheets on diseases and treatments, and a drug index. Visitors will also find comprehensive listings of Internet resources in categories such as diseases and conditions, medicine, public health, women's health, and allied health. Unique to the site are "Bid for Surgery" and "Bid for Rx" centers where consumers enter their requirements for cosmetic procedures or prescriptions and physicians or pharmacists respond with their qualifications, location, and price. Directories of physicians, hospitals, and vendors are provided, and a link to MOL.net takes the visitor to a portal offering a customizable home page for professionals with access to "Bid for surgery," reference information, message boards, and information on laboratory management. By accessing the "Health Topics" menu, viewers are taken to large selections of general resources and links for the chosen topic.

(free registration) http://www.medicineonline.net/

MedicineNet.com   Described as "100 percent doctor-produced healthcare information," this Web page offers fact sheets written in laymen's terms on a variety of health-related topics. Areas covered include allergies, arthritis, asthma, cancer, cholesterol, depression, diabetes, digestion, high blood pressure, HIV, thyroid, and women's health. Alphabetized indices on diseases and conditions, procedures and tests, medications, and healthy living (nutrition and fitness) are also available, as well as a medical dictionary and an online drugstore. The home page features news, updates, and information on commonly requested conditions such as acne, asthma, cancer, and diabetes. Also on the home page is quick reference information such as first aid, poison control, and product recalls. http://www.medicinenet.com/Script/Main/hp.asp

MEDLINEplus   Sponsored by the National Library of Medicine, the world's largest medical library, and the National Institutes of Health, this site provides up-to-date, high-quality healthcare information. Resources on this Web page cover an array of health information for professionals and consumers. The "Health Topics" section offers more than 30 broad topics, each with several subsections leading to additional links to information such as overviews, clinical trials, diagnosis and symptoms, specific conditions, policy, organizations, statistics, and Spanish publications. The site also features drug information, with a guide to more than 9,000 prescription and over-the-counter medications. There are several medical dictionaries, along with directories of physicians and hospi-

tals. Information found under the "Other Resources" section includes organizations, libraries, publications, databases, and access to MEDLINE.
http://www.medlineplus.gov/

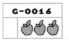

MedMark: Medical Bookmarks Designed by a physician, this Web page is a comprehensive directory of thousands of health-related sites with information for both the professional and consumer. Sites are categorized under more than 30 specialties such as endocrinology, immunology, and pediatrics. Clicking on a specialty brings up a list of Internet sites organized in categories such as associations, centers, departments, education and training, consumer information, guidelines, journals, and programs. There are also links for free access to MEDLINE (registration required), as well as a list of related sites that contain large directories of resources. At the top of the site, there is a link for sites in Korea.
http://members.kr.inter.net/medmark/

MedNets This international research site uses proprietary search engines for accessing information on specialties in medicine. Users select from one of four areas including a research engine and communities geared toward professionals, patients, and the health industry. The community for professionals covers nearly 50 topics of interest to clinicians, including anesthesiology, family medicine, managed care, pathology, practice guidelines, and telemedicine. Within each topic are links to associations, clinical information, centers of excellence, and news and research.
http://www.mednets.com

Medscape Medscape offers a directory of Web sites that provide information on a wide range of medical specialties. Information in each specialty includes news items, conference summaries and schedules, treatment updates, practice guidelines, articles, and patient resources. Medscape also offers resources for medical students, medical office managers, nurses, and pharmacists.
(free registration) http://www.medscape.com

Medscout The Medscout Web page offers a directory of health-related Web sites. More than 50 broad topics are listed such as clinical alerts, CME, diseases, employment, guidelines, hospitals, informatics, journals, medical supplies, and telemedicine, and each topic is broken down into further subtopics with hyperlinks. The site also includes extensive information on the Health Insurance Portability and Accountability Act (HIPAA), as well as several fee-based tools for securely connecting healthcare professionals to payers, pharmacies, and each other. (some features fee-based) http://www.medscout.com/

Megasite Project: A Metasite Comparing Health Information Megasites and Search Engines The Megasite Project, created by librarians at Northwestern University, the University of Michigan, and Pennsylvania State University, evaluates and provides direct links to 25 of the largest health information Internet sites. Criteria for evaluation and comparison include administration and quality control, content, and design. Users can access results of site evaluations, tips for successful site searches, unique features of particular sites, lists of the best general and health information search engines reviewed, and site comparisons listed by evaluation criteria. A bibliography of articles on Web design and Internet resource evaluation is found at the address, as well as descriptions of other aspects of the project.

http://www.lib.umich.edu/megasite/toc.html

G-0022

National Library of Medicine (NLM) The National Library of Medicine, the world's largest medical library, collects materials in all areas of biomedicine and healthcare and focuses on biomedical aspects of technology; the humanities; and the physical, life, and social sciences. This site contains links to government medical databases, including MEDLINE and MEDLINEplus, information on funding opportunities at the National Library of Medicine and other federal agencies, and details of services, training, and outreach programs offered by NLM. Users can access NLM's catalog of resources (LOCATORPlus), as well as NLM publications, including fact sheets, published reports, and staff publications. NLM research programs discussed at the site include topics in computational molecular biology, medical informatics, and other related subjects. The Web site features 15 databases, covering journal searches via MEDLINE; AIDS information via AIDSLINE, AIDSDRUGS, and AIDSTRIALS; bioethics via BIOETHICSLINE; and numerous other important topics. The NLM Gateway—a master search engine—searches MEDLINE using the user-friendly retrieval engine called PubMed. There are over 11-million citations in MEDLINE and PreMEDLINE and the other related databases. Additionally, the NLM provides sources of health statistics, serials programs, and services maintained through a system called SERHOLD.

http://www.nlm.nih.gov

G-0023

New York Online Access to Health (NOAH): Health Topics and Resources The entire NOAH Web page is available in English and Spanish and offers a broad array of health information. Visitors can browse by subject or alphabetically. The home page features more than 30 health topics such as AIDS, arthritis, cancer, kidney diseases, and nutrition. By clicking on a topic, a long list of links appears for in-depth information such as a description of the disease or condition along with diagnosis, symptoms, and treatment. There is also a resource section for more information including patient rights, medications, support groups, and New York City and county healthcare and community services resources.

http://www.noah-health.org/english/qksearch.html

G-0024

University of Iowa: Virtual Hospital A service of the University of Iowa Health Care system, this Web page features the Virtual Hospital, a digital library with more than 350 peer-reviewed books and booklets. Separate sections are available for healthcare providers and patients. The provider section is organized by categories such as specialty, department, organ system, and by type of information, including multimedia, textbooks, journals, and guidelines. The patient section contains categories such as problem, department, organ system, and FAQs. The "Common Problems" link provides a comprehensive alphabetical list of the site's contents, with separate professional and patient links. The home page also features a link to the Virtual Children's Hospital, as well as CME online courses. http://www.vh.org

WebMD   High-quality consumer health information and resources are available at this address. Consumer resources include information on conditions, treatments, and drugs; medical news and articles; a forum for obtaining answers to health questions; online chat events with medical experts; and articles and expert advice on general health topics. Consumers can also join a "community" for more personalized information and forums. A section for health teachers offers lesson guides and teacher supports for improving school-based health education. Physician services, available for a fee, include access to medical news, online journals, and reference databases; online insurance verification and referrals; e-mail, voice mail, fax, and conference call capabilities; practice management tools; online trading; financial services; and other resources. The site offers a preview tour of the service for interested professionals. (some features fee-based) http://www.webmd.com

14.2 ABBREVIATIONS

Acronym and Abbreviation List   This site offers a database of acronyms and abbreviations. Visitors can search for an acronym and see what it means, or search for a word and its related acronym.
http://www.ucc.ie/info/net/acronyms/index.html

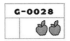

Common Medical Abbreviations   Several hundred major medical abbreviations are defined in an alphabetical listing at this educational information site.
http://courses.smsu.edu/jas188f/690/medslpterm.html

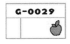

How to Read a Prescription   A guide to interpreting a prescription is offered on this Web page, directed to healthcare professionals. More than 20 common abbreviations are listed along with their interpretation.
http://www.dallas.net/~stonemik/sigs.html

National Council for Emergency Medicine Informatics   The National Council for Emergency Medicine Informatics provides a database for medical abbreviations and acronyms. By clicking on "Abbreviation Translator" and entering the letters to be identified, single or multiple definitions will be returned.
http://www.ncemi.org

14.3 ABSTRACT, CITATION, AND FULL-TEXT SEARCH TOOLS

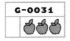

EMBASE: Medical Abstracts Database   Produced by Elsevier Science, the EMBASE database contains more than 13-million citations from the biomedical and pharmacological literature. Entries from 1974 to the present also contain abstracts. A distinction noted from the site asserts that EMBASE is "renowned for its comprehensive international coverage." The database is updated daily, and a free demo is available from this site.

(fee-based) http://www.embase.com/

Google Particularly hard to find resources can often be located with the Google search engine, which returns pages that include all search terms listed. Medical and other scientific materials on the Web are especially easy to locate and often include a wide selection of online textbook pages, scholarly reference material, online tutorials, and medical journal entries. http://www.google.com/

Ingenta A searchable bibliographic database—featuring more than 25,000 publications—is offered on this site for several subject areas, including medicine and nursing. Search results yield a citation with the option to purchase the full-text article. For those with a subscription to a specific journal, access to the full-text article is free. In addition, each medical specialty has links to news, conferences, clinical trials, and practice guidelines.

(some features fee-based) http://www.ingenta.com

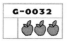

Infomine: Scholarly Internet Resources Infomine offers biological, agricultural, and medical Internet Web site collections, primarily consisting of university-level research and education. There are close to 20,000 links, including databases, electronic journals, textbooks, and conference proceedings. Web sites can be browsed by author, title, subject, or keyword. Recently added sites are stored in a separate section. The site also offers links to additional Internet medical resources.

http://infomine.ucr.edu/search/bioagsearch.phtml

InfoTrieve: Article Finder A database of more than 20-million citations drawn from over 30,000 scientific, technical, and medical journals can be searched on this site, dating back to 1966. Users can order reprints of articles through the site for a fee.

(some features fee-based) http://www4.infotrieve.com/search/databases/newsearch.asp

MEDLINE/PubMed at the National Library of Medicine (NLM) PubMed is a free MEDLINE search service providing access to 11-million citations with links to the full text of articles of participating journals. Probably the most heavily used and reputable free MEDLINE site, PubMed permits advanced searching by subject, author, journal title, and many other fields. It includes an easy-to-use "citation matcher" for completing and identifying references, and its PreMEDLINE database provides journal citations before they are indexed, making this version of MEDLINE more up-to-date than most.

http://www.ncbi.nlm.nih.gov/PubMed

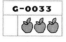

National Cancer Institute (NCI): Literature and Bibliographic Database of Cancer Information The NCI offers this Web page with links to a broad array of cancer literature. Visitors can search CancerLit, NCI's bibliographic database with more than 1.5 million citations and abstracts. NCI publications for professionals and the public are available online; categories include types of cancer, treatment options, clinical trials, genetics, coping with cancer, testing for cancer, and risk factors. A general category encompasses clinical research and statistics. Peer-reviewed summaries on treatment, screening, prevention, genetics, and supportive care are available through a link to PDQ, NCI's cancer database. There are separate sections for professionals and patient information in PDQ, as well as directories of physicians and cancer care organizations. The *Journal of the National Cancer Institute* is available online to subscribers. In addition, there are links to other cancer literature Internet sites. (some features fee-based) http://cnetdb.nci.nih.gov/cancerlit.html

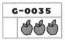

National Library of Medicine (NLM): Online Databases This site offers links to and descriptions of the databases and electronic information sources provided by the National Library of Medicine. Topics covered include bioethics, biotechnology, cancer information, clinical trials, consumer information, HIV/AIDS resources, history of medicine, population information, and toxicology and environmental health information. Links provided include MEDLINE via PubMed; MCA/MR; a multiple congenital anomaly/mental retardation database; and MEDLINEplus, information for consumers. Hyperlinks on each topic offer further information on the resources available and how to access them. http://www.nlm.nih.gov/databases/databases.html

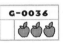

National Library of Medicine (NLM): PubMed PubMed is a free MEDLINE search service, from the National Library of Medicine, providing access to over 11-million citations with links to the full text of articles from more than 4,000 biomedical journals. Probably the most heavily used and reputable free MEDLINE site, PubMed permits advanced searching by subject, author, journal title, and many other fields. It includes an easy-to-use "citation matcher" for completing and identifying references, and its PreMEDLINE database provides journal citations before they are indexed, making this version of MEDLINE more up-to-date than most.
http://www.ncbi.nlm.nih.gov/PubMed

National Library of Medicine Gateway Designed as a "one-stop shopping" portal for Internet users seeking information in the extensive National Library of Medicine collections, the NLM Gateway offers an extremely convenient and powerful search tool to simultaneously search multiple retrieval systems at NLM. Information for both professionals and consumers is drawn from MEDLINE, a bibliographic database containing more than 11-million journal citations from 1966 to the present; OLDMEDLINE, journal citations from 1958 to 1965; MEDLINEplus, consumer health information on more than 400 topics; and MEDLINEplus drug information covering more than 9,000 drugs. Additional resources at NLM include LOCATORPlus, a catalog of records for books, serials, and audiovisual materials; DIRLINE, a directory of health organizations, research resources, projects, and databases; meeting abstracts from AIDS meetings and health services research (HSR) meetings; as well as information on HSR projects in progress. Links on the site direct visitors to information on ordering documents, clinical trials, clinical alerts, TOXNET (a toxicology database), and the health services/technology assessment text (HSTAT) database. http://gateway.nlm.nih.gov/gw/Cmd

14.4 FEDERAL HEALTH AGENCIES

GENERAL RESOURCES

Federal Web Locator This is a useful search engine for links to federal government sites and information on the World Wide Web. The locator maintains separate sections of latest additions, quick jumps, and Web servers. Users can also search by agency name.
http://www.infoctr.edu/fwl

HEALTH AND HUMAN SERVICES

Department of Health and Human Services This site lists Department of Health and Human Services agencies and provides links to the individual agency sites. It offers news, press releases, and information on accessing HHS records and contacting HHS officials. It also provides a search engine for all federal HHS agencies and access to HealthFinder.
http://www.os.dhhs.gov

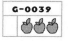

Administration for Children and Families This site provides descriptions of, resources for, and links to ACF programs and services. These sites detail programs and services that relate to areas such as welfare and family assistance, child support, foster care and adoption, Head Start, and support for Native Americans, refugees, and the developmentally disabled. Updated news and information are provided as well.
http://www.acf.dhhs.gov

Administration on Aging (AOA) This site provides resources for seniors, practitioners, and caregivers. Resources include news on aging, links to Web sites on aging, statistics about older people, consumer fact sheets, retirement and financial planning information, and help finding community assistance for seniors.
http://www.aoa.dhhs.gov

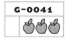

Agency for Healthcare Research and Quality (AHRQ) The Agency for Healthcare Research and Quality (AHRQ) site offers healthcare professionals clinical information, research findings, quality assessment, and information on funding opportunities. In the clinical information section there are evidence-based practice reports, outcomes research findings, technology assessments, preventive services, and clinical practice guidelines. Users may also access data and surveys such as the medical expenditure panel survey and an interactive tool

for hospital statistics, a publications catalog, and an electronic reading room. A section of the site is dedicated to consumers and offers fact sheets on health conditions, health plans, prescriptions, prevention, quality of care, smoking cessation, and surgery. Some fact sheets are available in Spanish.
http://www.ahrq.gov/

Agency for Toxic Substances and Disease Registry The mission of this agency is "to prevent exposure and adverse human health effects and diminished quality of life associated with exposure to hazardous substances from waste sites, unplanned releases, and other sources of pollution present in the environment." To this end, the site posts national alerts and health advisories. It provides answers to frequently asked questions about hazardous substances and lists the minimal risk levels for each of them. The site offers the HazDat database, developed to provide access to information on the release of hazardous substances from Superfund sites or from emergency events as well as to information on the effects of hazardous substances on the health of human populations. The quarterly *Hazardous Substances and Public Health Newsletter* is available at the site, as are additional resources for children, parents, and teachers. http://www.atsdr.cdc.gov/atsdrhome.html

Centers for Medicare & Medicaid Services Formerly the Health Care Financing Administration (HCFA), Information on Medicare, Medicaid, and child health insurance programs is provided at this site. Statistical data on enrollment in the various programs as well as analysis of recent trends in healthcare spending, employment, and pricing is also provided. The site offers consumer publications and program forms which are available for download.
http://www.hcfa.gov

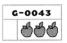

Food and Drug Administration (FDA) The FDA is one of the oldest consumer protection agencies in the United States, monitoring the manufacture, import, transport, storage, and sale of about $1 trillion worth of products each year. This comprehensive site provides information on the safety of foods, human and animal drugs, blood products, cosmetics, and medical devices. The site also contains details of field operations, current regulations, toxicology research, medical products reporting procedures, and answers to frequently asked questions. Users can search the site by keyword and find specific information targeted to consumers, industry, health professionals, patients, state and local officials, women, and children.
http://www.fda.gov

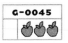

Indian Health Service The Indian Health Service provides federal health services to American Indians and Alaskan Natives. Information of interest to physicians is primarily contained in the "About the IHS" section. This section offers access to the Native Health Research bibliographic database, with some entries containing full-text articles. There is also a Native Health History database covering the years 1652-1970. Clinical practice guideline information is provided, including IHS patient education protocols. Also within this section is

an IHS facility locator. The site also describes their programs under the "Medical Programs" section, relating to such topics as AIDS, child health, diabetes, and elder care. In addition, there is information on health professional jobs, scholarships, and office locations.
http://www.ihs.gov

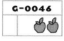

National Center for Toxicological Research Charged with supporting the U.S. Food and Drug Administration's regulatory needs by researching the effects of toxicity and improving human exposure and risk assessment methods, the National Center for Toxicological Research describes their activities on this site. Under the "Science" section, there are descriptions of NCTR research projects, a bibliography of related NCTR publications, and the full text of the report on each year's activities.
http://www.fda.gov/nctr/index.html

National Guideline Clearinghouse (NGC) The National Guideline Clearinghouse (NGC) is a database of evidence-based clinical practice guidelines and related documents produced by the Agency for Healthcare Research and Quality, in partnership with the American Medical Association and the American Association of Health Plans. Users can search the database by keyword or browse by disease category.
http://www.guidelines.gov/index.asp

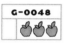

Public Health Service The Public Health Service is an umbrella organization consisting of many health service agencies and programs. Their site offers links to public health service agencies such as the National Institutes of Health, the Centers for Disease Control and Prevention, and the U.S. Food and Drug Administration. Links to offices dedicated to public health include the Office of Minority Health and the Office of Women's Health. In addition, Health and Human Services' vacancy announcements are available at the site. The site is linked directly to the Office of the Surgeon General, providing transcripts of speeches and reports, a biography of the current Surgeon General, and a history and summary of duties associated with the position.
http://www.hhs.gov/phs/

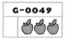

Substance Abuse and Mental Health Services Administration Examining substance abuse and mental illness, the Substance Abuse and Mental Health Services Administration site offers resources dedicated to the prevention, treatment, and rehabilitation of these conditions. The site features SAMHSA programs and centers, namely the Center for Mental Health Services, the Center for Substance Abuse Prevention, and the Center for Substance Abuse Treatment. Information clearinghouses on the site feature online booklets, fact sheets, and conference proceedings from these three centers. There is also information on their managed care initiative, including reports on quality improvement, policy studies, and technical assistance and training. Grant opportunities, along with data and statistics on substance abuse and mental illness, are included. A public information section offers easy-to-understand publications as well as directories of service providers. http://www.samhsa.gov

NATIONAL INSTITUTES OF HEALTH (NIH)

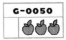

National Institutes of Health (NIH) The NIH is one of eight health agencies of the Public Health Service which, in turn, is part of the U.S. Department of Health and Human Services. The NIH mission is to uncover new knowledge that will lead to better health for everyone. NIH works toward that mission by conducting research in its own laboratories; supporting the research of non-federal scientists in universities, medical schools, hospitals, and research institutions throughout the country and abroad; helping in the training of research investigators; and fostering communication of biomedical information. The site provides employment and summer internship program information, science education program details, and a history of the NIH. A site search engine and links to the home pages of all NIH institutes and centers are available. http://www.nih.gov

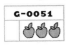

Center for Information Technology The Center for Information Technology incorporates the power of modern computers into the biomedical programs and administrative procedures of the NIH by conducting computational biosciences research, developing computer systems, and providing computer facilities. The site provides information on the activities and organization of the center, as well as links to many useful information technology sites. http://www.cit.nih.gov/home.asp

Center for Scientific Review The Center for Scientific Review is the focal point at NIH for the conduct of initial peer review, the foundation of the NIH grant and award process. The center carries out a peer review of the majority of research and research training applications submitted to the NIH. The center also serves as the central receipt point for all Public Health Service applications and makes referrals to scientific review groups for scientific and technical merit review of applications and to funding components for potential award. To this end, the center develops and implements innovative, flexible ways to conduct referral and review for all aspects of science. The site contains transcripts of public commentary panel discussions, news and events listings, grant applications, peer review notes, and links to additional biomedical and government sites. http://www.drg.nih.gov

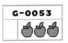

Fogarty International Center The Fogarty International Center for Advanced Study in the Health Sciences leads NIH efforts to advance the health of the American public and citizens of all nations through international cooperation on global health threats. Resources at the site include the center's publications, regional information on programs and contacts, research and training opportunities, a description of the center's Multilateral Initiative on Malaria

(MIM), details of the NIH Visiting Program for Foreign Scientists, and news and vacancy announcements.
http://www.nih.gov/fic

National Cancer Institute (NCI) The National Cancer Institute (NCI) leads a national effort to reduce the burden of cancer morbidity and mortality, ultimately to prevent the disease. Through basic and clinical biomedical research and training, the NCI conducts and supports programs to understand the causes of cancer; prevent, detect, diagnose, treat, and control cancer; and disseminate information to the practitioner, patient, and public. The site provides visitors with many informational resources related to cancer, including Cancer-Trials for clinical trials resources and CancerNet for information on cancer tailored to the needs of health professionals, patients, and the general public. Additional resources relate to funding opportunities as well as to events and research at NCI.
http://www.nci.nih.gov

National Center for Biotechnology Information (NCBI) A comprehensive site that provides a wide array of biotechnology resources, the center includes sources such as a genetic sequence database (GenBank); links to related sites, a newsletter, and genetic sequence search engines; information on programs, activities, and research projects; seminar and exhibit schedules; and database services. Databases available through this site include PubMed for free access to MEDLINE searches and the Online Mendelian Inheritance in Man (OMIM) for an extensive catalog of human genes and genetic disorders.
http://www.ncbi.nlm.nih.gov

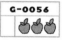

National Center for Complementary and Alternative Medicine (NCCAM) The National Center for Complementary and Alternative Medicine identifies and evaluates unconventional healthcare practices; supports, coordinates, and conducts research and research training on these practices; and disseminates information. The site describes specific program areas; answers common questions about alternative therapies; and offers news, research grants information, and a calendar of events. Information resources include a citation index related to alternative medicine obtained from MEDLINE; a bibliography of publications; the NCCAM clearinghouse of information for the public, media, and healthcare professionals; and a link to the National Women's Health Information Center. http://nccam.nih.gov

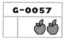

National Center for Research Resources The National Center for Research Resources creates, develops, and provides a comprehensive range of human, animal, technological, and other resources to support biomedical research advances. The center's areas of concentration are biomedical technology, clinical research, comparative medicine, and research infrastructure. The site offers specific information on each of these research areas, grants information, news, current events, press releases, publications, and research resources.
http://www.ncrr.nih.gov

National Eye Institute (NEI)   The National Eye Institute (NEI) conducts and supports research, training, health information dissemination, and other programs with respect to blinding eye diseases, visual disorders, mechanisms of visual function, preservation of sight, and the special health problems and requirements of the visually impaired. Information at the site is tailored to the needs of researchers, health professionals, the general public and patients, educators, and the media. Resources include a clinical trials database, intramural research information, funding, grants, a news and events calendar, publications, and an overview of the NEI offices, divisions, branches, and laboratories.
http://www.nei.nih.gov

National Heart, Lung, and Blood Institute (NHLBI)   The National Heart, Lung, and Blood Institute (NHLBI) provides leadership for a national research program in diseases of the heart, blood vessels, lungs, and blood, and in transfusion medicine through support of innovative basic, clinical, and population-based health education research. The site provides health information; scientific resources; research funding information; news and press releases; details of committees, meetings, and events; clinical guidelines; notices of studies seeking patient participation; links to laboratories at the NHLBI; and technology transfer resources. Highlights of the site include cholesterol, weight, and asthma management resources.
http://www.nhlbi.nih.gov

National Human Genome Research Institute   The National Human Genome Research Institute supports the NIH component of the Human Genome Project, a worldwide research effort designed to analyze the structure of human DNA and determine the location of the estimated 50,000-100,000 human genes. The NHGRI Intramural Research Program develops and implements technology for understanding, diagnosing, and treating genetic diseases. The site provides information about NHGRI, the Human Genome Project, grants, intramural research, policy and public affairs, workshops and conferences, and news items. Resources include links to the institute's Ethical, Legal, and Social Implications Program and the Center for Inherited Disease Research, genomic and genetic resources for investigators, and a glossary of genetic terms.
http://www.nhgri.nih.gov

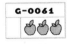

National Institute of Allergy and Infectious Diseases (NIAID)   The National Institute of Allergy and Infectious Diseases provides support for scientists conducting research aimed at developing better ways to diagnose, treat, and prevent the many infectious, immunologic, and allergic diseases that afflict people worldwide. This site provides NIAID news releases, a calendar of events, links to related sites, a clinical trials database, grants and technology transfer information, and current research information including meetings, publications, and research resources. Fact sheets are available for different immunological disorders, allergies, asthma, and infectious diseases.
http://www.niaid.nih.gov

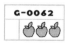
G-0062

National Institute of Arthritis and Musculoskeletal and Skin Diseases (NIAMS) NIAMS conducts and supports a broad spectrum of research on normal structure and function of bones, muscles, and skin, as well as the numerous and disparate diseases that affect these tissues. NIAMS also conducts research training and epidemiologic studies in addition to disseminating information. The site provides details of research programs at the institute and offers personnel and employment listings, news, and an events calendar. Health information is provided in the form of fact sheets, brochures, health statistics, and other resources. Scientific resources include bibliographies of publications, consensus conference reports, grants and contracts applications, grant program announcements, and links to scientific research databases. Information on current clinical studies and transcripts of NIAMS advisory council, congressional, and conference reports are also available at the site.
http://www.nih.gov/niams

G-0063

National Institute of Child Health and Human Development (NICHD) The institute conducts and supports laboratory, clinical, and epidemiological research on the reproductive, neurobiologic, developmental, and behavioral processes that determine and maintain the health of children, adults, families, and populations. Research in the areas of fertility, pregnancy, growth, development, and medical rehabilitation strives to ensure that every child is born healthy and wanted and grows up free from disease and disability. The site provides general information about the institute; funding and intramural research details; information about the Division of Epidemiology, Statistics, and Prevention Research; a publications bibliography; fact sheets; reports; employment and fellowship listings; and research resources. http://www.nichd.nih.gov

G-0064

National Institute of Dental and Craniofacial Research (NIDCR) The National Institute of Dental and Craniofacial Research (NIDCR) provides leadership for a national research program designed to understand, treat, and ultimately prevent the infectious and inherited craniofacial-oral-dental diseases and disorders that compromise millions of human lives. General information about the institute, news and health information, details of research activities, and NIDCR employment opportunities are all found at the site.
http://www.nidr.nih.gov

G-0065

National Institute of Diabetes and Digestive and Kidney Diseases (NIDDK) The National Institute of Diabetes and Digestive and Kidney Diseases conducts and supports basic and applied research and also provides leadership for a national program in diabetes, endocrinology, and metabolic diseases; in digestive diseases and nutrition; and in kidney, urologic, and hematologic diseases. Information at the site includes a mission statement, history, organization description, and employment listing. Additional resources include news; a database for health information; clinical trials information, including a patient recruitment section; and information on extramural funding and intramural research at the institute. http://www.niddk.nih.gov

National Institute of Environmental Health Sciences (NIEHS) The National Institute of Environmental Health Sciences (NIEHS) reduces the burden of human illness and dysfunction from environmental causes by defining how environmental exposures, genetic susceptibility, and age interact to affect an individual's health. News and institute events, research information, grant and contract details, fact sheets, employment and training notices, teacher support, and an online resource for kids are all found at this site. Library resources include a book catalog, electronic journals, database searching, NIEHS publications, and reference resources. Visitors can use search engines at the site to find environmental health information and news, publications, available grants and contracts, and library resources.

http://www.niehs.nih.gov

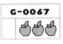

National Institute of General Medical Sciences (NIGMS) The National Institute of General Medical Sciences (NIGMS) supports basic biomedical research that is not targeted to specific diseases but that increases the understanding of life processes and lays the foundation for advances in disease diagnosis, treatment, and prevention. Among the most significant results of this research has been the development of recombinant DNA technology, which forms the basis for the biotechnology industry. The site provides information about NIGMS research and funding programs, information for visitors, news, a publications list, reports, grant databases, employment listings, and links to additional biomedical resources.

http://www.nigms.nih.gov/

National Institute of Mental Health (NIMH) The National Institute of Mental Health (NIMH) provides national leadership dedicated to understanding, treating, and preventing mental illnesses through basic research on the brain and behavior as well as through clinical, epidemiological, and services research. Resources available at the site include information for visitors to the campus, employment opportunities, NIMH history, and publications from activities of the National Advisory Mental Health Council and Peer Review Committees. News, a calendar of events, information on clinical trials, funding opportunities, and intramural research are also provided. Pages tailored specifically for the public, health practitioners, and researchers contain mental disorder information, research fact sheets, statistics, science education materials, news, links to NIMH research sites, and patient education materials.

http://www.nimh.nih.gov

National Institute of Neurological Disorders and Stroke (NINDS) The National Institute of Neurological Disorders and Stroke supports and conducts research and research training on the normal structure and function of the nervous system and on the causes, prevention, diagnosis, and treatment of more than 600 nervous system disorders including stroke, epilepsy, multiple sclerosis, Parkinson's disease, head and spinal cord injury, Alzheimer's disease, and brain tumors. The site provides visitors with an organizational diagram, links to advisory groups, the mission and history of NINDS, employment and training opportunities, and information on research at NINDS. Information is available for patients, clinicians, and scientists. It includes publications, details of current clinical trials, links to other health organizations, and research funding information. http://www.ninds.nih.gov

National Institute of Nursing Research (NINR) The National Institute of Nursing Research (NINR) supports clinical and basic research to establish a scientific basis for the care of individuals across the life span, from management of patients during illness and recovery to the reduction of risks for disease and disability and the promotion of healthy lifestyles. NINR accomplishes its mission by supporting grants to universities and other research organizations as well as by conducting research intramurally. Visitors to this site can find the NINR mission statement and history, employment listings, news, conference details, publications, speech transcripts, answers to frequently asked questions, information concerning legislative activities, research program and funding details, health information, highlights and outcomes of current nursing research, and links to additional Web resources.
http://www.nih.gov/ninr

National Institute on Aging (NIA) The National Institute on Aging (NIA) leads a national program of research on the biomedical, social, and behavioral aspects of the aging process. The goals of the institute include the prevention of age-related diseases and disabilities and the promotion of a better quality of life for all older Americans. The site presents recent announcements and upcoming events, employment opportunities, press releases, and media advisories of significant findings. Research resources include news from the National Advisory Council on Aging, links to extramural aging research conducted throughout the United States, and funding and training information. Health professionals and the general public can access publications on health and aging topics or order materials online.
http://www.nih.gov/nia

National Institute on Alcohol Abuse and Alcoholism (NIAAA) The National Institute on Alcohol Abuse and Alcoholism (NIAAA) conducts research focused on improving the treatment and prevention of alcoholism and alcohol-related problems to reduce the enormous health, social, and economic consequences of this disease. General resources at the site include an introduction to the institute, extramural and intramural research information, an organizational flowchart, details of legislative activities, Advisory Council roster and minutes, information on scientific review groups associated with the institute, and employment announcements. Institute publications, data tables, press releases, conferences and events calendars, answers to frequently asked questions on the subject of alcohol abuse and dependence, and links to related sites are also available. The ETOH Database, an online bibliographic database containing over 100,000 records on alcohol abuse and alcoholism, can be accessed from the site, as can the National Library of Medicine's MEDLINE database.
http://www.niaaa.nih.gov:80

National Institute on Deafness and Other Communication Disorders (NIDCD)   The National Institute on Deafness and Other Communication Disorders (NIDCD) conducts and supports biomedical research and research training in the normal and disordered processes of hearing, balance, smell, taste, voice, speech, and language. The institute also conducts and supports research and research training related to disease prevention and health promotion; addresses special biomedical and behavioral problems associated with people who have communication impairments or disorders; and supports efforts to create devices that substitute for lost and impaired sensory and communication function. The site provides visitors with fact sheets and other information resources on hearing and balance; smell and taste; voice, speech, and language; hearing aids; otosclerosis; vocal abuse and misuse; and vocal cord paralysis. Other resources include a directory of organizations related to hearing, balance, smell, taste, voice, speech, and language; a glossary of terms; an online newsletter; information for children and teachers; and clinical trials details. Information on research funding and intramural research activities, a news and events calendar, and general information about NIDCD are also available.
http://www.nidcd.nih.gov

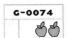

National Institute on Drug Abuse (NIDA)   The National Institute on Drug Abuse (NIDA) site offers resources for healthcare professionals, featuring news, events, research updates, and special NIDA Web sites covering common drugs of abuse, such as steroids and club drugs. There are also sections on drug abuse research and prevention, grant funding, international opportunities, and legislative issues. The publications section offers online publications as well as items for purchase. Research training at NIDA, as well as the proceedings from their scientific meetings, can also be found. A comprehensive list of related resources is provided.
http://www.nida.nih.gov/

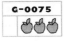

National Library of Medicine (NLM)   The National Library of Medicine (NLM), the world's largest medical library, collects materials in all areas of biomedicine and healthcare and focuses on biomedical aspects of technology; the humanities; and the physical, life, and social sciences. This site contains links to government medical databases, including MEDLINE and MEDLINE-plus; information on funding opportunities at the NLM and other federal agencies; and details of services, training, and outreach programs offered by NLM. Users can access NLM's catalog of resources (LOCATORPlus), as well as NLM publications, including fact sheets, published reports, and staff publications. NLM research programs discussed at the site include topics in computational molecular biology, medical informatics, and other related subjects. The Web site features 15 searchable databases, covering journal searches via MEDLINE; AIDS information via AIDSLINE, AIDSDRUGS, and AIDSTRIALS; bioethics via BIOETHICSLINE; and numerous other important topics. The NLM Gateway—a master search engine—searches MEDLINE using the user-friendly retrieval engine called PubMed. There are more than 11-million citations in MEDLINE and PreMEDLINE and the other related databases. Additionally, the

NLM provides sources of health statistics, serials programs, and services maintained through a system called SERHOLD.
http://www.nlm.nih.gov

G-0076

Warren Grant Magnuson Clinical Center The Warren Grant Magnuson Clinical Center is the clinical research facility of the National Institutes of Health, supporting clinical investigations conducted by the NIH. The clinical center was designed to bring patient-care facilities close to research laboratories, allowing findings of basic and clinical scientists to move quickly from the laboratory to the treatment of patients. The site provides visitors with news, events, details of current clinical research studies, patient recruitment resources, links to departmental Web sites, and information resources for NIH staff, patients, physicians, and scientists. Topics discussed in the center's Medicine for the Public Lecture Series and resources in medical and scientific education offered by the center are included at the site.
http://www.cc.nih.gov:80

CENTERS FOR DISEASE CONTROL AND PREVENTION

G-0077

Centers for Disease Control and Prevention (CDC) The mission of the Centers for Disease Control and Prevention is to promote health and quality of life by preventing and controlling disease, injury, and disability. The site provides users with links to nearly a dozen associated centers, institutes, and offices; a Web page devoted to travelers' health; publications, software, and other products; data and statistics; training and employment opportunities; and subscription registration forms for online CDC publications. Highlighted publications include the *Emerging Infectious Disease Journal* and the *Morbidity and Mortality Weekly Report,* both of which can be received by e-mail on a regular basis. The CDC offers a comprehensive, alphabetical list of general and specific health topics as well as links to additional CDC resources and state and local agencies concerned with public health issues. Visitors can also search the site by keyword and read spotlights on current research and information.
http://www.cdc.gov

G-0078

Epidemiology Program Office Information and resources on public health surveillance are provided by the Epidemiology Program Office at this Web address. Publications and software related to epidemiology are available for download. Updated news, events, and international bulletins are also featured at the site. http://www.cdc.gov/epo/index.htm

G-0079

National Center for Chronic Disease Prevention and Health Promotion Maintained by the CDC, this site focuses on many different aspects of chronic disease prevention. Intended for healthcare professionals, the site provides facts on the economic burden of chronic disease, risk prevention, and comprehensive approaches to prevention. Resources available in the chronic diseases section include information on the center's programs; reports; and fact

sheets for arthritis, cancer, cardiovascular disease, diabetes, epilepsy, and oral diseases. Additional links provide information on specific populations such as pregnant women and minorities.
http://www.cdc.gov/nccdphp/index.htm

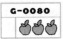

National Center for Environmental Health   The National Center for Environmental Health Web page offers information on the center's programs and activities related to the prevention of health problems from environmental hazards. The health topics section offers an A-to-Z listing of topics covered on the site, including such issues as the prevention of birth defects by the use of folic acid. The publications section offers fact sheets, brochures, and scientific publications on issues such as lead poisoning and the indoor use of pesticides. There is also an index of articles from the *Morbidity and Mortality Weekly Report*. In addition, the site offers current employment opportunities and information on training programs. Spanish and child-oriented versions of the NCEH site are also available.
http://www.cdc.gov/nceh/default.htm

National Center for Health Statistics (NCHS)   The National Center for Health Statistics Web page features health data and statistics on a broad array of topics including AIDS, chickenpox, divorce, and obstetrical procedures. Visitors can read descriptions of the NCHS survey and data collection systems; healthcare professionals can learn how to include their patients in the surveys. A "Data Warehouse" section offers tabulated data on the national and state level, as well as an international classification of diseases. A link to FASTATS A-to-Z provides national statistics, along with links for more comprehensive data. There is also information on NCHS research and development.
http://www.cdc.gov/nchs/default.htm

National Center for HIV, STD, and TB Prevention   Part of the CDC, the National Center for HIV, STD, and TB Prevention offers general information for professionals and the public on the control and prevention of HIV/AIDS, sexually transmitted diseases, and tuberculosis. The home page highlights news and CDC updates. Information of interest to professionals is accessed by clicking on the link for "Site Highlights" in the sidebar menu; among the highlights is a link to the National Prevention Information Network, which offers information on HIV/AIDS, STD, and TB and the connections between them. By clicking on a disease, visitors will find resources, related links, a bulletin board, distance learning, publications, and FAQs. The site also features a database of organizations that provide HIV/AIDS, STD, and TB prevention, education, healthcare, and social services. CDC laboratory research is accessible including disease information and reports, and the top of the home page has a link for funding opportunities.   http://www.cdc.gov/nchstp/od/nchstp.html

National Center for Infectious Diseases   Dedicated to the study of infectious diseases, the National Center for Infectious Diseases Web page provides an A-to-Z listing of disease information with links to fact sheets, laboratory assistance information, and related articles. Visitors can access the NCID online journal, *Emerging Infectious Diseases,* with full-text articles. There are also articles, booklets, and a video on preventing emerging infectious diseases. Data and reports on diseases can also be found under "Surveillance Resources." A link to "DPDx" features reviews on parasites and parasitic diseases, diagnostic procedures, diagnostic assistance, and an image library. A travel section covers region-specific issues, diseases, recommended vaccinations, and tips. In addition, the publications section offers many free online brochures. A short list of related links is provided.

http://www.cdc.gov/ncidod/index.htm

National Center for Injury Prevention and Control Healthcare professionals and the public will find a broad array of information on injury prevention on this Web page. The site offers fact sheets on injuries and safety such as child passenger safety, fireworks injury prevention, suicide, and fall prevention programs for seniors. The data section features WISQARS, an interactive database of injury-related mortality data. There is also a list of publications, viewable online, as well as information on research funding. Facts and data in categories such as injury care, violence, and unintentional injury are also available. Consumers can click on the SafeUSA link to access safety tips.

http://www.cdc.gov/ncipc/ncipchm.htm

National Immunization Program The National Immunization Program of the CDC offers a wide range of immunization information resources directed to healthcare professionals and consumers. The site features clinical information in categories such as vaccine recommendations; advances in immunization; educational resources, including training for professionals, and vaccine safety. Information on grants and funding, as well as data and statistics. Under the category of "Subsites," visitors can find information on the development of immunization registries, along with downloadable clinical assessment software (CASA) to track immunization practices within an office. Links at the top of the page are provided to publications for both the professional and consumers and to the Web site's Dictionary of Immunization Terms.

http://www.cdc.gov/nip/

National Institute for Occupational Safety and Health (NIOSH) Created to conduct research on work-related illnesses and injuries, the National Institute for Occupational Safety and Health (NIOSH) describes the organization's activities and recommendations on this site. A topic index provides articles and guidelines on issues such as chemical safety, indoor air quality, and latex. The publications section features fact sheets, brochures, and bulletins, with some available online. In addition, there is information on NIOSH research activities, funding opportunities, and training.

http://www.cdc.gov/niosh/homepage.html

National Prevention Information Network Designed to provide information on HIV/AIDS, STDs, and TB, the CDC's National Prevention Information Network site offers useful resources for the healthcare professional and consumer. A bulletin board, distance learning, FAQs, mortality and morbidity reports, and related links are provided in each disease category. A large list of publications is found, along with a database of organizations. Information on the CDC's prevention research is also available with links to numerous reports and journal articles.

http://www.cdcnpin.org/

OTHER HEALTH AGENCIES

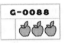

Center for Nutrition Policy and Promotion The Center for Nutrition Policy and Promotion, within the U.S. Department of Agriculture (USDA), conducts research on the nutritional needs of Americans and disseminates their findings. The center's site provides statistical information and resources for educators, contains dietary guidelines for Americans, and offers official USDA food plans. A database on the nutrient content of the U.S. food supply (on a per capita basis) is provided. In addition, there is a 76-page booklet available that offers recipes and tips for healthy meals.

http://www.usda.gov/cnpp

Food and Nutrition Service The Food and Nutrition Service (FNS) of the U.S. Department of Agriculture "reduces hunger and food insecurity in partnership with cooperating organizations by providing children and needy families access to food, a healthful diet, and nutrition education in a manner that supports American agriculture and inspires public confidence." The site provides details of FNS nutrition assistance programs such as food stamps, WIC, and child nutrition. Research, in the form of published studies and reports, is also available at the site.

http://www.fns.usda.gov/fns

Food Safety and Inspection Service The Food Safety and Inspection Service, part of the U.S. Department of Agriculture, is dedicated to food safety. Its site offers news, recall notification on meat and poultry products, a newsletter, and related links. A consumer education section offers fact sheets on the safe handling and cooking of meat, poultry, and eggs. Technical publications and a video library can be accessed under the publications section. Also of interest to professionals is a fellowship program related to food safety, which can be found in the drop-down menu under "Featured Topics." In addition, information on distance learning at the Food Safety Virtual University is provided.

http://www.fsis.usda.gov

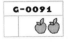

National Bioethics Advisory Commission The National Bioethics Advisory Commission (NBAC) studies bioethical issues related to genetics and the protection of humans as research subjects and directs their reports to the National Science and Technology Council. The NBAC also advises on the applications of their research, including clinical applications. This site lists meeting

dates, full-text transcripts of meetings, and news. Reports they have produced are available for such topics as ethical issues in human stem cell research, research involving persons with mental disorders, and cloning human beings. A list of links to related sites is provided.
http://bioethics.gov/cgi-bin/bioeth_counter.pl

National Science Foundation (NSF): Directorate for Biological Sciences The Division of Integrative Biology and Neuroscience (IBN), part of the National Science Foundation (NSF), supports research aimed at understanding the living organism—plant, animal, or microbe—as a unit of biological organization. Current scientific emphases include biotechnology, biomolecular materials, environmental biology, global change, biodiversity, molecular evolution, plant science, microbial biology, and computational biology, including modeling. Research projects support the education and training of future scientists, including doctoral dissertation research, research conferences, workshops, symposia, Undergraduate Mentoring in Environmental Biology (UMEB), and a variety of NSF-wide activities. This site describes in detail the activities and divisions of IBN and offers award listings and deadline dates for funding applications. http://www.nsf.gov/bio/ibn/start.htm

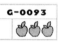

Office of National Drug Control Policy This site states the missions and goals of the ONDCP. It has a clearinghouse of drug policy information with a staff that will respond to the needs of the general public, providing statistical data, topical fact sheets, and information packets. There is information on related science, medicine, and technology. There are also resources on prevention, education, and treatment programs. Information on the enforcement of the policies is provided for the national, state, and local levels.
http://www.whitehousedrugpolicy.gov

14.5 FULL-TEXT ARTICLES

Amedeo Amedeo is a free medical literature service that allows users to select topics and journals in specific areas of interest. Visitors can browse among more than 20 health-related topics for new articles and preselected recommended journals. For each article, links are provided to its abstract and to related articles in PubMed. The service also offers a weekly e-mail with an overview of new articles reflecting specifications indicated by the user, with the option to create a personal home page with abstracts of relevant articles. The site allows registered users to access a network center, which facilitates literature exchange among users with similar interests. This service is supported through educational grants by numerous pharmaceutical companies.
(free registration) http://www.amedeo.com

BioMed Central: Online Journals Produced by the commercial publisher, Current Science Group, BioMed Central makes full-text peer-reviewed articles available on this Web page. The site's content is grouped by subject into journals

published by BMC including *BMC Cancer, BMC Infectious Diseases, BMC Surgery,* and *BMC Pediatrics.* Each journal's articles are available for download in PDF format. http://www.biomedcentral.com/browse/medicine/

CatchWord   There are more than 1,100 journals on a variety of subjects available on this Web page. Visitors can view the journal's table of contents and abstracts, then purchase full-text articles online. Institutions can utilize the services of CatchWord to provide a single interface to their online journal collections. Approximately 20 specialties of medicine are found, including cardiology, oncology, and psychiatry.

(some features fee-based) http://www.catchword.co.uk/

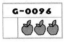

EurekAlert   This site allows professionals and consumers to search the archives for the latest articles, press releases, news items, events, awards, and grants in broad areas of science, including chemistry and physics. The "Medicine and Health" section covers nearly 70 topics including Alzheimer's disease, diabetes, fertility, and sleep disorders. Under each heading, press releases are categorized by date and provide the source and contact information.

http://www.eurekalert.org

Free Medical Journals.com: Full-Text Articles Healthcare professionals will find more than 550 free medical journals on this site with access to full-text articles. The site organizes the journals into categories that indicate whether the journal is free, free one to six months after publication, free one year after publication, or free two years after publication. However, the home page only shows a fraction of what is available; visitors should click on "Journals Sorted by Specialty" on the left side of the page to view all of the journals. Specialties include AIDS, cardiology, dermatology, hematology, oncology, infectious diseases, psychiatry, rheumatology, and pediatrics. Some journals are available in other languages. Visitors can register for an alert service that will e-mail information on new free online journals as they become available.

http://www.freemedicaljournals.com/

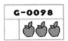

HighWire Press: Full-Text Articles   Stanford University's HighWire Press, developer of the Web versions of many important biomedical journals, maintains this extensive listing of links to full-text journal archives. A list of journals offering free access is provided at this site, with a notation indicating whether a title is free, free for a trial period, or free for back issues. More than 100 journals are listed, and a link on the left side of the page brings up a list of full-text science archives on the Web. http://highwire.stanford.edu/lists/freeart.dtl

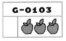

Ingenta   This enormous database of medical and nonscientific journals' tables of contents permits searching by keyword, journal title, or author. Full articles can be obtained by fax or e-mail for a fee. As the result of a merger between Ingenta and UnCover, an integrated service provides tables of contents for specific journals as they are published and added to the database. Ingenta UnCover users can log in to Ingenta using their UnCover profile ID and password.

(some features fee-based) http://www.ingenta.com

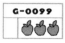

Journal Watch Online Subscribers to the Journal Watch service can access summaries, written by physicians, of the most recent clinical research literature for many subspecialties at this Web site. Produced by the Massachusetts Medical Society, publishers of the *New England Journal of Medicine,* Journal Watch updates its summaries four times a week in the areas of dermatology, cardiology, psychiatry, women's health, infectious diseases, neurology, and gastroenterology. Research summaries and commentary are drawn from approximately 50 journals, including general medical and specialty journals, to provide a broad range of coverage. Sample summaries are also available.
(fee-based) http://www.jwatch.org/

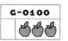

MD Consult Physicians can access the full text of nearly 40 major medical textbooks and nearly 50 core medical journals on this Web site. Journals available on the site include *Arthritis and Rheumatism,* the *Cancer Journal, Chest,* and the *Journal of the American Academy of Dermatology.* The site also offers the ability to search MEDLINE and other key databases simultaneously in order to locate full-text articles. Other features include clinical practice guidelines, CME modules, patient education handouts, and prescription information. A 10-day free trial of full site access is available for physicians.
(fee-based) http://www.mdconsult.com/

MEDLINE Journal Links to Publishers Through the National Library of Medicine, MEDLINE provides direct access to hundreds of medical journals in all fields, listed alphabetically by name, with direct links to their respective publishers. Upon accessing an individual publication, the reader can view the current issue table of contents and abstracts for the articles. Some articles are available without charge while others require a fee. Each page explains the available information and the conditions for access since policies vary by publisher and journal. http://www.ncbi.nlm.nih.gov/entrez/journals/loftext_noprov.html

Medscape Visitors to this site can access more than 25,000 full-text articles from more than 40 journals and medical news periodicals. Medical journals include *Chest, American Heart Journal,* and *Southern Medical Journal.* The site also features "Journal Scan," clinical summaries of the latest literature for specialties such as cardiology, dermatology, infectious diseases, psychiatry, and respiratory care. There are also several online textbooks available. (free registration)
http://www.medscape.com/Home/Topics/
multispecialty/directories/dir-MULT.JournalRoom.html

PubList: Health and Medical Sciences This site contains a list of links to thousands of medical journals, divided by subject areas. Information such as frequency, publisher, and format is included for each publication, as well as links to the publication. A search engine can be used to identify titles of interest.
http://www.publist.com/indexes/health.html

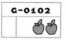

PubMed Central: Full-Text Article Archive PubMed Central is a digital library with archives of life sciences literature. It was developed and is managed by the National Center for Biotechnology Information and the National Library

of Medicine. Currently, eight journals with full-text articles and archives are found on the site with 10 more slated for addition in the future. Available journals include all BioMedCentral journals (see separate write-up of this site), *Arthritis Research, Breast Cancer Research,* and the *British Medical Journal.* Many of these journals delay release of their full-text content to this site, with the most current content available at their own sites on a subscription basis.
http://www.pubmedcentral.nih.gov/

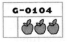

University of Georgia: Science Library An A-to-Z listing of science journals available on the Internet is provided on this site. The list can be navigated by clicking on the appropriate letter at the bottom of the site. Some journals can only be accessed by faculty and students at the University of Georgia.
http://www.libs.uga.edu/science/fullalph.html

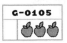

WebMedLit WebMedLit provides access to the latest medical literature on the Web by indexing medical Web sites daily and presenting articles from each site organized by subject categories. All WebMedLit article links are from the original source document at the publisher's Web site, and most articles are available in full text.
http://webmedlit.silverplatter.com/index.html

14.6 GOVERNMENT INFORMATION DATABASES

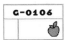

Agency for Healthcare Research and Quality (AHRQ): Search Tool This site offers a search tool to find information located on the Agency for Healthcare Research and Quality Web page. There is information appropriate to professionals and the public.
http://www.ahcpr.gov/query/query.htm

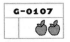

Centers for Disease Control and Prevention (CDC): Web Search Both healthcare professionals and consumers can find useful information using the search tool provided on the CDC site. Visitors have the opportunity to search all CDC Web sites by keyword and to search state health departments. By checking the box next to the state health department of interest, one can search one or more of them or all of them at once.
http://www.cdc.gov/search.htm

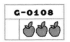

Combined Health Information Database Designed as a bibliographic database, the Combined Health Information Database (CHID) draws upon health information from health-related federal agencies. The database is categorized under nearly 20 health topics such as Alzheimer's, cancer, diabetes, and weight control. Searches can be limited to individual subtopics, or the database can be searched in its entirety. Access to information is only available through a keyword search, which can be done with a simple or detailed search. Results include health promotion and educational materials aimed at consumers and not indexed elsewhere.
http://chid.nih.gov/

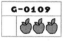

CRISP: Computer Retrieval of Information on Scientific Projects

Funded by the NIH, CRISP is a database of federally funded biomedical research projects conducted at universities, hospitals, and other research institutions. Users, including the public, can use CRISP to search for scientific concepts, emerging trends, and techniques or to identify specific projects and/or investigators. http://www-commons.cit.nih.gov/crisp

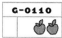

Department of Energy: Comprehensive Epidemiologic Data Resource

Compiled by the U.S. Department of Energy, this site features a collection of resources on health and radiation exposure data related to DOE installations. Included are data from epidemiologic studies performed by DOE-funded investigators on health and mortality, classic radiation, and dose reconstruction. The site also covers studies of populations living near DOE installations and other studies on radiation effects, such as those on atomic bomb survivors. http://cedr.lbl.gov/

FedWorld Information Network

Information from many federal agencies can be accessed through this Web page. By clicking on the database section at the top of the page, visitors will find links to 20 databases encompassing a variety of information such as Supreme Court decisions, EPA Clean Air Act data, and U.S. Customs Headquarter's rulings. The home page features search tools for the entire FedWorld network, U.S. government reports, and U.S. government Web sites. (some features fee-based) http://www.fedworld.gov/

Government Databases in Health

Maintained by St. Mary's University of San Antonio, Texas, this site features a list of more than 25 selected government sites dealing with health and medicine. Sites covered include those on clinical trials, Congressional Research Service reports, food composition data, and MEDLINE; each site listed has a description of its contents. (free registration) http://library.stmarytx.edu/acadlib/doc/electronic/dbhealth.htm

Government Information Locator Service

Visitors to this site can search for government information across several federal agencies, such as the Department of Health and Human Services and the Environmental Protection Agency, at the same time. The agencies listed on the site have compiled their public information on the same server for easy access to a wide variety of information. http://www.access.gpo.gov/su_docs/gils/index.html

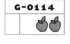

Healthfinder

Healthfinder provides links to public medical or health sciences libraries on the Internet. Directories of libraries are also available to find local facilities, library organizations, and research and reference resources. http://www.healthfinder.gov/scripts/SearchContext.asp?topic=14332&section=5

MEDLINEplus

A comprehensive database of health and medical information, MEDLINEplus serves a different purpose from its sister service, MEDLINE, which is a bibliographic search engine to locate citations and abstracts in medical journals and reports. MEDLINEplus offers the ability to search by topic and obtain full information rather than citations. One can search body systems, disorders and diseases, treatments and therapies, diagnostic procedures, side effects, and numerous other important topics related to personal health and the field of medicine in general.

http://www.nlm.nih.gov/medlineplus/medlineplus.html

14.7 HEALTH AND MEDICAL HOTLINES

Toll-Free Numbers for Health Information A categorized list of hundreds of toll-free health information hotlines is provided by this site. Each hotline provides educational materials for patients.

http://www.health.gov/nhic/NHICScripts/
Hitlist.cfm?Keyword=Toll%2DFree%20Information%20Services

14.8 HEALTH INSURANCE PLANS

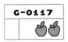

HealthPlanDirectory.com Produced by a commercial marketing company, DoctorDirectory.com, this site contains a directory of health insurance plans, listed by state. Contact information for each plan is provided.

http://www.doctordirectory.com/healthplans/directory/default.asp

14.9 HEALTHCARE LEGISLATION AND ADVOCACY

American Medical Association (AMA): AMA in Washington The purpose of this site is to encourage physicians around the country to get involved in the AMA's grassroots lobbying efforts. It covers information on legislation relevant to the medical profession, the AMA's congressional agenda, and educational programs available through the AMA on political activism for physicians. The Web site is updated regularly with the latest news on medical issues in the government.

http://www.ama-assn.org/ama/pub/category/4015.html

American Medical Group Association: Public Policy and Political Affairs The AMGA provides legislative advocacy to medical groups, addressing current political debates in the medical community. Updated legislative and media alerts, an electronic newsletter for members, and comments and testimony on several subjects affecting healthcare providers are offered. Relevant Web sites of interest are accessible. (some features fee-based)

http://www.amga.org/AMGA2000/PublicPolicy/index_publicPolicy.htm

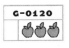

American Medical Student Association: Health Policy AMSA is an organization that attempts to improve healthcare and medical education. Its "Health Policy" department contains news of legislation that affects medical education, educational information on how to be a health policy activist, and a

listing of printable documents concerning relevant health policy issues such as gene patents and prescription drug coverage.
http://www.amsa.org/hp/hpindex.cfm

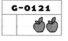

American Medical Women's Association AMWA promotes issues related to women's health and professional development for female physicians. The site's advocacy and actions sections contain articles on news and legislation that are relevant to these issues and also give advice on how to get involved.
http://www.amwa-doc.org/index.html

THOMAS: U.S. Congress on the Internet Within THOMAS, one can find information on bills, laws, reports, or any current U.S. federal legislation. *Congressional Record*, the official record of the proceedings of the U.S. Congress, and committee information are also available. The site's search engine can be used to find current congressional bills by keyword or bill number.
http://thomas.loc.gov

14.10 HOSPITAL RESOURCES

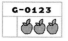

American Hospital Association An extremely broad range of resources pertaining to hospitals is available either at this site or at a link from this site, including advocacy, health insurance, hospital information, research and education, health statistics, and valuable links to the National Information Center for Health Services Administration as well as other organizations and resources.
http://www.aha.org

HospitalDirectory.com This useful site provides a listing of states and territories, each of which is a direct link to a further listing of cities in the state or territory. By clicking on a city, the database provides a listing of hospitals in that area including name, address, and telephone numbers. The site also offers other links pertaining to health plans, doctors, health news, insurance, and medical products for physicians.
http://www.doctordirectory.com/hospitals/directory

HospitalWeb This site is a guide to hospitals throughout the world that have sites established on the World Wide Web. Under each country, the names of a number of hospitals in that country are listed. By clicking on the hospital name, the user is taken to the hospital's Web site which provides further information.
http://neuro-www2.mgh.harvard.edu/hospitalwebworld.html

14.11 INTERNET MEDICAL NEWSGROUPS

Internet newsgroups are places where individuals can post messages on a common site for others to read. Many newsgroups are devoted to medical topics, and these groups are listed below. To access these groups you can either use a newsreader program (often part of an e-mail program) or search and browse using a popular Web site, groups.google.com

On the Google site, visitors can look for one of the newsgroup names listed below, such as sci.med, by either browsing the list of newsgroups or searching by the group name. Once there, the forum appears as a bulletin board with a posting on a particular topic, followed by responses to it. One can navigate the discussion by clicking on the postings of interest or post a reply.

Since newsgroups are mostly unmoderated, there is no editorial process or restrictions on postings. The information at these groups is therefore neither authoritative nor based on any set of standards.

sci.med	sci.med.nutrition	sci.med.vision
sci.engr.biomed	sci.med.occupational	alt.image.medical
sci.med.aids	sci.med.orthopedics	alt.med
sci.med.cardiology	sci.med.pathology	alt.med.allergy
sci.med.dentistry	sci.med.pharmacy	alt.med.cfs
sci.med.diseases.cancer	sci.med.physics	alt.med.ems
sci.med.diseases.hepatitis	sci.med.prostate.bph	alt.med.equipment
sci.med.diseases.lyme	sci.med.prostate.cancer	alt.med.fibromyalgia
sci.med.diseases.viral	sci.med.prostate.prostatitis	alt.med.outpat.clinic
sci.med.immunology	sci.med.psychobiology	alt.med.phys-assts
sci.med.informatics	sci.med.radiology	alt.med.urum-outcomes
sci.med.laboratory	sci.med.telemedicine	alt.med.veterinary
sci.med.nursing	sci.med.transcription	alt.med.vision.improve

14.12 LOCATING A PHYSICIAN

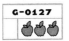

American Medical Association (AMA): Physician Select Online Doctor Finder The AMA is the primary "umbrella" professional association of physicians and medical students in the United States. The AMA Physician Select system provides information on virtually every licensed physician, including more than 690,000 physicians and doctors of osteopathy. According to the site, physician credentials have been certified for accuracy and authenticated by accrediting agencies, medical schools, residency programs, licensing and certifying boards, and other data sources. The user can search for physicians by name or by medical specialty. http://www.ama-assn.org/aps/amahg.htm

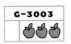

DoctorDirectory.com This commercial site contains a directory of physicians, organized by specialty. Within the specialties, visitors can click on the state and city of interest. Results include the physician's name, gender, graduation year, specialties, and address.
http://www.doctordirectory.com/doctors/directory/default.asp?newSession=true

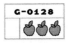

HealthPages This search tool allows visitors to locate doctors in their area by specialty and location. Over 500,000 physicians and 120,000 dentists are listed. Doctors may update their profiles for free. Local provider choices are displayed to consumers in a comparative format. They can access charts that compare the training, office services, and fees of local physicians; the provider networks and quality measures of area managed care plans; and the size, services, and fees of local hospitals. Patients can post ratings and comments about their doctors. http://www.thehealthpages.com

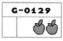

Physicians' Practice   This site allows the user to search for doctors in many specialty areas. Searches are performed by specialty and zip code. Physicians must pay a fee to be listed but enjoy benefits such as referrals, Internet presence, and a newsletter. http://www.physicianpractice.com

14.13   MEDICAL AND HEALTH SCIENCES LIBRARIES

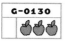

Medical Libraries at Universities, Hospitals, Foundations, and Research Centers   This site includes an up-to-date listing of libraries that can be accessed through links produced by staff members of the Hardin Library at the University of Iowa. Libraries are listed by state, enabling easy access to hundreds of library Web sites. Numerous foreign medical library links are also provided. http://www.lib.uiowa.edu/hardin-www/hslibs.html

National Institutes of Health (NIH): Library Online   Information on the NIH Library is presented on this site, including current exhibits, hours, materials available to NIH personnel and the general public, current job vacancies, maps for visitors, and answers to frequently asked questions about the library. Users can search the library's catalog of books, journals, and other periodicals; access public and academic medical databases; and find seminar and tutorial information as well as links to related sites. http://nihlibrary.nih.gov

National Library of Medicine (NLM)   The National Library of Medicine, the world's largest medical library, collects materials in all areas of biomedicine and healthcare and works on biomedical aspects of technology, the humanities, and the physical, life, and social sciences. This site contains links to government medical databases, including MEDLINE and MEDLINEplus; information on funding opportunities at the National Library of Medicine and other federal agencies; and details of services, training, and outreach programs offered by NLM. Users can access NLM's catalog of resources (LOCATORPlus), as well as NLM publications, including fact sheets, published reports, and staff publications. NLM research programs discussed at the site include topics in computational molecular biology, medical informatics, and other related subjects. The Web site features 15 searchable databases, covering journal searches via MEDLINE; AIDS information via AIDSLINE, AIDSDRUGS, and AIDSTRIALS; bioethics via BIOETHICSLINE; and numerous other important topics. The NLM Gateway, a master search engine, searches MEDLINE using the retrieval engine called PubMed. It is very user-friendly. There are over 11-million citations in MEDLINE and PreMEDLINE and the other related databases. Additionally, the NLM provides sources of health statistics, serials programs, and services maintained through a system called SERHOLD. http://www.nlm.nih.gov

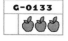

National Network of Libraries of Medicine   Composed of eight regional libraries, the NN/LM provides access to numerous other health science libraries

in each region, located at universities, hospitals, and institutes. The Web site enables the user to link directly to each of the libraries in any region of the United States. These libraries have access to the NLM's SERHOLD system database of machine-readable holdings for biomedical serial titles. There are approximately 89,000 serial titles that are accessible through SERHOLD-participating libraries. http://nnlm.gov/

14.14 MEDICAL CONFERENCES AND MEETINGS

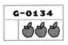

Doctor's Guide: Medical Conferences and Meetings This address lists several hundred conferences and meetings, including continuing medical education programs worldwide, organized by date, meeting site, and subject. Location and other details are provided. http://www.docguide.com/crc.nsf/web-byspec

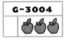

EventOnline.org Sponsored by Excerpta Medica, this site offers a comprehensive database of medical, biotechnical, and scientific events. Search results yield contact information, as well as a basic description of the event. Some events have links to the sponsor's Web page. In addition, there are links for weather, hotels, and maps to assist in planning a visit. http://www.eventonline.org/

Medical Conferences.com A broad range of medical conference listings is covered on this site, including meetings related to many different areas of healthcare, such as pharmaceuticals and hospital supplies, as well as the clinical medical specialties. An easy-to-use search mechanism provides access to the numerous listings, each of which links to details concerning each conference. The site is updated daily, providing details on over 7,000 forthcoming conferences. http://www.medicalconferences.com

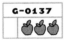

MediConf Online This site categorizes conferences by medical subject and provides information on conference dates, location, and organizer, mostly covering meetings to be held in the next month or two. The listings include research conferences, seminars, annual meetings of professional societies, medical technology trade shows, and opportunities for CME credits. The information provided free on the Internet is only a small percentage of the complete fee-based database, which includes more than 60,000 listings of meetings to be held through 2014 and is available through the information vendors, Ovid or Dialog. (some features fee-based) http://www.mediconf.com/online.html

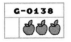

Medscape: Multispecialty Conference Schedules Medical conference schedules are posted on this Web page, courtesy of Medscape. The schedules are listed chronologically and categorized by specialties such as family medicine, pediatrics, nursing, and radiology. Conference dates, addresses, Web site links, and contact information are provided. http://www.medscape.com/Home/Topics/ multispecialty/directories/dir-MULT.ConfSchedules.html

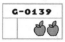

Physician's Guide to the Internet Dates and locations for major national medical meetings are listed alphabetically by association at this site. There are also hyperlinks to association pages for additional information.
http://www.physiciansguide.com/meetings.html

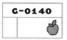

Princeton Medicon: The Medical Conference Resource Details regarding worldwide major medical conferences of interest to medical specialists and primary care professionals are featured on this site. It is also periodically published in printed form. Access to lists of meetings is provided through a search engine that permits searching by specialty, year, and geographic region.
http://www.medicon.com.au

14.15 MEDICAL DATABASE SERVICES

American Chemical Society: SciFinder This site provides information on the SciFinder research database, designed for scientists to use for searching Chemical Abstracts and MEDLINE. The database system contains more than 16-million abstracts, with links to full-text articles. Users can search by company name, chemical reactions, substructure, or keyword. Subscription information for research organizations is provided.
(fee-based) http://www.cas.org/SCIFINDER/scicover2.html

Cambridge Scientific Abstracts: Internet Database Service More than 50 bibliographic databases and electronic journals can be searched through this site. Databases include MEDLINE, TOXLINE, and other science/technology databases such as Biotechnology & Bioengineering. CSA-published electronic collections of abstracts, called "journals," such as *Genetics Abstracts, Medical & Pharmaceutical Biotechnology Abstracts,* and *Virology and AIDS Abstracts,* are also included.
(fee-based) http://www.csa.com/csa/ids/ids-main.shtml

Cochrane Library An international working group of experts has developed the Cochrane Library database with evidence-based medicine reviews by specialty and a bibliography of controlled trials. Searching, browsing, and displaying of abstracts is available free of charge; full access is available only to subscribers. (fee-based) http://www.cochranelibrary.com/enter/

Database of Abstracts of Reviews of Effectiveness Quality-assessed reviews of the literature are compiled in the Database of Abstracts of Reviews of Effectiveness (DARE) database of evidence-based medicine, courtesy of the University of York. Reviews included have been assessed and selected for their high methodological value. Searches return structured abstracts that state the author's objective, intervention, participants included, and outcomes assessed. Additional information includes the sources searched, methods by which data was extracted, and results. A complete guide to searching the DARE database is provided. http://agatha.york.ac.uk/darehp.htm

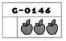

EBSCO Information Services EBSCO information services provides subscription services for biomedical libraries plus access to numerous electronic journals and databases, some with full-text articles, such as Alternative Medicine, CancerLit, International Pharmaceutical Abstracts, and MEDLINE. (fee-based) http://www.epnet.com/database.html

Electric Library The Electric Library is an online database containing full-text articles from more than 150 newspapers; hundreds of magazines; national and international news wires; 2,000 books; photos; maps; television, radio, and government transcripts; and a free, complete encyclopedia. There is a 10-day free trial period. (fee-based) http://wwws.elibrary.com

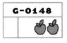

Information Quest Information Quest seeks to link publishers, libraries, and the research audience electronically. The database is divided into libraries including life sciences, medicine, and physical sciences. Each library offers access to hundreds of journals and their abstracts; some have full-text articles. (fee-based) http://www.informationquest.com/

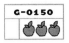

Institute for Scientific Information A list of the bibliographic databases and research information available to Institute for Scientific Information (ISI) subscribers is provided on this site. Database topics include biotechnology, clinical medicine, and neuroscience. In addition, many of these databases provide citation searching capabilities through the ISI search tool, Web of Science, the unique search feature for which ISI is known. Users can find all of the published materials that have cited a particular work, regardless of discipline. (fee-based) http://www.isinet.com/isi/products/index.html

International Digital Electronic Access Library The International Digital Electronic Access Library (IDEAL) offers users access to the full text of journals published by Academic Press, Churchill Livingstone, W. B. Saunders, Bailliere Tindall, and Mosby. There are also full-text reference encyclopedias related to immunology, human nutrition, virology, food microbiology, spectroscopy and spectrometry, and forensic sciences. Subscriptions are available for libraries; individuals can access articles on a pay-per-view basis. (fee-based) http://www.idealibrary.com

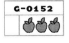

LINK: Online Library: Medicine The LINK online library, dedicated to medicine, lists more than 100 journals, many containing full-text articles. The site can be searched and abstracts viewed free of charge; access to full-text articles requires a subscription. (some features fee-based) http://link.springer.de/ol/medol/index.htm

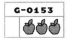

Manual, Alternative, and Natural Therapy (MANTIS) Database The MANTIS database contains citations and abstracts for healthcare disciplines such as acupuncture, alternative medicine, chiropractic, herbal medicine, homeopathy, naturopathy, osteopathic medicine, physical therapy, and traditional Chinese medicine. The database covers domestic and international sources for more than 1,000 journals. (fee-based) http://www.healthindex.com/MANTIS.asp

G-0154

Ovid Medical Databases Bibliographic databases available through Ovid include MEDLINE and EMBASE for medicine and allied health, CINAHL for nursing, and BIOSIS for bioscience. Ovid's clinical products include resources on evidence-based medicine and drug information as well as decision support reference texts and journals. In total, there are more than 80 commercial bibliographic databases available. The Ovid interface offers many advanced search features, including links to full-text articles, and for most databases it incorporates database-specific thesauri to promote retrieval of relevant results. (fee-based) http://www.ovid.com/products/databases/index.cfm

 G-0155

ScienceDirect Described as the "largest online full-text platform for scientific, technical, and medical information," the ScienceDirect database offers more than one million full-text articles from more than 1,200 journals, most published by Elsevier Science. Subject areas include biochemistry, clinical medicine, microbiology and immunology, pharmacology and toxicology, and neurosciences. Subscriptions are available only to libraries. (fee-based) http://www.sciencedirect.com/science/page/static/scidir/static_scidir_splash_about.html

 G-0156

SilverLinker A new service from SilverPlatter.com, SilverLinker offers more than 2.5 million Internet links to over 6,500 journals and 2-million articles from more than 90 SilverPlatter databases. The SilverLinker database Internet links take visitors directly from citations to full-text articles. (fee-based) http://www.silverplatter.com/silverlinker/index.htm

 G-0157

SilverPlatter: Medical and Pharmaceutical Collection Full-text access to research, clinical findings, policy issues, and practice is available through this collection of databases. The databases include MEDLINE, EMBASE, International Pharmaceutical Abstracts, Patient Education Library, Biological Abstracts, and Drug Information Fulltext. (fee-based) http://www.silverplatter.com/hlthsci.htm

 G-0158

STNEasy This site provides subscribers with a user-friendly interface for searching a variety of databases covering bioscience, health, medicine, and pharmacology. More than 30 databases are listed under "Medicine." A new feature called eScience provides relevant Web content by automatically entering the user's search terms into the Google or Chemindustry.com search engines. Users are charged by the length of time spent searching for information. (fee-based) http://stneasy.fiz-karlsruhe.de/html/english/login1.html

 G-0159

SwetsnetNavigator More than 5,000 journals related to medicine are found in the SwetsnetNavigator database, some with access to full-text articles. This tool is designed to help institutions organize access to the tables of contents and full text for the titles to which they subscribe. Journals published by major biomedical publishers, such as Academic Press, Elsevier, and Kluwer, are included. (fee-based) http://www.swetsnet.nl/cgi-bin/SB_main

14.16 MEDICAL EQUIPMENT AND MANUFACTURERS

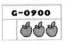
G-0900

Medical Equipment and Pharmaceutical Companies An A-to-Z listing of medical equipment and pharmaceutical manufacturers is provided on this site, courtesy of the Andrews School of Medical Transcription. The list is comprehensive with hyperlinks to hundreds of companies.
http://www.mtdesk.com/mfg.shtml

14.17 MEDICAL GLOSSARIES

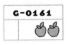
G-0161

Boston University: Pharmacology Glossary Provided by the Boston University School of Medicine, this Web page features a glossary of terms and symbols used in pharmacology. Each word has a definition and related terms.
http://www.bumc.bu.edu/www/busm/pharmacology/Programmed/framedGlossary.html

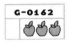
G-0162

CancerWEB: Online Medical Dictionary This site offers a comprehensive medical dictionary online for clinical, medical student, and patient audiences. It is a convenient source for a quick definition of an unfamiliar term.
http://www.graylab.ac.uk/omd/index.html

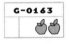
G-0163

drkoop.com: Insurance This site provides descriptions of both terms and phrases relating to health insurance. Terms are listed alphabetically.
http://www.drkoop.com/hcr/insurance/glossary.asp

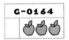
G-0164

HealthAnswers.com: Disease Finder A wide range of diseases is listed in this alphabetical directory of information for patients and consumers. Visitors can search by keyword or browse the directory for information. Details include alternative names, definitions, causes, incidence, risk factors, prevention, symptoms, signs and tests, treatment, prognosis, and complications. Many helpful diagrams or representative photographs related to the condition are also provided. http://www.healthanswers.com/Library/library_fset.asp

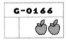
G-0166

Immunology Glossary A glossary of immunology is featured on this Web page, courtesy of the University of Leicester, Department of Microbiology and Immunology, in the United Kingdom. The entire glossary can be browsed at once since it is all located on this one page.
http://www-micro.msb.le.ac.uk/MBChB/ImmGloss.html

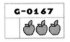
G-0167

InteliHealth: Vitamin and Nutrition Resource Center InteliHealth offers this comprehensive glossary of vitamins and minerals, listed under fat-soluble vitamins, water-soluble vitamins, and minerals. Information provided under each entry includes important facts about the vitamin or mineral, daily intake recommendations for men and women, benefits, food sources, amounts of the substance present in various food sources, and cautions in terms of health consequences of the overuse or deficiency of the substance.
http://www.intelihealth.com/IH/ihtIH/WSIHW000/325/20932.html

Don't type in long URLs – add the site number to the eMedguides URL: www.eMedguides.com/**G-1234**.

MedicineNet.com: Medications An index of medications is featured on this Web page, produced by MedicineNet. Of interest to both professionals and consumers, the index consists of an A-to-Z listing of prescription and over-the-counter drugs. Each drug has information such as its generic name, brand names, drug class and mechanism, storage, reasons for use, dosing, drug interaction, and side effects. In addition, each drug has links to further information such as related diseases, medications, and health facts.
http://www.medicinenet.com/Script/Main/Alphaldx.asp?li=MNI&p=A_PHARM

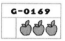

MedicineNet.com: Procedures and Tests Index By clicking on "Procedures and Tests" at the top of the MedicineNet.com Web page, visitors will find a comprehensive, user-friendly index to common and not-so-common diagnostic tests and treatment procedures. Each diagnostic and treatment mini-forum contains a main article for general information, outlining the purpose and safety of the procedure, related diseases and treatments, articles written by physicians on related topics of interest, and interesting related consumer health facts. http://www.medicinenet.com

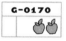

National Human Genome Research Institute: Genetics Glossary The National Human Genome Research Institute has developed this online glossary of genetic terms. The glossary can be browsed alphabetically or searched by keyword. Each term comes with a definition, an audio clip explaining the term, and a list of related terms.
http://www.nhgri.nih.gov/DIR/VIP/Glossary/

Spellex Development: Medical Spell Spellex Medical and Spellex Pharmaceutical online spelling verification allows visitors to check the spelling of medical terms. The search returns possible correct spellings if the word entered was not found.
http://www.spellex.com/speller.htm

Stedman's Shorter Medical Dictionary (1943): Poisons and Antidotes Posted as an item of historical interest only, this site features poisons and their antidotes from *Stedman's Shorter Medical Dictionary* (1943). An alphabetical listing of poisons is provided; each has a description of symptoms and appropriate treatment.
http://www.botanical.com/botanical/steapois/poisonix.html

University of Texas: Life Science Dictionary This free online dictionary designed for the public and professionals contains terms that deal with biochemistry, biotechnology, botany, cell biology, and genetics. The dictionary also contains some terms relating to ecology, limnology, pharmacology, toxicology, and medicine. The search engine allows the user to search by a specific term or by a term contained within a definition.
http://biotech.icmb.utexas.edu/search/dict-search.html

14.18 MEDICAL JOURNALS & PUBLISHERS

 MedBioWorld: Medical Journals Main Index Visitors to this address will find comprehensive listings of online journals, categorized by specialty topic. Major broad-coverage medical journals, nursing journals, science journals, and books on medical writing are also listed through the site, as well as links to many publishers' Web sites.

http://www.medbioworld.com/journals/medicine/med-bio.html

 Academic Press This site lists a variety of journals published by Academic Press, a Harcourt Science and Technology Company. By clicking on "Biomedical Sciences" in the "Subject Categories" drop-down box, a listing of journals is presented including *Epilepsy and Behavior, Experimental Neurology, Seminars in Cancer Biology,* and *Virology.* A table of contents, along with abstracts, is available at no charge. Full-text articles can be purchased individually online or viewed by subscribers.

(some features fee-based) http://www.academicpress.com/journals/

 Annual Reviews: Biomedical Sciences Volumes of the *Annual Reviews* for biomedical sciences are listed on this site; each review offers in-depth analysis and commentary on current topics from the previous year. Subjects include genomics and human genetics, immunology, and medicine. Visitors can access abstracts of articles from the current and past volumes. Full-text articles are available online to subscribers.

(some features fee-based) http://arjournals.annualreviews.org/biomedicalhome.dtl

 Ashley Publications Ltd. The Ashley publishing group offers journals related to pharmacology, including *Expert Opinions* on biological therapy, pharmacotherapy, emerging drugs, investigational drugs, therapeutic patents, and therapeutic targets. In addition to free sample issues, visitors can access tables of contents and abstracts from back issues of each journal. Subscribers can access full-text articles.

(some features fee-based) http://www.ashley-pub.com/html/journals.asp

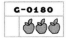 **Blackwell Science** This site offers online access to information regarding over 200 Blackwell Science publications. Journals are sorted alphabetically by title and are available in all major fields of science and medicine. Blackwell Science provides a good general overview regarding the content and aim of each of its journals. Tables of contents are available for current and back issues of each title. Access to abstracts and articles requires a fee.

(some features fee-based) http://www.blackwell-science.com/uk/journals.htm

 Brookwood Medical Publications of PJB Publications Five journals related to clinical research are described on this site: the *Journal of Drug Assessment,* the *Journal of Clinical Research,* the *Journal of Outcomes Research, Good Clinical Practices Journal,* and the *Journal of Medical Economics.* Abstracts of selected articles are available on the site. There is also a link to PharmaProjects, a leading pharmaceutical intelligence database available only on a subscription basis. http://www.pjbpubs.co.uk/pjb5a.htm

Cambridge University Press   Journal titles available from Cambridge University Press are listed at this address. Topics encompass all subject areas, but many are devoted to medical specialties. The journals can be browsed alphabetically, by subject, and by online availability; tables of contents are provided. Visitors can browse both current and archived issues and journals can be ordered online. http://www.cup.org/journal/

Carden Jennings Publishing Co, Ltd.   The Carden Jennings medical multimedia publishing division offers journals, online publications, CD-ROMs, and books. Abstracts and free full-text articles (in Adobe Acrobat PDF format) are available online for journals including the *Biology of Blood and Marrow Transplantation, Laboratory Hematology,* and the *Heart Surgery Forum.* http://www.cjp.com/stories/storyReader$6

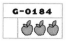

Elsevier Science   Covering all Reed-Elsevier publications related to medicine, this site includes a subject index for access to individual journals in a variety of specialties including cardiology, obstetrics and gynecology, and psychiatry. Free sample copies of the journals are available online. Information is also included on Elsevier's books, CD-ROMs, and related products. http://www.elsevier.com

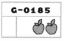

Gordon and Breach Publishing Group   This section of the Gordon and Breach Web page offers books, journals, and magazines related to medical and life sciences. Journals are available in anesthesiology, cardiology, general medicine, hematology, nuclear medicine, oncology, pediatrics, and surgery. Tables of contents are available for current and past issues. Some journals have a link to online full-text articles for subscribers. (some features fee-based) http://www.gbhap-us.com/medical.htm

Guilford Press   A publisher of psychology, psychiatry, and behavioral health publications, Guilford Press offers PDF samples of each of its journals. Information includes a list of titles available online and ordering details. http://www.guilford.com/cartscript.cgi?page=home.html&cart_id=202303.24572

Hanley & Belfus   A list of over 10 medical journals published by Hanley & Belfus is provided on this site. Titles include *Academic Medicine, Journal of Cancer Education,* and *Prehospital Emergency Care.* Tables of contents and article abstracts are available online. Subscribers can read full-text articles. (some features fee-based) http://www.hanleyandbelfus.com/browse.asp?category=5

Harcourt Health Sciences   Information on journals published by the Harcourt Health Sciences group, which includes Churchill Livingstone, IMNG, JEMS Communications, Mosby, and W. B. Saunders, is presented on this site. By clicking on "Find a Journal by Specialty," visitors can access journals related

to topics such as cardiology, endocrinology, and oncology. Tables of contents and subscription information are provided.
http://www.harcourthealth.com/scripts/om.dll/serve?action=home

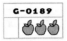

Harcourt International   International medical journals published by Harcourt are provided on this site, sorted into more than 75 specialties. Topics covered include clinical cancer, gastroenterology, midwifery, and surgery. Visitors can access the tables of contents and abstracts to current and back issues of the journals. Full-text articles are available for a fee.
(some features fee-based) http://www.harcourt-international.com/journals/jsbrowse.cfm

Haworth Medical Press   Information on the Haworth Medical Press, an imprint of the Haworth Press, is provided at this site including a listing of its 15 medical journals. The online catalog provides additional information on the journals, including a section for reader reviews.
http://www.haworthpressinc.com/imprints/details.asp?ID=HMP

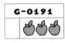

HighWire Press   HighWire Press presents a list of its biomedical journals, organized alphabetically or by subject, including detailed information regarding the features available at no charge for each title. For each journal there is a link to its home page, where tables of contents and abstracts are available. The full text of entire journals or back issues is available for many titles.
http://highwire.stanford.edu

Karger   Medical journals published by Karger are listed alphabetically on this site. The abstracts and tables of contents of current and back issues are available online. Subscribers can access full-text articles. A free sample copy of each journal is available online.
(some features fee-based) http://www.karger.com/journals/index.htm

Kluwer Academic Publishers   Journals of interest in medicine and related subjects are listed on this page. Journal categories include cardiology, internal medicine, neurology, oncology, and urology. Visitors can browse through the table of contents of each publication for current and archived issues or conduct searches by keyword for returns of specific articles.
http://kapis.www.wkap.nl/jrnlsubject.htm/E+0+0+0

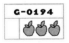

Lippincott Williams & Wilkins   Medical and scientific journals published by Lippincott Williams & Wilkins can be browsed by specialty on this site. There are more than 80 specialties and subspecialties represented. A table of contents, abstracts, and subscription information are provided for each journal, including full-text access options and links. http://www.lww.com/periodicals.htm

Marcel Dekker   Scientific, technical, and medical journals published by Marcel Dekker are listed on this site. By clicking on "Medicine," journals and other types of publications can be searched. There are more than a dozen journals related to medicine, including the *Journal of Toxicology, Immunopharmacology and Immunotoxicology,* and the *Journal of Asthma.* The tables of contents and abstracts are free. Many full-text articles are available online to subscribers. (some features fee-based) http://www.dekker.com/index.jsp

Mary Ann Liebert, Inc. This site offers more than 50 journals and 25 books published by Mary Ann Liebert, Inc., in the field of biotechnology. Journal titles include *AIDS Patient Care and STDs, Microbial Drug Resistance,* and *Thyroid.* General information on each journal is provided, as well as the table of contents for current and archived issues, and a free sample copy.
http://www.liebertpub.com/journals/default1.asp

Medical Economics Company The Medical Economics Company site offers healthcare professionals journals and newsletters related to the diagnosis and treatment of disease. Journals include *Contemporary OB/GYN, Contemporary Urology, Contemporary Pediatrics,* and the *Journal of the American Academy of Physician Assistants.* Journals have their own Web sites and some include full-text articles. In addition, there are clinical newsletters.
(some features fee-based) http://www.medec.com/

Munksgaard New titles, along with an alphabetical index of more than 70 scientific, technical, and medical journals, are provided on this site, which also allows visitors to view journals by subject. The journals are international in scope. General information on each journal is provided, along with a sample issue. Subscribers can access some of the journals online.
(some features fee-based) http://journals.munksgaard.dk/

Nature Publishing Group of Macmillan Publishers, Ltd. An alphabetical list of more than 25 specialist medical journals is provided on this Web site, along with the *Nature* scientific specialty journals. Titles include the *European Journal of Human Genetics, Leukemia,* and the *Hematology Journal.* Tables of contents and abstracts are available online. There is also an online sample copy. Full-text articles are available only to subscribers.
(some features fee-based) http://www.naturesj.com/sj/journals/journals_index.html

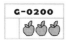

Oxford University Press Medical journals from Oxford University Press are listed on this site. There are over 20 journals listed; each publication offers tables of contents and abstracts. Subscribers can access full-text articles. A free e-mail alert service is available to receive, in advance, the table of contents for new issues. (some features fee-based) http://www.oup.co.uk/medicine/journals/

Parthenon Publishing Group Links to more than a dozen journals published by Parthenon are featured on this Web page. Titles include *Gynecological Endocrinology,* the *Aging Male,* the *Journal of Drug Evaluation,* and the *Journal of Maternal-Fetal Medicine.* The table of contents from the most recent issue of each journal is posted. In addition, a catalog of the group's books, slides, videos, and CD-ROMs is provided.
http://www.parthpub.com/journal.html

Pulsus Group   The Pulsus Group offers information at this site on journals published by the group for specialties such as plastic surgery, cardiology, gastroenterology, infectious diseases, and pediatrics. Visitors can access abstracts and full-text articles in some of the journals.
http://www.pulsus.com/

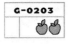

SLACK Inc.   In addition to journals, this site lists books, Internet resources, and symposia on the Web for a variety of medical specialties, allied health, and nursing subspecialties. A sample table of contents along with general information about each journal is provided. Visitors must scroll down the page to view the entire index of publications.
http://www.slackinc.com/areas.asp

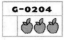

Springer   Covering the large list of journals published by Springer-Verlag, this site primarily contains abstracts rather than full-text articles. Full-text articles are available for individuals or institutions who maintain print subscriptions. The site covers a broad range of biomedical titles, all of which provide tables of contents from the most recent years.
(some features fee-based) http://link.springer.de/ol/medol/index.htm

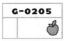

Swets & Zeitlinger   The journal catalog of Swets & Zeitlinger is featured on this Web site. Journals related to health can be found under life sciences, neuroscience, ophthalmology, and psychology. The list of journals includes *Pharmaceutical Biology, Neuro-Ophthalmology,* and the *Clinical Neuropsychologist.* Tables of contents and abstracts for the current issue, as well as back issues, of each journal are available.
http://www.swets.nl/sps/journals/jhome.html

Taylor & Francis Group   Journals are listed by subject on this site and include the behavioral sciences, biomedical sciences, and biosciences. The journals are international in nature. Although the table of contents is free, access to the articles is by subscription only.
(some features fee-based) http://www.tandf.co.uk/journals/sublist.html

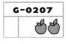

Thieme   There are over 30 medical journals listed on this Web page published by the German publisher Thieme. Topics covered include pediatric surgery, reproductive medicine, liver disease, and perinatology. Selected article citations are provided.
http://www.thieme.com/SID1997012758581/journals/index.html

VSP: International Science Publishers   A listing of more than 40 VSP journals is offered on this site. The journals cover a broad array of sciences; titles of interest to healthcare professionals include *Gene Therapy and Regulation, Haematologia, Inflammopharmacology,* and *Trauma Quarterly.* The tables of contents from previous issues are online. A free sample issue of any journal can be requested through the Web site.
http://www.vsppub.com/journals/index.html

Wiley Interscience This site is maintained by John Wiley and Sons, Inc., and provides a subject index to all Wiley journals. More than 90 journals are listed under the "Life and Medical Sciences" section. Free registration allows access to tables of contents and abstracts published within the last 12 months. Full-text access is available via registration to both individual and institutional subscribers of the print counterparts of the Wiley online journals.

(some features fee-based) http://www3.interscience.wiley.com/journalfinder.html

14.19 MEDICAL NEWS

1st Headlines: Health The "Health" section of this news information site offers a keyword search engine for access to nationwide health news derived from more than 70 daily publications and reputable broadcast and online networks, including *USA Today's* health section, Reuters Health, MSNBC, and drkoop.com. News coverage includes treatment discoveries, pharmacological updates, the latest in managed care, product recalls, and hundreds of other breaking news bulletins.

http://www.1sthealthnews.com/index.htm

American Medical Association (AMA): American Medical News Published by the American Medical Association, *American Medical News* is "the newspaper for America's physicians." The site offers free access to the latest issue online, with each electronic publication providing coverage of top stories, legislative updates, and professional issues. Business information and the ability to read a mobile edition on any handheld device are provided, as well as archived issues and e-mail headline alerts.

http://www.ama-assn.org/public/journals/amnews/amnews.htm

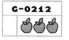

CNN: Health News Health News from CNN is produced in association with WebMD. Specific articles are available in featured topics, ethics matters, research, and home remedies, and an allergy report is also provided. National and international health news is presented, and users can access specific articles on AIDS, aging, alternative medicine, cancer, children's health, diet and fitness, men's health, and women's health. Visitors can also access patient questions and answers from doctors, chat forums, and special community resources available through WebMD. Information and articles are also offered by Mayo Clinic and AccentHealth.com.

http://www.cnn.com/HEALTH

Doctor's Guide: Medical and Other News This site provides current medical news and information for health professionals. Visitors can search the Doctor's Guide medical news database and access medical news Webcasts within the past week or the past month. News items organized by subject, first-hand conference communiques, and journal club reviews are also available at this informative news site.

http://www.pslgroup.com/MEDNEWS.HTM

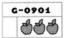

MDLinx MDLinx offers daily medical journal articles organized by sub-specialty. There are nearly 25 medical fields as well as areas in allied health represented in the menu at this home page. Each field is further categorized into subspecialties, providing articles in each area. Article selections are updated daily to reflect the release of new issues of monthly journals.
http://www.mdlinx.com

Medical Breakthroughs Daily news updates are posted and can be delivered to individual e-mail addresses from this site. Visitors can also search archived articles by keyword, read weekly general interest articles, find links to related sites, and watch videos related to current health issues. The site is sponsored by Ivanhoe Broadcast News, Inc., a medical news gathering organization providing stories to television stations nationwide.
(free registration) http://www.ivanhoe.com/#reports

Reuters Health The Reuters Health Web page provides breaking medical news, updated daily, as well as a subscription-based database of the news archives of reuters news service. Visitors can access MEDLINE and a database of drug information from the site.
(some features fee-based) http://www.reutershealth.com

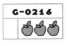

UniSci: Daily University Science News This site offers current articles related to all branches of science, including medicine. Many medical articles are available, and special archives offer additional medical resources. Users can access news from the past 10 days and perform searches for archived material.
http://unisci.com

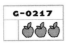

USA Today: Health *USA Today's* feature stories and headline archives are directly accessible at this Web site where visitors can view some of the best in nationwide medical news coverage. Articles are listed by topic, including addiction, AIDS, allergies, alternative medicine, arthritis, cancer, diabetes, genetics, hepatitis, mental health, surgery, and vision. Visitors will also find the latest in medical and pharmacotherapeutic research.
http://www.usatoday.com/life/health/archive.htm

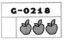

Yahoo!: Health Headlines Updated several times throughout the day, "Health Headlines" at Yahoo offers full news coverage and Reuters news with health headlines from around the globe. Earlier daily and archived stories may be accessed, and the site's search engine allows viewers to browse, with full color, the latest in photographic coverage of news and events.
http://dailynews.yahoo.com/headlines/hl

14.20 MEDICAL SEARCH ENGINES

Additional resources can be found under the General Medical Supersites.

Achoo Healthcare Online   A directory of Web sites in three main categories—human health and disease, business of health, and organizations and sources—is featured on this Web page. Extensive subcategories and short descriptions are provided for each site. Daily health news of interest to patients, the public, and medical professionals is available at the site, as well as links to journals, databases, employment directories, and discussion groups.
http://www.achoo.com

AlltheWeb   Visitors can search the Web in more than 25 languages using this search tool. The option to search for pictures, videos, MP3 files, or FTP files is also featured.   http://www.alltheweb.com

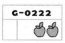

Biocrawler: The Life Science Search Engine   Described as a life science search engine, this Web page contains a large directory with thousands of Internet sites. The directory can be searched by keyword or by clicking on a particular topic such as anthropology, biotechnology, genetics, bioinformatics, and biomedicine. There is also a directory of biology-related jobs that have been posted on the Internet.
http://www.biocrawler.com/

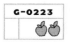

Citeline.com Search Tool   The search tool on this Web page allows visitors to search the Web by keyword and, if desired, to limit the search to any or all of the following categories: disease and treatment, organizations, news and journals, and research and trials.
(free registration) http://www.citeline.com/C1SE/search

CliniWeb International   CliniWeb, a service of Oregon Health Sciences University, provides an index and table of contents for clinical resources available on the World Wide Web. Information found at the site is of particular interest to healthcare professional students and practitioners. Search terms can be entered in five different languages: English, German, French, Spanish, and Portuguese. The site offers links to additional search resources and is linked directly to MEDLINE.   http://www.ohsu.edu/cliniweb

Galen II: The Digital Library of the University of California, San Francisco (UCSF)   This online library directory includes UCSF and UC resources and services, links to the AMA Directory, Drug Info Fulltext, Harrison's Online (requires a password), the *Merck Manual,* Consumer Health, and a database of additional resources and publications including electronic journals. Visitors can search the Galen II database or the World Wide Web using a variety of search engines.
http://galen.library.ucsf.edu

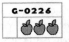 **Google** Google offers a comprehensive search tool, integrating resources from several smaller search engines. Several subject areas are available for more specific queries, including health and related subtopics. Visitors can enter a search term, view Google results, and try the same query through AltaVista, Excite, HotBot, Infoseek, Lycos, and Yahoo through the site.
http://www.google.com

 Health On the Net (HON) Foundation: MedHunt The Health On the Net Foundation provides several widely used medical search engines including MedHunt, HONselect, and MEDLINE. Users can access databases containing information on newsgroups, LISTSERVs, medical images and movies, upcoming and past healthcare-related conferences, and daily news stories on health-related topics. Topical searches yield brief site descriptions, which are ranked by relevance. http://www.hon.ch/MedHunt

 InfoMedical.com: Medical Search Engine This site features a directory with hundreds of medical sites categorized as companies, distributors, products, organizations, services, and Web resources. The directory can be searched or browsed by category. Of interest to physicians, the Web resources section contains clinical trial postings, job postings, online libraries, online medical discussions, and online medical multimedia. Each site has a company profile and a list of their products and services.
http://www.infomedical.com/

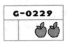 **MDchoice.com** MDchoice.com is a privately held company founded by academic physicians with the goal of making access to health and medical information on the Internet as efficient and reliable as possible. The site features an UltraWeb search with all content selected by board-certified physicians. In addition, users have access to MEDLINE, drug information, health news, and a variety of clinical calculators. Also offered are several interactive educational exercises, online journals and text books, and employment opportunities.
http://www.mdchoice.com

 Med411.com: Medical Research Portal This site offers separate links to a variety of comprehensive search tools, allowing users to search medical libraries, professional associations, online health manuals, peer-reviewed journals, health services, images, and clinical trials. Linked institutions include the National Library of Medicine, the Combined Health Information Database (CHID), CancerNet, the National Institute of Diabetes and Digestive and Kidney Diseases, HealthFinder, and WebPath.
http://www.med411.com/resources.html

 MedExplorer MedExplorer is a comprehensive medical and health directory. Short descriptions of each site are provided. The site also lists related newsgroups and has information on conferences and employment.
http://www.medexplorer.com

Medscape   Medscape provides several databases from which users can search the Web. Resources that can be accessed include articles, news, information for patients, MEDLINE, AIDSLINE, TOXLINE, drug information, a dictionary, a bookstore, the Dow Jones Library, and medical images. There is a wealth of additional information provided including articles, case reports, conference schedules and summaries, CME resources, job listings, journals, news, patient information, practice guidelines, treatment updates, and links to medical specialty sites. Access requires free online registration.
(free registration) http://www.medscape.com

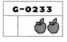

Metacrawler   At the Metacrawler site users can search for Web resources through a directory or a search engine. The search engine offers extensive coverage in the field of medicine.
http://www.metacrawler.com

Search Taxi.com: Health   A directory dedicated to health is featured on this site. There are thousands of sites listed under categories such as alternative medicine, conditions and diseases, medicine, and mental health. These categories are broken down further into topics such as employment, health insurance, men's health, and substance abuse.
http://www.searchtaxi.com/dir/Health/

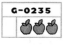

Stanford University: MedBot   Offered by Stanford University, this site allows users to search medical and health resources on the Web using major general and medical search engines. More specific searches can be performed within topics such as education and learning, news and information, and medical images, as well as multimedia resources.
http://www-med.stanford.edu/medworld/medbot

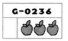

Yahoo!   Yahoo offers visitors the opportunity to search the Web and browse sites listed in multiple categories including health and science. Within each category are more specific subcategories that indicate the number of entries available. Most sites are suggested by users. Additionally, Yahoo offers a wealth of services such as free e-mail, shopping, people search, news, travel, weather, and stock reports.
http://www.yahoo.com/health

14.21   MEDICAL STATISTICS

Centers for Disease Control and Prevention (CDC): Biostatistics/Statistics   This address provides visitors with links to sources of national and regional statistics. Resources include federal, county, and city data, as well as statistics related to labor, current population, public health, economics, trade, and business. Sources for mathematics and software information are also found through this site.
http://www.cdc.gov/niosh/biostat.html

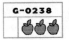

Health Sciences Library System: Health Statistics The University of Pittsburgh's Falk Library of the Health Sciences developed this site to provide information on obtaining statistical health data from Internet and library sources. Resources include details on obtaining statistical data from U.S. population databases, government agencies collecting statistics, organizations and associations collecting statistics, and other Web sites providing statistical information. The site explains specific Internet and library tools for locating health statistics and offers a glossary of terms used in statistics.
http://www.hsls.pitt.edu/intres/guides/statcbw.html

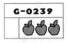

National Center for Health Statistics (NCHS) The National Center for Health Statistics, part of the Centers for Disease Control and Prevention, provides an extensive array of health and medical statistics for the medical, research, and consumer communities. This site provides express links to numerous surveys and statistical sources at the NCHS. http://www.cdc.gov/nchs/default.htm

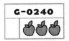

University of Michigan: Statistical Resources on the Web: Health Online sources for health statistics are cataloged at this site, including comprehensive health statistics resources and sources for statistics by topic. Topics include abortion, accidents, births, deaths, disability, disease experimentation, hazardous substances, health insurance, HMOs, hospitals, mental health, nutrition, occupational safety, pregnancy, prescription drugs, risk behaviors, sleep, smoking, substance abuse, surgery, transplants, and vital statistics. Users can also access an alphabetical directory of sites in the database and a search engine for locating more specific resources.
http://www.lib.umich.edu/libhome/Documents.center/sthealth.html

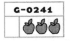

World Health Organization (WHO): Statistical Information System The Statistical Information System of the WHO is intended to provide access to both statistical and epidemiological data and information from this international agency in electronic form. The site provides health statistics, disease information, mortality statistics, AIDS/HIV data, immunization coverage and incidence of communicable diseases, and links to statistics from other countries as well as links to the Centers for Disease Control and Prevention. This site is the premier resource for statistics on diseases worldwide. The WHO main site, http://www.who.int, provides additional disease-related statistics.
http://www.who.int/whosis

14.22 ONLINE TEXTS AND TUTORIALS

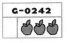

eMedicine: World Medical Library A medical library is featured on this Web page, with online textbooks for professionals and consumers, courtesy of eMedicine. Professionals can read *Emergency Medicine,* and they have access to Gold Standard Multimedia online books. The Gold Standard books focus on basic science such as clinical pharmacology, human anatomy, and immunology. A Gold Standard link provides access to their Web site, where specific books can

be selected from a drop-down menu. Books for consumers include *Consumer Treatment Guidelines* and *Wilderness Emergencies*.
(free registration) http://www.emedicine.com/

Harrison's Online   Directed to physicians, this Web page features the online text of *Harrison's Principles of Medicine*. Each chapter includes information such as diagnosis, prevalence, pathogenesis, clinical features, treatment, complications, and a bibliography. Links are also provided on each topic for related sites, updates, clinical trial information, and self-assessment quizzes.
(fee-based) http://www.harrisonsonline.com/

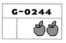

Medical Textbooks Online   Professionals will find a directory of links to online medical textbooks on this Web page maintained by medic8.com. Close to 30 specialties are represented, including geriatric medicine, neurosurgery, microbiology, and pediatrics.
http://www.medic8.com/MedicalTextbooksOnline.htm

Medical Texts on the Internet   This list of medical texts, arranged by specialty, includes access to a variety of medical papers and articles in over 25 areas. Links to documents in cardiology, dermatology, oncology, and urology are included, with each listing a series of related tutorials and texts.
http://members.tripod.com/gustavo_01/textmed.html

Merck Manual of Diagnosis and Therapy   Hosted by Merck, this site features the *Merck Manual of Diagnosis and Therapy*. Primarily of interest to healthcare professionals, the site offers a table of contents with links to a broad range of disorders categorized in sections such as nutritional disorders, gastrointestinal disorders, pulmonary disorders, and pediatrics. In total, there are 23 sections with 308 chapters. Typical chapters provide a detailed clinical discussion of the disorder including an overview, etiology, symptoms and signs, and treatment information. Within the chapter, links are provided to related topics.
http://www.merck.com/pubs/mmanual/sections.htm

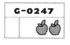

University of Illinois: Atlases and Other Medical Texts   Maintained by the University of Illinois at Urbana-Champaign, this Web page features more than 50 links for atlases and online medical textbooks. At the bottom of the page, there are hyperlinks to general medical information and medical education sites.   http://alexia.lis.uiuc.edu/~buenker/atlases.html

University of Iowa: Family Practice Handbook   The *University of Iowa Family Practice Handbook* is featured on this Web page, primarily of interest to physicians. This searchable textbook has 20 chapters covering topics such as cardiology, pulmonary medicine, gynecology, pediatrics, and dermatology. Chapters typically cover diseases and conditions by providing an overview, along with causes, diagnosis, and treatment information. In addition to disorders, office and hospital procedures, as well as drug doses of commonly prescribed medications, are covered.
http://www.vh.org/Providers/ClinRef/FPHandbook/FPContents.html

Virtual Hospital: Multimedia Textbooks Intended for healthcare providers, a list of multimedia textbooks is featured on this Web page, hosted by the University of Iowa Virtual Hospital. All textbooks listed are drawn from the Virtual Hospital and include more than 40 topics such as anatomy, dermatology, pediatrics, the human brain, and pathology. Along with text, there are also video clips, photomicrographs and photographs, and radiographic images.
http://www.vh.org/Providers/Textbooks/MultimediaTextbooks.html

14.23 PHARMACEUTICAL INFORMATION

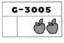

CenterWatch: Newly Approved Drug Therapies For many researchers and physicians, information about FDA drug approvals is of central concern. A concise summary of such approvals by medical specialty and condition from 1995 to the present is featured on this Web page.
http://www.centerwatch.com/patient/drugs/druglist.html

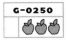

Doctor's Guide: New Drugs and Indications The Doctor's Guide provides an ongoing source of new drug information, including FDA approvals and drug indications. Drug articles are presented in order of article datelines, with the most current stories listed first. Information for drug releases for the past 12 months is provided. http://www.pslgroup.com/NEWDRUGS.HTM

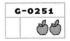

drkoop.com: Drug Interactions Search Visitors can enter drug names into a search tool for general information as well as access to Drug Checker information on warnings, side effects, pharmacology, lactation, and pregnancy. The Drug Checker also provides information on interactions between two or more drugs.
http://www.drugchecker.drkoop.com/apps/drugchecker/DrugMain?cob=drkoop

Drug InfoNet Information and links to areas on the Web concerning healthcare and pharmaceutical-related topics are available at this site. The drug information is available by brand name, generic name, manufacturer, and therapeutic class. Visitors can also obtain pharmaceutical manufacturer information.
http://www.druginfonet.com/phrminfo.htm

DrugFacts.com Library Described as the "most comprehensive source of free and premium drug, interaction, and herbal information on the Internet," this site offers information drawn from *Drug Facts,* courtesy of the Wolters Kluwer International Health and Science companies. An "A-to-Z Drug Facts" section offers more than 4,500 drugs, along with information such as action, indication/contraindication, dosage, interactions, adverse reactions, precautions, and patient education tips. An abridged version for professionals is available after a free registration process. Other highlights include information drawn from *Drug Interaction Facts* and from a guide to 125 herbal products. Patients can access "Med Facts" for easy-to-read information on more than 4,000 drugs.
http://www.drugfacts.com/DrugFacts/tabs/library.jhtml?pf=&ps=&cr=&si=#druginfo

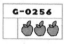

Food and Drug Administration (FDA): Approved Drug Products
The U.S. Food and Drug Administration's *Electronic Orange Book* for approved drug products is posted on this Web site. The book can be searched by active ingredient, proprietary name, applicant holder, or application number. The results for a search provide all of this information as well as the dosage form, route, and strength.
http://www.fda.gov/cder/ob/default.htm

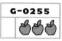

Food and Drug Administration (FDA): Center for Drug Evaluation and Research The Center for Drug Evaluation and Research provides information on prescription, consumer, and over-the-counter drugs at this address. Resources include alphabetical lists of new and generic drug approvals, new drugs approved for cancer indications, the *Electronic Orange Book* listing all FDA-approved prescription drugs, a national drug code directory, labeling notices, patient information, and alerts of new indications. Links are available to many resources related to drug safety and side effects, public health alerts and warnings, and pages offering information on major drugs. Reports and publications, special projects and programs, and cancer clinical trials information are also found through this address.
http://www.fda.gov/cder/drug/default.htm

MedicineNet.com: Medications Index This pharmacological database from MedicineNet provides a mini-forum for each prescription and nonprescription medication, including a brief main article pertaining to the medication, related medications, related news and updates, diseases associated with the medication, and a listing of articles pertinent to the pharmacological agent's usage. http://www.medicinenet.com/Script/Main/AlphaIdx.asp?li=MNI&d=51&p=A_PHARM

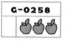

MedWatch: The FDA Medical Products Reporting Program MedWatch, the FDA Safety Information and Adverse Event Reporting Program, is designed to educate health professionals about the importance of being aware of, monitoring for, and reporting adverse events and problems to the FDA and/or the product manufacturer. The program is also intended to disseminate new safety information rapidly within the medical community, thereby improving patient care. To these ends, the site includes an adverse event reporting form and instructions as well as safety information for health professionals, including "Dear Health Professional" letters and notifications related to drug safety. It also includes relevant full-text continuing education articles and reports regarding drug and medical device safety issues.
http://www.fda.gov/medwatch

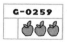

PDR.net PDR.net publishes health-related articles geared toward specific groups including physicians, pharmacists, physician assistants, oncologists, nurse practitioners, nurses, and consumers. Sections dedicated to each type of audience present articles from sources that include professional journals, CenterWatch, MEDLINE, Cancerfacts.com, the Centers for Disease Control and Prevention, the Government Clinical Trial Website, and the Mayo Health Clinic

Oasis. Physicians can access "PDR Online" and obtain extensive information on drugs, herbal medicine, multidrug interactions, and drug pricing. Online CME materials are also provided for physicians, nurses, pharmacists, and veterinarians. (free registration) http://www.pdr.net

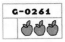

Pharmaceutical Research and Manufacturers of America   This association Web site includes a "New Medicines in Development" database; a publications section containing reports relating to the pharmaceutical industry; various links for facts and figures on pharmaceutical research and innovation; and an issues and policies section covering many current topics of interest to pharmaceutical companies, such as genetics research and healthcare liability reform.   http://www.phrma.org

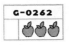

RxList: The Internet Drug Index   This site allows users to search for drug information by name, imprint code, or keyword. The top 200 prescribed drugs for the previous six years are listed alphabetically or by rank. Patient monographs are available for a wide range of drugs, and one section is devoted to alternative medicine information and answers to frequently asked questions. The site also provides a forum for drug-specific discussions.
http://www.rxlist.com

Virtual Library Pharmacy   This library of pharmacy information contains resources for professionals in all medical areas. The site provides information on pharmacy schools, associations, companies, journals and books, Internet databases relating to pharmaceutical topics, conferences, hospital sites, government sites, pharmacy LISTSERVs, and news groups. Hundreds of site links are provided for the above areas.
http://www.pharmacy.org

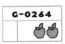

World Standard Drug Database   Information on pharmaceutical products at this address includes ingredients, dosage, routes of administration, and products with the same ingredients and/or strengths. Visitors can search for relevant information by drug, ingredient, indications, contraindications, or side effects.
http://209.235.4.229/drugcgic.cgi/START

14.24 PHYSICIAN BACKGROUND

American Board of Medical Specialties   This verification service contains the names of all physicians certified by an American Board of Medical Specialties (ABMS) member board. It permits the public to verify the credentials and certification status of any physician, searching by name, city, state, and specialty within the 24 member board specialty areas. There is no fee for this service.
http://www.abms.org

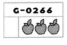

Healthgrades.com   This resource specializes in healthcare ratings, providing hospital ratings by procedure or diagnosis, physician ratings by specialty and geographic area, and ratings of health plans. Directories of hospitals, physicians, health plans, mammography facilities, fertility clinics, assisted-living facilities, home health agencies, hospice programs, cancer centers, dentists, and chiropractors are also available. Visitors can access tips on choosing a hospital, physician, or health plan, as well as a glossary of terms and health news articles. http://www.healthgrades.com

Physician Background Information Service Searchpointe.com offers background information on doctors and chiropractors licensed in the United States, such as name of medical school and year of graduation, residency training record, ABMS certifications, states where certified, and records of sanctions or disciplinary actions. There is a fee for license and sanction reports.
(some features fee-based) http://www.searchpointe.com

14.25 STATE HEALTH DEPARTMENTS

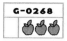

State Health Departments A list of links to U.S. state health departments is featured on this site maintained by the Centers for Disease Control and Prevention. A search tool enables the visitor to search state health departments for certain information. In addition, links to related international resources can be found on the left side of the page, such as the Pan American Health Organization and the World Health Organization.
http://www.cdc.gov/mmwr/international/relres.html

15

PROFESSIONAL TOPICS
AND CLINICAL PRACTICE

15.1 ANATOMY AND PHYSIOLOGY

G-0269

American Medical Association (AMA): Atlas of the Body The Atlas of the Body is a site offered by the American Medical Association that provides detailed information and labeled illustrations of the various systems and organs of the human body. The site also provides descriptions of disorders that affect these systems and organs.
http://www.ama-assn.org/insight/gen_hlth/atlas/atlas.htm

G-0270

Health On the Net (HON) Foundation: Medical Images Part of a larger Health On the Net Foundation Web page, this site features a medical image and video library on anatomy. There are more than 750 images related to topics such as the cardiovascular system, digestive system, musculoskeletal system, and nervous system. In addition to organ systems, other categories include organisms, diseases, chemicals and drugs, techniques, and biological sciences. Each image has a hyperlink to its source for additional information.
http://www.hon.ch/Media/anatomy.html

G-0271

Karolinska Institutet: Anatomy and Histology Resources available on this site directed to physicians include more than 50 links on anatomy and nearly 20 on histology. Many of the sites contain numerous illustrations and photographs, and some have video. The sites are drawn primarily from universities around the world.
http://www.mic.ki.se/Anatomy.html

G-0272

Martindale's Health Science Guide: Virtual Medical Center: Anatomy and Histology Center This "Virtual Medical Center" offers links to examinations, tutorials, and associations. It lists numerous atlases and sites with anatomical images, including some on embryology and developmental anatomy. The center which also provides links to general medical dictionaries, glossaries, and encyclopedias, as well as sites containing information on metabolic pathways and genetic maps.
http://www-sci.lib.uci.edu/HSG/MedicalAnatomy.html

G-0275

MedBioWorld: Anatomy and Physiology Journals More than 65 journals related to anatomy and physiology are listed on this Web page. Hyperlinks are provided to the online versions of the journals; some are for subscribers only. http://www.medbioworld.com/journals/medicine/anatomy.html

MedNets: Anatomy Dedicated to anatomy, this site features links for information such as associations, databases, and journals. Some journals are for subscribers only. General resources include information on specific parts of the anatomy, as well as 3-D anatomy for students.

(some features fee-based) http://www.mednets.com/anatomy.htm

Purdue University: Anatomy Links A list of links on human anatomy and resources for medical students is featured on this Web page, courtesy of Purdue University. The links are accessed in a sidebar menu where there are more than a dozen categories including cardiology, clinical information, embryology, histology, gross anatomy, lumen, neuroscience, ophthalmology, radiology, the reproductive system, sports medicine, and surgery. Medical students will find a section dedicated to them with links for general resources.

http://www.vet.purdue.edu/bms/ai/frames/intlink_00.htm

University of Arkansas for Medical Sciences: Anatomy Tables Maintained at the University of Arkansas for Medical Sciences, this site features anatomy tables. The tables are organized by system such as arteries or bones and by region of the body. Each table includes the proper name of the anatomical part and a description.

http://anatomy.uams.edu/HTMLpages/anatomyhtml/medcharts.html

Whole Brain Atlas Administered by the Harvard Medical School, this site shows imaging of the brain using magnetic resonance imaging (MRI), roentgenray computed tomography (CT), and nuclear medicine technologies. Structures within the images are labeled. Normal brain images are provided, as well as images of brains subjected to cerebrovascular disease, neoplastic disease, degenerative disease, and inflammatory or infectious disease. The entire atlas is available free of charge online or can be ordered on CD-ROM for a fee.

http://www.med.harvard.edu/AANLIB/home.html

15.2 BIOMEDICAL ETHICS

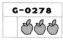

American Society of Bioethics and Humanities The American Society of Bioethics and Humanities is an organization that promotes scholarship, research, teaching, policy development, and professional development in the field of bioethics. The site offers information on the society, the annual meeting, position papers, and awards. There is also a large list of resource links covering academic centers, education, ethics and philosophy, law, medicine and the humanities, online texts, organizations, and science and technology.

http://www.asbh.org

American Society of Law, Medicine, and Ethics This site offers information on the American Society of Law, Medicine, and Ethics; the *Journal*

of Law, Medicine, and Ethics; and the *American Journal of Law and Medicine.* Also provided are details on research projects; a news section that gives updates on recent developments in law, medicine, and ethics; and information on future and past conferences held by the society. A comprehensive listing of related resources is also provided in categories such as bioethics, cancer, genetics, geriatrics, health law, managed care, and nursing.

http://www.aslme.org

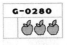

Bioethics Discussion Pages   This page is a discussion forum for people to share their views on selected topics in the field of biomedical ethics. There are also polls and articles on ethical issues.

http://www-hsc.usc.edu/~mbernste/#Welcome

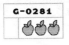

Bioethics.net   Produced by the Center for Bioethics of the University of Pennsylvania and hosted by the *American Journal of Bioethics Online,* Bioethics.net contains a host of resources pertaining to biomedical ethics. Included are sections on cloning and genetics, emergency room bioethics, surveys for pay, and assisted suicide. The site also provides news updates, book reviews, articles, and tables of contents of other journals. "Bioethics for Beginners" contains material that is meant to educate the general public and people interested in the field about bioethics, its meaning, and its applications. At this beginner's site, there are resources for students and educators, including a list of biomedical ethics associations.

http://www.med.upenn.edu/bioethics/index.shtml

Human Genome Project: Ethical, Legal, and Social Issues (ELSI)
With funding from the U.S. Department of Energy and the National Institutes of Health, this site describes and explores the ethical, legal, and social issues surrounding availability of genetic information. A link to "Privacy and Legislation" gives more detail on who should have access to genetic information and how it can be used. Gene testing and gene therapy links feature the risks and limits of genetic technology, as well as the implementation of standards. A section on behavioral genetics examines conceptual and philosophical implications. In addition, a section on patenting covers who owns genes and other pieces of DNA.

http://www.ornl.gov/hgmis/elsi/elsi.html

Medical Ethics: Where Do You Draw the Line?   Interactive scenarios on ethical decisions are featured on this site. Visitors can answer multiple choice questions about living with cancer, understanding cloning, or handling headaches. The site also provides a summary of visitors' responses. Links at the end of each section lead to an ethics forum, a bulletin board discussion, and related sites on cancer, cloning, and headaches.

http://www.learner.org/exhibits/medicalethics

National Bioethics Advisory Commission   In addition to providing information on current research trends in the biotechnology industry, the commission explores the ethical implications of technological advances. The site acts as a forum for the ethical concerns of the public regarding rapidly advancing technology. Transcripts from its meetings are available on the site, as well as reports on topics such as ethical issues in human stem cell research and cloning human beings. A short list of bioethics-related links is provided.

http://bioethics.gov/cgi-bin/bioeth_counter.pl

National Reference Center for Bioethics Literature Linked to the Kennedy Institute of Ethics at Georgetown University, this center holds a large collection of literature on biomedical ethics. Serving as a resource for both the public and scholars of ethics, the site also provides access to free searching of the world's literature in bioethics using BIOETHICSLINE or the Ethics and Human Genetics Database. Other relevant links are provided in the areas of educational and teaching resources, the center's library, bibliographies, and Internet resources for bioethics.

http://www.georgetown.edu/research/nrcbl

The Hastings Center The Hastings Center is a major center for the study of biomedical ethics. Its Web site provides information about current research activities in medicine and biomedical research, values and biotechnology, healthcare policy and healthcare systems, and humans and nature. Other resources include information on educational opportunities at the center, a catalog of publications, and a list of related links.

http://www.thehastingscenter.org

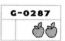

UNESCO: International Bioethics Committee The International Bioethics Committee of the United Nations Educational, Scientific, and Cultural Organization (UNESCO) created this Web site to inform the public of their work on human rights in relation to advances made in genetics and molecular biology. The site outlines their activities, along with proceedings from their meetings. The Universal Declaration on the Human Genome and Human Rights resolution is available on the site. Under the "Ethical Issues" section, visitors can read IBC reports on subjects such as the teaching of bioethics, neuroscience, the human genome, bioethics and human rights, and genetics. The site can also be viewed in French.

http://www.unesco.org/ibc

University of Buffalo Center for Clinical Ethics and Humanities in Health Care Information about the center, news and events notices, a library of bioethics and medical humanities documents, and the Ethics Committee Core Curriculum are available at this address. Links are presented to Internet resources on featured topics including bioethics education, hospice and palliative care, advance directives, philosophy of mind, medical record privacy, genetics, and ethics. http://wings.buffalo.edu/faculty/research/bioethics/nav.html

15.3 BIOTECHNOLOGY

Bio Online Bio Online is a comprehensive Web site for the life sciences and the biotechnology industry. This site provides general information, current news, an industry guide, academic and government links, and an extensive career center. It is an informative resource for seeking information on the biotechnology industry and related sciences.
http://www.bio.com

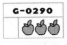

Biofind.com Biofind.com provides insight into the biotechnology industry and is a resource for general information, news, and developments in emerging technologies. The site also contains a job search database, a chat room, the "Biotech Rumor Mill" for anonymous public discussion of current events in the field, an events database, a secure "Innovations" database for posting projects needing venture capital or corporate funding, and press releases from biotechnology companies. A subscription service, available for a fee, provides daily e-mail updates on jobs, candidates, business opportunities, innovations, and press releases. http://www.biofind.com

BioInfoSeek.com Infobiotech is a collaboration of government, academic, and private sector resources. This Canadian-based site provides general information, resources, and links to both North American and international sources. In addition, it offers career information, events, and a large list of related sites providing current information on advances in the biotechnology industry.
http://www.cisti.nrc.ca/ibc/home.html

BioPortfolio.com A database of biotechnology companies, technology, and products worldwide is featured on this Web site. More than 11,000 companies are included in the database. Some have detailed profiles, as well as hyperlinks for investor information and news. Subscribers can search the database by keyword, category, organization name, or region. The site allows a limited search on a free trial basis.
(fee-based) http://www.bioportfolio.com/bio/

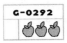

Bioresearch Online Bioresearch Online is a virtual community, forum, and marketplace for biotechnology professionals. Users have access to the latest headlines, product information, and industry analyses, as well as career information. There are also specific pages devoted to pharmaceutical research and laboratory science.
http://www.bioresearchonline.com/content/homepage

Biotechnology Industry Organization This industry-sponsored Web site provides weekly news updates on developing technology and world news. The site also offers general information, links to corporate Web sites, an online library, and a number of other educational resources.
http://www.bio.org/welcome.html

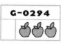

Biotechnology: An Information Resource   Dedicated to providing current information in all areas of biotechnology, this site is a subsidiary of the National Agricultural Library and the U.S. Department of Agriculture. The site catalogs press releases and offers an exhaustive listing of links to other Web-based resources from around the world, especially in the area of agricultural biotechnology. http://www.nal.usda.gov/bic

BioWorld Online   BioWorld Online tracks the growth of the biotechnology market. In addition to providing stock and financial information, the site provides access to current industry headlines, job search resources, forums, and news worldwide. http://www.bioworld.com

CorpTech Database   This comprehensive database provides details on companies involved in high-tech industries, including biotechnology and pharmaceutical companies. Basic information such as each company's description, annual sales, and CEO name is available free; however, more in-depth financial and business data is only accessible to fee-paying subscribers. Searches for products or names of company officers are also available, with some information provided at no cost.
(some features fee-based) http://www.corptech.com

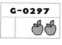

Enzyme Nomenclature Database   The database at this Web site provides access to enzyme information by Enzyme Commission (EC) number, enzyme class, description, chemical compound, and cofactor. There is also an accompanying user manual for the enzyme database, report forms for new enzyme entry, and links to resources on biochemical pathways and protein databases.
http://www.expasy.ch/enzyme

International Food Information Council   The International Food Information Council (IFIC) collects and disseminates scientific information on food safety, nutrition, and health by working with experts to help translate research findings into understandable and useful language for opinion leaders and consumers. This site provides information and news on food safety and nutrition in categories such as functional foods, agriculture and food production, and food biotechnology. The site also offers publications including IFIC's journal *Food Insight*, recent news articles, government guidelines and regulations, and links to other resources on the Internet.
http://ificinfo.health.org

MedWebPlus: Biotechnology   MedWebPlus contains an extensive guide to online resources in biotechnology, organized alphabetically and in focused subsets, cataloging hundreds of Internet resources containing many forms of information. Links are provided to journals, online publications, and recent articles of interest.
http://www.medwebplus.com/subject/Biotechnology.html

National Center for Biotechnology Information (NCBI)   A collaborative effort produced by the National Library of Medicine and the National In-

stitutes of Health, NCBI is a national resource for molecular biology information. The center creates public databases, conducts research in computational biology, develops software tools for analyzing genome data, and disseminates information in an effort to improve the understanding of molecular processes affecting human health and disease. In addition to conducting and cataloging its own research, NCBI tracks the progress of important research projects worldwide. The site provides access to public molecular databases containing genetic sequences, structures, and taxonomy; literature databases; catalogs of whole genomes; tools for mining genetic data; teaching resources and online tutorials; and data and software available to download. Research performed at NCBI is also discussed at the site.
http://www.ncbi.nlm.nih.gov

Recombinant Capital ReCap acts as a "centralized industry 'filing cabinet'" for public resources relevant to biotechnology, serving as a database for biotechnology executives and investors. *Signals,* the online magazine, provides analysis of the biotechnology industry and is particularly appropriate for those seeking to invest in companies on the forefront of this rapidly growing industry. Although much of the information presented is from a financial perspective, the site gives an overview of the entire industry and provides daily news updates.
http://www.recap.com

WWW Virtual Library: Biotechnology A directory of sites in the field of biotechnology is featured on this Web page. This site catalogs hundreds of reviewed links including publications, educational resources, products, genomics, software, pharmaceutical companies, clinical trials and regulatory affairs, and government links. There is also a rating system used by the editor of the site to point out links of specific importance.
http://www.cato.com/biotech

15.4 CLINICAL PRACTICE MANAGEMENT

GENERAL RESOURCES

Cut to the Chase This site offers information for healthcare management in the form of a list of over 30 categories relevant to a variety of work settings. Topics covered include accreditation, billing, career development, health policy, legal issues, medical records, practice management, and telemedicine. Within each category are subheadings containing articles, abstracts, and additional links. http://www.cuttothechase.com

Guide to Clinical Preventive Services This guide is a comprehensive online reference source covering recommendations for clinical practice on more than 150 preventive interventions, including screening tests, counseling interven-

tions, immunizations, chemoprophylactic regimens, and other preventive medical tools. Approximately 60 target conditions are discussed in the report.
http://cpmcnet.columbia.edu/texts/gcps/gcps0000.html

Health Services/Technology Assessment Text This electronic resource provides access to consumer brochures, evidence reports, reference guides for clinicians, clinical practice guidelines, and other full-text documents useful in making healthcare decisions. Users can download documents from the site, access general information about the system, and browse links to additional sources for information. Searches can be comprehensive or limited to specific databases within the HSTAT system, and users can also search by keyword.
http://text.nlm.nih.gov

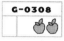

Medsite.com Described as an e-services portal for the medical community, this site offers books, medical software, and supplies at discounted prices; financial resources; a scheduling tool geared for medical professionals; and free e-mail accounts. Also available are daily health news updates, interactive grand rounds and other online courses, and links to medical textbooks and journals. Some areas require registration or subscription.
(some features fee-based) http://www.medsite.com

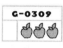

PDR.net PDR.net is a medical and healthcare Web site created by the Medical Economics Company, publisher of healthcare magazines and directories including the *Physicians' Desk Reference*. The site has specific areas and content for physicians, pharmacists, physician assistants, nurses, and consumers. Access to the full-text reference book is free for U.S.-based M.D.s, D.O.s, and P.A.s in full-time practice. There is a fee for other users of this service, but most of the site's features are free.
(some features fee-based) http://www.PDR.net

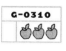

Physician's Guide to the Internet A directory of Web sites for physicians is offered on this site. Features include physician lifestyle resources, such as sites offering suggestions on stress relief; news items; clinical practice resources, including access to medical databases and patient education resources; and postgraduate education and new physician resources. Other resources include links to sites selling medical books, products, and services for physicians; links to Internet search tools; and Internet tutorials.
http://www.physiciansguide.com

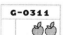

State Medical Boards Directory This directory provides the names, addresses, telephone numbers, and e-mail or Web site information for each of the state medical boards. Physicians can contact a board for information on licensing in that state or for other information regarding medical regulation or standards. http://www.fsmb.org/members.htm

CLINICAL CALCULATORS

MedCalc 3000 Medical Calculator MedCalc 3000 offers several hundred online medical calculator tools at this site. It combines various equations, clinical criteria scores, and decision trees used in healthcare. In addition, there is a quick converter to convert value units easily and a math calculator. Alphabetical lists of the medical equations and clinical criteria topics are presented, with links to the actual calculators.
http://calc.med.edu/

Medical Tools, Calculators and Scores Medic8.com provides clinicians with 60 medical calculators to measure blood oxygen content, body mass, opioid drug dosage, and numerous other factors. Scores such as coronary disease probability, the geriatric depression scale, the Glasgow coma scale, and the TWEAK alcoholism score are also included. A sidebar menu offers links to reference information on medical subjects, specialties, medical news, books, software, and services.
http://www.medic8.com/MedicalTools.htm

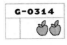

Online Clinical Calculators: Medstudents Medstudents.com hosts this site providing visitors with nearly 25 online clinical calculators for various measurements, including arterial oxygen content, oxygen consumption, water deficit, and pulmonary shunt. By filling in spaces for critical measurements, then clicking on the result box, the desired results are produced.
http://www.medstudents.com.br/calculat/index2.htm

EVIDENCE-BASED MEDICINE

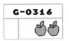

Cochrane Collaboration The Cochrane Collaboration is an international working group of experts who catalog and maintain information on evidence-based medicine by specialty. The site explains the history of the collaboration, along with descriptions of the Cochrane library site, which contains a database of systematic reviews and a controlled trials register. Abstracts are available on the library site free of charge; full access is available only to subscribers.
(some features fee-based) http://www.cochrane.org/default.html

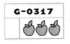

Evidence-Based Medicine Resource Center Resources offered on the New York Academy of Medicine's evidence-based medicine site may be useful to both teaching and practicing physicians. There are links to databases, publications, teaching tools, education resources, and tips on searching for evidence-based medicine. The "Practicing" section includes clinical guidelines, clinical trials, and systematic reviews. There are also organizations, glossaries, journals, LISTSERV discussion groups, and related links.
(some features fee-based) http://www.ebmny.org/thecentr2.html

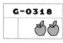

Medscout: Evidence-Based Medicine Guidelines Targeted to physicians, this site offers a comprehensive list of evidence-based medicine guidelines available on the Internet. There are more than 30 sites drawn mostly from universities and journals around the world.
http://www.medscout.com/guidelines/evidence_based/

New York Online Access to Health (NOAH): Evidence-Based Medicine Patients seeking information on evidence-based medicine (EBM) will find this site from NOAH very useful. There are more than 55 sites listed offering information on types of evidence, research methods, statistical terms in EBM, and a basic overview of EBM.
http://www.noah-health.org/english/ebhc/ebhc.html

MEDICAL ETHICS

American Medical Association (AMA): Ethics Standards Reports of the Council on Ethical and Judicial Affairs, an organization that sets ethics policy for the AMA, are accessible from this site. Visitors can access an online policy finder, which can be browsed alphabetically, or get answers to frequently asked questions about the role of the council, the Code of Medical Ethics, and the End-of-Life Care Project. The Institute for Ethics at the AMA, functioning as an independent research organization, provides news from its task force and information about the E-Force program. Other AMA ethics Web sites and pages of professional standards are available.
http://www.ama-assn.org/ama/pub/category/2416.html#ethics

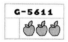

American Society of Law, Medicine, and Ethics The search engine at this site allows visitors to access a variety of educational information related to law, medicine, and ethics. Details about the organization's peer-reviewed journals, access to research projects on pain undertreatment, and a news section offering up-to-date information on recent developments in the field are offered. A multimedia educational link connects visitors to more than 50 streaming audio presentations in the fields of genetics, health law, and end-of-life decision making. http://www.aslme.org/

Karolinska Institutet: Ethics in Biomedicine A comprehensive listing of more than 100 links related to ethics is offered on this Web page. The links are categorized as bioethics, professional ethics, institutional ethics, scientific misconduct, humanism, and morals. The sites are drawn from Internet sources around the world.
http://www.mic.ki.se/Diseases/k1.316.html

Medscout: Medical Ethics Over 100 medical ethics resources are presented at this site from Medscout. Examples of resources are the American Society of Bioethics and Humanities, the Center for Ethics and Professionalism, the Center for Clinical Ethics and Humanities in Health Care, and the National Human Genome Research Institute. Visitors to this site will also find topical links to resources in areas such as diseases, government, immunizations, journals, and health policy. http://www.medscout.com/ethics/

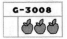

The Hastings Center This independent, interdisciplinary research and education center explores the ethical issues surrounding health, medicine, and the environment. Examination of the moral issues arising from advances in medicine can be found at the site's project pages on medicine and biomedical research, values and biotechnology, and health policy. Several relevant online resources for bioethics-related information are offered. http://www.thehastingscenter.org/

MEDICAL INFORMATICS

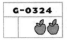

Agency for Healthcare Research and Quality (AHRQ): Healthcare Informatics Healthcare informatics is featured on this Web site, courtesy of the Agency for Healthcare Research and Quality (AHRQ). The site provides data and survey reports covering public health, standard activities for federal agencies, medical informatics and health services research data, and the use of computers to advance healthcare. In addition, there are links to research findings, funding opportunities, consumer health, clinical information, and medical news. http://www.ahcpr.gov/data/infoix.htm

American Health Information Management Association Directed to health information managers, the American Health Information Management Association Web page offers details about the association and the field. "Hot Topics" in health information management covers more than a dozen areas such as accreditation, data quality management, and information security. Within each category are articles, position statements, seminars/events, and research and benchmarks. A resource center for patients includes information on accessing and protecting personal medical records. (some features fee-based) http://www.ahima.org/

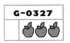

American Medical Informatics Association With the proliferation of medical information, the growth of medical research, the development of medical information systems, and the creation of management systems for computerized patient data, the medical informatics field has grown substantially. Major themes of the association are privacy and confidentiality of medical records, public policy development for legislation in the field, conferences of medical informatics professionals, and the issuance of papers and publications covering various aspects of the medical information field. The site features publications, including the *Journal of the American Medical Informatics Association,* and related reports and videos. Other resources include information on the various working and special interest groups, a job bank, and links to related sites. http://www.amia.org

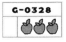

American Telemedicine Association Dedicated to promoting access to medical care for consumers and professionals through the use of telecommunications technology, the American Telemedicine Association promotes education, research, and advocacy in the field. Visitors to the site can learn more about the association, its member groups, and meetings. Information under the "News and Resources" section includes bulletin boards, a comprehensive list of related links, and a job bank. In the same section is a library containing a member directory, telemedicine news updates, and proceedings from their annual meetings. (some features fee-based) http://www.atmeda.org

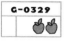

Duke University: Medical Informatics Links   Maintained by the Division of Clinical Informatics of Duke University Medical Center, this Web page offers more than 50 links related to medical informatics. The Web pages listed are drawn from associations and universities around the world.
http://dmi-www.mc.duke.edu/dukemi/misc/links.html

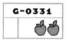

Galaxy: Medical Informatics Resources   This site provides links to more than 20 U.S. and international centers and medical departments dealing with medical informatics. Included in this list are centers at Oregon Health Sciences University, Stanford University, Columbia University, and European institutions. There are also articles, directories, and discussion group links for further resources on medical informatics.
http://www.galaxy.com/cgi-bin/dirlist?node=25091

International Medical Informatics Association   The International Medical Informatics Association's (IMIA) Web site features the association newsletter, along with information on IMIA working groups and member societies. A report on the recommendations of the IMIA on education in health and medical informatics is provided. There is also an extensive list of related resources that includes institutions and organizations, medical resources, and health informatics resources.
http://www.imia.org

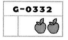

Medscout: Medical Informatics   For those interested in medical informatics, this Web page contains a comprehensive list of Internet resources. The sites are categorized as national information associations, newsletters and journals, and medical informatics on the Internet. In total, there are more than 85 sites from both domestic and international sources.
http://www.medscout.com/informatics/index.htm

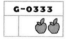

Telemedicine   More than 20 telemedicine resources are provided at this site from Galaxy, a medical portal. Featured resources include the Center for Telemedicine Law, Cyberspace Telemedical Office, MediaStation 5000, and telemedicine initiatives by state. Links are provided to access remote consultation, telepathology, and teleradiology resources.
http://www.galaxy.com/galaxy/Medicine/Medical-Informatics/Telemedicine.html

Medical Law

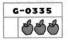

American Medical Association (AMA): Legal Issues for Physicians
Healthcare providers can access information regarding legal issues in the areas of business and management, patient-physician relationships, and compliance at this Web site, maintained by the AMA. Various medical case summaries are provided, as well as a Compliance Interactive Tutorial System offering online assistance with fraud and abuse regulations for members of the association.
(some features fee-based) http://www.ama-assn.org/ama/pub/category/4541.html

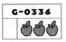

MedNets: Medical Law Links to more than 30 medical law resources, including the American Bar Association Health Law Section, AMA Statements on Advanced Directives, Expert Witness Net, the Health Care Liability Alliance, Medical Care Law, the U.S. States Abortion Laws, and the Law and Legislative Center are offered at this site from MedNets. Visitors can also access medical law databases, health law journals, news, and resources related to medical ethics through this site.
http://www.mednets.com/medlaw.htm

Medical Licensure

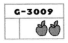

Administrators in Medicine: Association of State Medical Board Executive Directors A list of participating state licensing authorities is compiled at this page, maintained by DocFinder. The list is not exhaustive but contains many connections to state medical examiners' home pages and tools that allow visitors to search for physicians by name or license number.
http://www.docboard.org/

Federation of State Medical Boards The Federation of State Medical Boards (FSMB) site provides visitors with policy documents, details on post-licensure assessment, a credentials verification service, and state medical board information. A publications catalog is provided, which includes the *Journal of Medical Licensure and Discipline* and the *FSMB Handbook*. The FSMB library is accessible to members of the organization. There is also information on their database of board actions taken against physicians.
(some features fee-based) http://www.fsmb.org/

Practice Guidelines and Consensus Statements

Medscout: Medical Specialty Guidelines Sponsored by Medscout, this Web page offers a comprehensive listing of more than 50 clinical guidelines plus links to other guidelines sites available on the Internet. The guidelines are drawn primarily from American and Canadian sources.
http://www.medscout.com/guidelines/medical_specialty/

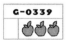

National Guideline Clearinghouse (NGC) The National Guideline Clearinghouse is a comprehensive database of evidence-based clinical practice guidelines and related documents produced by the Agency for Healthcare Research and Quality, in partnership with the American Medical Association and the American Association of Health Plans. The guidelines can be searched by keyword or browsed by category such as disease and condition, treatment and intervention, and issuing organization. Each guideline has a brief summary and information for obtaining the full text. A useful tool on the site is the "Compare Guidelines," feature which allows users to add guidelines on a specific topic to their collection and then select a comparison button to produce a report that compares them. In addition, there are guideline syntheses on certain topics such as asthma treatment and childhood immunizations in which all the guidelines written on the topic are combined into one report.
http://www.guideline.gov/index.asp

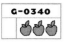

Primary Care Clinical Practice Guidelines Clinical practice guidelines for primary care providers are offered on this Web page, courtesy of the University of California San Francisco. The guidelines can be searched by keyword, browsed alphabetically, or selected through clinical content categories such as mental disorders, cardiovascular system, and pregnancy. Each category has many subtopics listed, along with hyperlinks to the appropriate guideline. Also of interest is the resources section, which offers an enormous list of online textbooks, journals, superlists of links, and other related resources.
(some features fee-based) http://medicine.ucsf.edu/resources/guidelines/

PRACTICE MANAGEMENT TOOLS

Medical Group Management Association Primarily targeted to healthcare administrators, the Medical Group Management Association focuses on practice management solutions and tools. The site contains information on the association's research activities and on policy issues, as well as a job bank and career services. A catalog of survey reports features medical group practice performance data.
(some features fee-based) http://www.mgma.com/

Medscape: The Journal of Medical Practice Management Abstracts and full-text articles are available to registered users at this online journal site of Medscape. Available content includes current feature articles and archived issues that address software systems, managed care, economic trends in healthcare delivery, and billing and coding topics.
(free registration) http://managedcare.medscape.com/JMPM/public/JMPM-journal.html

15.5 CLINICAL TRIALS

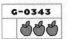

CenterWatch This clinical trials listing service offers both patient and professional resources. Patient resources include a listing of clinical trials by disease category, a notification and matching service, links to current NIH trials, drug directories including a clinical trials results database and drugs currently in clinical research, listings of new FDA drug therapy approvals, and current research headlines. Background information on clinical research is also available to patients unfamiliar with the clinical trials process. Industry professional resources include research center profiles, industry provider profiles, industry news, and career and educational opportunities. Links to related sites of interest to patients and professionals are also available.
http://www.centerwatch.com/main.htm

ClinicalTrials.gov The National Institutes of Health and the National Library of Medicine provide access to information about clinical trials through ClinicalTrials.gov. Visitors can search the database by entering keywords or phrases into the search engine; by using a focused search by disease, location, treatment, or sponsor; or by browsing alphabetical listings of thousands of conditions and sponsors. Links to information on studies recruiting patients offer additional details on study purpose, protocol, and researcher contact.
http://clinicaltrials.gov/ct/gui/c/b

15.6 DISSERTATION ABSTRACTS

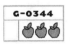

Dissertation Abstracts Database A database of more than 1.6 million citations and abstracts from doctoral dissertations and master's theses is provided on this site. Visitors are offered free access to the most current two years of citations, which includes an abstract and a 24-page preview. Subscriber institutions are able to download the entire dissertation in PDF format for the years 1997 to the present. Subscribers can also search for citations dating back to 1861. (some features fee-based) http://wwwlib.umi.com/dissertations/about_pqdd

15.7 ENVIRONMENTAL HEALTH

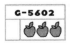

Agency for Toxic Substances and Disease Registry Environmental and occupational public health hazards and risks are the focus of this division of the U.S. Department of Health and Human Services. A variety of resources can be accessed, including national alerts, health advisories, answers to frequently asked questions about hazardous substances, and relevant legislation. Databases available from the site provide information on specific hazardous waste sites, as well as information on those exposed to such substances. Scientific papers published by the agency, sites addressing issues specific to children, and a calendar of events are included. http://www.atsdr.cdc.gov/atsdrhome.html

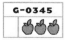

New York Online Access to Health (NOAH): Environmental Health

This NOAH site features a directory of environmental health links available on the Internet. There are more than 55 links categorized under environmental health topics such as air quality, chemical sensitivities, toxins and pesticides, and water quality. More than 45 sites are found under a resources section that includes advocacy, governmental agencies, and legal resources. The site can also be accessed in Spanish.

http://www.noah-health.org/english/illness/environment/environ.html

15.8 GENETICS AND GENOMICS

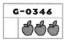

GeneClinics

Funded by the National Institutes of Health and developed by the University of Washington, GeneClinics is a knowledge base of expert-authored, up-to-date information relating genetic testing to the diagnosis, management, and counseling of individuals and families with inherited disorders. Directed at healthcare professionals, the site contains textbook-type genetic testing and counseling information on a large number of diseases. The disease profiles are peer-reviewed and continuously updated.

http://www.geneclinics.org

Genetics Jump Station

This site provides a comprehensive listing of Web-based resources for geneticists. Sites indexed here are technical in nature and intended for investigators. Resources include links to molecular biology, microbiology, and genetics jump sites, which contain catalogs of links; sites containing protocols on laboratory techniques; journals and other online publications; news groups and mail lists; institutes and organizations; conferences and meetings announcements; commercial sites; and sources for ordering technical books. The site is sponsored by Beckman, Horizon Scientific Press, the *Journal of Molecular Microbiology and Biotechnology,* and MWG-Biotech.

http://www.horizonpress.com/gateway/genetics.html

Genetics Virtual Library

A comprehensive listing of links to major Web sites on specific topics in genetics is featured on this site. Links are subdivided by organism, from yeast to humans, and by topic, including genetic testing, cloning, and pharmacogenomics. A list of human chromosomes by number is also provided, with links to information on gene markers, lineage maps, and animal models. The main site also features links to genome projects in a variety of organisms.

http://www.ornl.gov/TechResources/Human_Genome/genetics.html

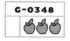

Genomics Lexicon

Part of a larger genomics site produced by the Pharmaceutical Research and Manufacturers of America and the Foundation for Genetic Medicine, Inc., this site features "Lexicon," a glossary of genomic terms. The glossary can be browsed alphabetically or by an index. Reference sources for the glossary are listed along with hyperlinks to the original source. The site

also features *Genomics Today*, a collection of links to genomics news at other Web sites; news is posted daily and an archive is available.
http://genomics.phrma.org/lexicon/r.html

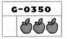

Genomics: A Global Resource   Presented by the Pharmaceutical Research and Manufacturers of America, this Web page offers a broad array of resources related to genomics and bioinformatics. Drawn from around the world and updated daily, the most recent news stories can be found in the "News & Tools" section. Also within this section are links to journals as well as education resources such as online textbooks, organizations, academic programs, and grants. "Lexicon" offers a glossary of terms. There are also links for legislative issues, controversial issues such as cloning, and biodiversity. A therapeutics section covers medical testing and bioethics. In addition, bioinformatic databases for microbials, plants, invertebrates, vertebrates, and humans can be accessed.
(some features fee-based) http://genomics.phrma.org/

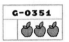

Kyoto Encyclopedia of Genomes and Genetics   The Kyoto Encyclopedia of Genes and Genomes attempts to computerize current knowledge of molecular and cellular biology in terms of information pathways consisting of interacting molecules or genes. The site also provides links to gene catalogs produced by genome sequencing projects. Information indexed at this site ranges from basic genetic information to technical descriptions of molecular pathways. Also provided is a listing of links to other major Internet sites containing information relevant to genetic research.
http://www.genome.ad.jp/kegg

MedBioWorld: Genetics, Genomics, and Biotechnology Journals
This site offers a comprehensive list of genetics, genomics, and biotechnology journals. There are more than 100 links to journals from the United States and abroad. http://www.medbioworld.com/journals/genetics.html

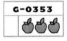

National Center for Biotechnology Information (NCBI): Online Mendelian Inheritance in Man (OMIM)   Dr. Victor A. McKusick, a researcher at Johns Hopkins University, and his colleagues have authored this database of human genes and genetic disorders. The database was developed for the World Wide Web by the center. Reference information, texts, and images are found, as well as links to the Entrez database of MEDLINE articles and sequence information. Visitors can search the OMIM Database, OMIM Gene Map, and OMIM Morbid Map (a catalog of cytogenetic map locations organized by disease). Information on the OMIM numbering system, details on creating links to OMIM, site updates, OMIM statistics, information on citing OMIM in literature, and the OMIM gene list are all available. The site also hosts links to allied resources, and the complete text of OMIM and gene maps can be downloaded from the site. http://www.ncbi.nlm.nih.gov/Omim

National Human Genome Research Institute   The National Human Genome Research Institute supports the NIH component of the Human Genome Project, a worldwide research effort designed to analyze the structure of

the human genome and determine the location of the estimated 50,000 to 100,000 human genes. The NHGRI Intramural Research Program develops and implements technology for understanding, diagnosing, and treating genetic diseases. The site provides information about NHGRI, the Human Genome Project, grants, intramural research, policy and public affairs, workshops and conferences, and news items. Resources include links to the institute's Ethical, Legal, and Social Implications Program and to the Center for Inherited Disease Research. The site also provides genetic resources for investigators and a glossary of genetic terms.

http://www.nhgri.nih.gov

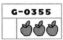

Office of Genetics and Disease Prevention   Created by the Centers for Disease Control and Prevention, this site offers access to current information on the impact of human genetic research and the Human Genome Project on public health and disease prevention. The site provides general information, indexes recent articles, lists events and training opportunities, and offers an extensive listing of links to other resources. Users can search the site by keyword and access the Human Genome Epidemiology Network (HuGENet), a global collaboration of individuals and organizations committed to the development and dissemination of population-based epidemiologic information on the human genome.   http://www.cdc.gov/genetics

Primer on Molecular Genetics   The U.S. Department of Energy presents a comprehensive resource for those seeking basic background information on genetics and genetic research at this site. Discussions include an introduction to genetics, DNA, genes, chromosomes, and the process of mapping the human genome. Mapping strategies, genetic linkage maps, and various physical maps are available, as well as links to mapping and sequence databases and a glossary of terms. The site also summarizes the predicted impact of the Human Genome Project on medical practice and biological research.

http://www.ornl.gov/hgmis/publicat/primer/intro.html

The Institute for Genomic Research (TIGR)   The Institute for Genomic Research is a not-for-profit research institute with interests in structural, functional, and comparative analysis of genomes and gene products in viruses, eubacteria, archaea, and eukaryotes. Information on recent advances in genetics and continuing research projects in the area of human genomics, an extensive database of previous research, and links to other genome centers worldwide are available at this site.

http://www.tigr.org

University of Kansas Medical Center: Genetics Education Center
Links are available at this address to Internet resources for educators interested in human genetics and the Human Genome Project. Sites are listed by topic, including the Human Genome Project, education resources, networking, genetic conditions, genetics programs and resources, and glossaries. Lesson plans are offered by the University of Kansas and other sources at the site. A description

of different careers in genetics is also available. This site provides access to useful genetics Internet resources for nonprofessionals and educators.
http://www.kumc.edu/gec

15.9 GERIATRIC MEDICINE

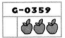

American Geriatrics Society (AGS) A national nonprofit association of geriatrics health professionals, research scientists, and other concerned individuals, the American Geriatrics Society is dedicated to "improving the health, independence, and quality of life for all older people." The site offers a description of the society, adult immunization information, AGS news, conference and events notices, legislation news, career opportunities, directories of geriatrics healthcare services in managed care, position statements, practice guidelines, awards information, and other professional education resources. Patient education resources, a selected bibliography in geriatrics, links to related organizations and government sites, and surveys are also found at this address.
(some features fee-based) http://www.americangeriatrics.org

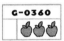

ElderWeb Designed as a research source for consumers and professionals, this Web page offers a broad array of resources related to the care of the elderly. In the "Finance and Law" section, more than 20 topics are listed such as drug costs, elder law, and Medicaid. Each topic lists resources that can be found on the site, in their newsletter, and on the Internet. Resources are listed in the same way under sections such as living arrangements and body and soul. There are also a regional directory of sites related to living arrangements, finance, and law; a list of association; and an eldercare locator that covers domestic and international sites. Visitors can access news on the home page or register for a free newsletter. (free registration) http://www.elderweb.com/

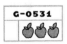

Hardin MD: Geriatrics and Senior Health The Hardin Meta Directory on this site features geriatrics and senior health. Categorized as large, medium, and small lists, there are links to Web pages that contain relevant Internet resources. The lists are drawn from both domestic and international sources and cover hundreds of sites. There are also links to additional directories of lists on Alzheimer's and Parkinson's disease.
http://www.lib.uiowa.edu/hardin/md/ger.html

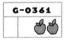

MedBioWorld: Geriatrics and Gerontology Journals A listing of geriatrics and gerontology journals available on the Internet is found on this site. There are more than 75 journals listed, some with full-text articles.
http://www.medbioworld.com/journals/medicine/geriatrics.html

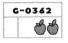

Medscout: Geriatric Medicine Resources on geriatric medicine can be found on this Web site maintained by Medscout. More than 60 sites are listed and categorized as geriatric news, associations, geriatric education, hospitals and medical centers, and geriatrics on the Internet.
http://www.medscout.com/specialties/geriatrics/

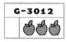

Merck Manual of Geriatrics The full text of the *Merck Manual of Geriatrics* is featured on this Web page. Sixteen chapters are provided for topics such as the basics of geriatric care; falls, fractures, and injury; surgery and rehabilitation; psychiatric disorders; neurologic disorders; and musculoskeletal disorders. In addition, disorders related to endocrinology, hematology/oncology, pulmonology, cardiology, urology/nephrology, infectious disease, dermatology, and gastroenterology are found. Each chapter contains numerous diseases and disorders with information on etiology, pathophysiology, symptoms, diagnosis, and treatment.
http://www.merck.com/pubs/mm_geriatrics/contents.htm

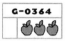

Resource Directory for Older People The National Institute on Aging and the Administration on Aging have compiled this directory of resources, serving older people and their families, health and legal professionals, social service providers, librarians, researchers, and others interested in the field of aging. The directory includes names of organizations and contact information. Visitors can search the directory by keyword or browse categories such as diseases and conditions, nutrition and fitness, and long-term-care planning from the table of contents.
http://www.aoa.dhhs.gov/aoa/dir/intro.html

15.10 GRANTS AND FUNDING SOURCES

Foundation Center The Foundation Center provides direct links to thousands of grant-making organizations, including foundations, corporations, and public charities, along with a search engine to enable the user to locate sources of funding in specific fields. In addition, the site provides listings of the largest private foundations, corporate grant makers, and community foundations. Other resources include information on funding trends, a newsletter, and grant-seeker orientation material. More than 900 grant-making organizations are accessible through this site. http://fdncenter.org

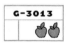

GrantSelect More than 10,000 funding opportunities are contained in the GrantSelect database for a variety of disciplines including biomedical and healthcare. The database is available to subscribers only; a free 30-day trial period is offered on the site. Subscribers can also receive an e-mail alert service for new additions to the database.
(fee-based) http://www.grantselect.com

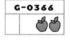

Mental Health Net: Grants and Funding Opportunities Part of a larger Mental Health Net Web page, this site features grant funding opportunities related to mental health and biomedicine in general that are available online. There are close to 20 sites listed with descriptions and ratings. The sites are categorized as Web resources; mailing lists; journals, publications, and research papers; professional organizations and centers; and other resources.
http://mentalhelp.net/guide/pro28.htm

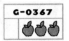

National Institutes of Health (NIH): Funding Opportunities Funding opportunities for research, scholarship, and training are extensive within the federal government. At this site for the National Institutes of Health, there is a grants page with information about NIH grants and fellowship programs, information on research contracts containing information on requests for proposals (RFPs), research training opportunities in biomedical areas, and an NIH guide for grants and contracts. The latter is the official document for announcing the availability of NIH funds for biomedical and behavioral research and research training policies. Links are provided to major divisions of the NIH that have additional information on specialized grant opportunities.
http://grants.nih.gov/grants

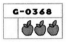

National Science Foundation (NSF): Grants and Awards Approximately 20 percent of the federal support to academic institutions for basic research comes from the National Science Foundation, making this site an important source of information for award opportunities, programs, application procedures, and other vital information. Forms and agreements may be downloaded as well, and regulations and policy guidelines are set forth clearly.
http://www.nsf.gov/home/grants.htm

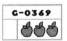

Society of Research Administrators: GrantsWeb The Society of Research Administrators has created this extremely useful grant information site with extensive links to government resources, general resources, private funding, and policy and regulation sites. The section devoted to U.S., Canadian, and other international resources provides links to government agency funding sources, the *Commerce Business Daily,* the Catalog of Federal Domestic Assistance, scientific agencies, research councils, and resources in individual fields, such as health, education, and business. Grant application procedures, regulations, and guidelines are provided throughout the site, and extensive legal information is provided through links to patent, intellectual property, and copyright offices. Associations providing funding and grant information are also listed, with direct links.
http://interchange.org/nsagislist/NL08249809.html

15.11 MEDICAL IMAGING AND RADIOLOGY

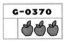

CT Is Us The CT (computed tomography) site offers information on medical imaging with a specific focus on spiral CT and 3-D imaging. Images of the body and various medical conditions are organized by region, and information on CME courses, teaching files, medical illustrations, and a 3-D vascular atlas are all available. The site also features protocols for multidetector CT and pediatric imaging, as well as teaching files and a gallery of medical illustrations.
http://www.ctisus.org

Dr. Morimoto's Image Library of Radiology This site provides users with access to images and videos collected by Dr. Ryuichi Morimoto, Depart-

ment of Radiology, Osaka National Hospital. Images were scanned and stored with JPEG and GIF format, and movies with QuickTime format. Ultrasonographic anatomy images related to the liver, pancreas, and bile duct include an illustration of portal anatomy, normal bile duct, tumor of liver hilum, bile duct cancer, pancreatic cancer, esophageal varix, and obstructive jaundice. Heart and major vessels images include a normal heart, major vessels of the body, and abdominal aortic aneurysm. Head images include a surface image of a human head and an image of an arachnoid cyst. Images related to the kidney and urinary tract include that of a renal cell carcinoma.
http://www.osaka-med.ac.jp/omc-lib/noh.html

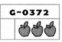

Health On the Net (HON) Foundation   This site provides links to radiological and surgical images on the Internet. Images are available of the abdomen, ankle, arm, full body, brain, elbow, eye, foot, hand, head, heart, hilum, hip, kidney, knee, leg, liver, lung, muscle, neck, pancreas, pelvis, shoulder, skin, skull, teeth, thorax, trachea, blood vessels, and wrist. The site can also be viewed in French.
http://www.hon.ch/Media/anatomy.html

Medical Imaging Resources on the Internet   Supported by the University of Leeds School of Computing in the United Kingdom, this Web page offers comprehensive resource lists for medical imaging. Visitors can view the list by geographic location, represented by the headings of Europe, North America, Asia, and Australasia. Within each region are subcategories such as universities, hospitals, research organizations, and the commercial sector. The list can also be viewed by content such as exhibits and publications, teaching aids, software, and general resources. There are also links for newsgroups, funding sources by region, and search engines.
http://www.comp.leeds.ac.uk/comir/resources/links.html

MedMark: Radiology   The professional resources provided on this site focus on the field of radiology. Hundreds of sites are listed in categories such as associations, centers, departments, education, imaging, journals, lists of resources, MRI/NMR, nuclear medicine, other organizations, PET, programs, research, and ultrasound. The sites are drawn from sources around the world and can be browsed in order or by using a drop-down menu to access the topic of interest. (some features fee-based) http://medmark.org/rad/rad2.html

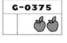

MultiDimensional Imaging   This Web site provides examples and applications of different techniques used in biomedical imaging. Multidimensional, multimodality, and multisensor applications are described in detail with methodology and specific examples of medical applications, along with discussions of new developments in this growing field.
http://www.expasy.ch/LFMI

Neurosciences on the Internet: Images   Hundreds of Internet sites are found through this address offering resources relating to human neuroanatomy and neuropathology, neuroscience images and methods, medical imaging cen-

ters, medical illustration, medical imaging indexes, and neuroanatomy atlases of animals.
http://www.neuroguide.com/neuroimg.html

Pediatric Radiology and Pediatric Imaging   Developed by Michael P. D'Alessandro, M.D., this Web page features a pediatric radiology digital library. The library contains common pediatric clinical problems with over 400 diseases represented by over 1,800 cases. There is a section on imaging approaches to common problems, as well as a section on performing common pediatric radiology procedures. Nearly 30 procedures are covered in a patient education section. There is also a link to pediatric radiology normal measurements and to musculoskeletal radiology of fractures. In addition to the library, the site lists hundreds of related links in categories such as textbooks, anatomy atlases, embryology, lectures, and patient education.
http://pediatricradiology.com/

University of Nebraska: Medical Images on the Web   A list of more than a dozen links is available at this address to Internet sources for medical images, maintained by the University of Nebraska Medical Center. Web pages listed include *Anatomy of the Human Body* by Henry Gray, a dermatology image library, a digital atlas of ophthalmology, the public health image library, the visible human project from the National Library of Medicine, and the whole brain atlas. All links are accompanied by short descriptions of resources at the site.   http://www.unmc.edu/library/eresources/medimage.html

15.12   MEDICAL SOFTWARE

Medical Software Reviews   The monthly newsletter found at this site publishes evaluations of medical software products for use by physicians and other health professionals. The contents of each issue are described, and information on Internet access for subscribers is provided. Categories of software include coding, databases, diagnosis, drug interactions, medical records, patient education, practice management, scheduling, and statistics. The table of contents for current and previous months can be viewed from the site's links; full reviews require a subscription. Subscriber information can be accessed by clicking on "Medical Software Reviews" at the bottom of the page.
(fee-based) http://www.crihealthcarepubs.com/msrmain.html

15.13   PAIN MANAGEMENT

American Academy of Pain Management   This site provides information about the academy and its activities, resources for finding a professional program in pain management, accreditation and continuing medical education resources, and a membership directory for locating a pain management professional. It also provides general information on pain management and a listing

of relevant links. Access to the National Pain Data Bank is available at the site, containing statistics on various pain management therapies based on an outcomes measurement system. The site is divided into two sections with information tailored to the needs of both patients and healthcare professionals.
http://www.aapainmanage.org

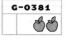

American Academy of Pain Medicine This site contains information about the academy's annual meeting, a member directory, FAQs, and related resources. Visitors can access an online newsletter, as well as a catalog of publications such as the academy's journal, *Pain Medicine,* pocket guides, and position papers. http://www.painmed.org/

American Pain Foundation The American Pain Foundation is dedicated to education and advocacy for patients and their families coping with pain. A patient information section features fact sheets on a variety of conditions such as arthritis and digestive diseases, as well as information in general on pain management and medication. There is also a section on policy and legislative issues, with links provided to related sites. On the home page, icons at the bottom lead visitors to the "Pain Care Bill of Rights" which outlines patient rights. The "You are Not Alone" section provides information on support groups, and personal stories can be read under the "Voices of People in Pain" section. In addition, there is a pain action guide and a section on finding help that contains both emotional and financial resources.
http://www.painfoundation.org/

American Pain Society The American Pain Society is a multidisciplinary, scientific organization that offers information on publications, advocacy, career opportunities, and upcoming events. A pain facility database allows the user to search for facilities by classifications, and additional resources for both patients and professionals provide contact information for related organizations. The American Pain Society site provides a search engine for abstracts in their database of pain-related topics.
http://www.ampainsoc.org/

New York Online Access to Health (NOAH): Pain Information on pain can be found through this large consumer health directory of Internet sites, maintained by the New York Online Access to Health project. The directory contains more than 100 sites categorized as the basics, types of pain, basic care, body-specific therapies, types of therapy, pain in children, and information resources. http://www.noah-health.org/english/illness/pain/pain.html

Pain.com This site is a comprehensive resource for seeking information on pain and pain management, with separate sections available for health professionals and consumers. For clinicians, information on meetings, free online CME courses, pain management standards, and full-text articles from pain journals are provided. Pages specifically addressing perioperative pain, cancer pain, interventional pain management, migraine and headache pain, and regional anesthesia are found and include information on related CME and discussion forums. Consumers can locate both a list of support groups and a directory of pain clinics. http://www.pain.com/index.cfm

15.14 PATENT SEARCHES

The following sites provide access to patent information for medical researchers and healthcare professionals interested in learning about the latest techniques, therapies, products, and drugs.

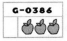

Intellectual Property Network   A spin-off of IBM, Delphion, Inc., provides this patent site which is ideal for physicians and researchers with an interest in patents. This service offers a database of patent information, titles and abstracts, and inventors and companies. The database displays patents on any topic, along with inventor information, dates of filing, application numbers, and an abstract of the patent. Users can search patent applications in the United States and Europe. The site also features a gallery of obscure patents.
(some features fee-based) http://www.delphion.com

U.S. Patent and Trademark Office   Access to the database of the U.S. Patent and Trademark Office is available through this site for detailed searching of patents by number, inventor, and topic. There are both a full-text database and a bibliographic database.
http://www.uspto.gov/patft/index.html

15.15 PATHOLOGY AND LABORATORY MEDICINE

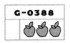

Hardin MD: Pathology and Laboratory Medicine Resources   Part of the Hardin Meta Directory from the University of Iowa, this site provides nearly 20 links to sites that each contain a list of other sites related to pathology and laboratory medicine. The sites are categorized as large, medium, or small lists.
http://www.lib.uiowa.edu/hardin/md/path.html

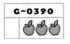

Indiana University: Pathology Image Library   An image library for pathology is featured on this Web page, maintained by Indiana University. The library is categorized by organ system such as bone and soft tissue, cardiovascular, gastrointestinal, endocrine, hepatobiliary, genitourinary, pulmonary, and renal. There is also a section for gross pathology observations. The library can be searched by keyword.
http://erl.pathology.iupui.edu/c604/Default.htm

MedBioWorld: Laboratory Science, Forensic Science, and Pathology Journals   Visitors to this Web page will find a listing of laboratory science, forensic science, and pathology journals available on the Internet. There are over 75 journals listed alphabetically.
http://www.medbioworld.com/journals/medicine/pathology.html

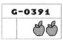

Pathology Images Developed by a group of physicians, this site features the "Lightning Hypertext of Disease," a database of pathology images with captions. The database is free to nonmembers but query results are limited to 30 images. Membership provides access to an alternate site where queries are returned with unlimited results. The results can be viewed in English, German, or Spanish. Other features include a spelling page for pathology terms, a precancer terminology page, and an abbreviations and acronyms page. There is also a section to help professionals study for their anatomic pathology and pathology specialty boards via a quiz that randomly selects questions from 6,000 multiple choice questions.

(some features fee-based) http://www.pathinfo.com/

Tulane University: Pathology Educational Resources Primarily for healthcare professionals, this site offers a listing of links related to pathology. More than 30 sites are listed under topics such as catalogs of pathology links, laboratory resources and images, and other Web resources. The sites are drawn mostly from American universities.

http://www.tmc.tulane.edu/classware/
pathology/medical_pathology/New_for_98/Resources.html

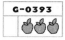

University of Illinois: The Urbana Atlas of Pathology The site provides a comprehensive collection of pathology images sectioned into general, cardiovascular, endocrine, pulmonary, and renal pathology. The general pathology section includes images of the kidney, heart, spleen, thyroid, testis, cervix, small intestine, lung, artery, pancreas, liver, lymph nodes, brain, colon, skin, mesentery, joints, uterus, and peritoneal cavity. Each image has an explanatory caption. http://www.med.uiuc.edu/PathAtlasf/titlepage.html

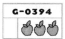

University of Michigan: Internet Resources for Pathology and Laboratory Medicine Hundreds of sites related to pathology and laboratory medicine are listed on this Web page, hosted by the University of Michigan Medical School Department of Pathology. The sites are listed in categories such as pathology departments (domestic and international), LISTSERVs, e-mail resources, databases and multimedia exhibits, regulatory and accreditation agencies, Usenet groups, job banks, organizations, and journals. There are also anatomic pathology and laboratory medicine resources. The entire list can be browsed or accessed quickly through a table of contents that lists the categories as well as subspecialty resources.

http://www.pathology.med.umich.edu/links

University of Utah: Pathology Image Library Intended for students and healthcare professionals, this site offers a pathology image library with more than 1,900 images. Maintained by the Department of Pathology at the University of Utah, the library is organized as general pathology and organ system pathology. There are also special sections with images and tutorials dedicated to AIDS pathology and anatomy/histology. A section on laboratory exercises offers case studies with images and questions. In addition, practice exams drawn from a bank of more than 1,600 questions are found. Mini-tutorials on a variety of conditions such as breast cancer, inflammatory bowel diseases, and tuberculosis are also provided. http://medstat.med.utah.edu/WebPath/webpath.html

15.16 PREVENTIVE MEDICINE

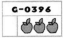

MedMark: Preventive Medicine Dedicated to preventive medicine, this site features a comprehensive listing of Internet resources. Hundreds of sites are found in categories such as associations, centers, departments, education, consumer resources, general, government, and guidelines. There are also journals, lists of resources, and programs. The site can be browsed in order or through hyperlinks found in the table of contents presented in a sidebar menu.
http://members.kr.inter.net/medmark/prevent/

15.17 PUBLIC HEALTH

American Public Health Association Health professionals may find the American Public Health Association site to be of interest. The site offers public health reports, abstracts from the *American Journal of Public Health,* and access to full-text articles from their newspaper, *The Nation's Health.* The site also has information on continuing education, legislative issues, and a publications catalog. Members will find funding opportunities under the "Programs/Projects & Practice" section. In addition, there are links for state public health associations, the World Federation of Public Health, and related public health resources.
(some features fee-based) http://www.apha.org/

National Health Service Corps After accessing the introductory page, visitors are taken to the table of contents for the National Health Service Corps Web site. General information is provided about the organization's public health mission in assisting underserved populations. Details on opportunities available to health professionals and a site on community assistance services are also available. Upcoming events and important dates, as well as other news items of the organization, are found.
http://www.bphc.hrsa.dhhs.gov/nhsc/

World Health Organization (WHO) A site index and search tool assist in navigation of this site, which is available for viewing in English, Spanish, or French. World Health Organization press releases are displayed at the main page, and connections to information resources, a press media center, and disease outbreak information are provided. Information on current emergencies by country is addressed, and a traveler's health advisory is found.
http://www.who.int/home-page/

16

MEDICAL STUDENT RESOURCES

16.1 GENERAL RESOURCES

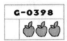
G-0398

American Medical Association (AMA): Medical Student Section The Medical Student Section of the AMA is dedicated to representing medical students, improving medical education, developing leadership, and promoting activism for the health of America. The site offers information about current issues and advocacy activities, meetings, chapter information, and leadership news. A community service link provides information on policy promotion, grant application, organ and tissue donation, and ideas for community service projects. http://amaMedstudent.org

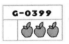
G-0399

American Medical Student Association Containing many useful resources for medical students, this site features daily health and medical news, legislative and policy issues, and LISTSERVs for special populations. A menu of topics lists issues such as community and public health, global health issues, health policy, humanistic medicine, and medical education, along with resources to get involved. This section also provides resources for positions, internships, and fellowships; leadership training information; and a list of related Internet sites. The "Resource Center" provides links for financial resources; interest groups in areas such as death and dying, psychiatry, and bioethics; and strategic priorities including diversity in medicine and medical student well-being. Additional resources include information on personal data assistants (PDAs), residency selection, and an AMSA catalog that offers many free online publications. Members can register for the career development program online and apply for financial resources such as loans and grants.
(some features fee-based) http://www.amsa.org/

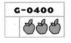
G-0400

American Medical Women's Association A national association, AMWA provides information and services to women physicians and women medical students, as well as promoting women's health and the professional development of women physicians. Resources include news, discussions of current issues, events, conferences, online publications, fellowship and residency information accessed through the Fellowship and Residency Electronic Interactive Database Access system (FRIEDA), general information and developments from AMWA staff members, advocacy activities, a listing of AMWA continuing edu-

cation programs, and links to sites of interest. A variety of topics related to women's health are discussed at the site.
http://www.amwa-doc.org

Association of American Medical Colleges This nonprofit association committed to the advancement of academic medicine consists of American and Canadian medical schools, teaching hospitals and health systems, academic and professional societies, and medical students and residents. News, membership details, publications, meeting and conference calendars, medical education Internet resources, research findings, and discussions related to healthcare are all found at the site. Employment opportunities at the AAMC are also listed.
http://www.aamc.org

Integrated Medical Curriculum This Web page integrates of major medical school courses, especially the first two years, with basic science and clinical program departments containing explanatory text, images, and cross-referenced hyperlinks. Anatomy is stressed, as well as basic clinical skills, clinical musculoskeletal pathology, and ethics. Other resources include a testing center with practice quizzes, a virtual student lounge, a faculty lounge, and related message boards.
(some features fee-based) http://www.imc.gsm.com

Internet Resources for Medical Students A comprehensive listing of links is offered on this Web page, courtesy of Lviv State Medical University, Ukraine. More than 150 links are found in categories such as associations, general sites, education, study help, multimedia, grants and funding, humor, and other resources. The sites are drawn from around the world; some are in Russian. http://www.meduniv.lviv.ua/inform/studlinks.html

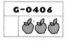

MedicalStudent.com This site contains an extensive medical textbook section organized by discipline. Features of the site included patient simulations, consumer health information, access to MEDLINE and medical journals online, continuing education sources, board examination information, medical organizations, and Internet medical directories.
http://www.medicalstudent.com

Stanford University: MedWorld MedWorld, sponsored by the Stanford Medical Alumni Association, offers information for students, patients, physicians, and the healthcare community. Resources include case reports and global rounds, links to quality medical sites and MEDLINE, doctor diaries and medical news, and newsgroups and discussion forums. Visitors can access Stanford's medical search engine, MEDBOT, to utilize several Internet medical search engines simultaneously.
http://medworld.stanford.edu/home

Student Doctor Network Hosted by the Student Doctor Network, this Web page offers medical students a broad array of resources. The SDN student forums offer discussion boards for medical and premedical students. There are

also medical student diaries, where five medical students post their thoughts and experiences as they go through medical school. "The Links Resource" features more than 740 links to information such as academic success, career choices, finance, dental resources, osteopathic resources, and medical resources. In addition, there is information on getting in and getting through medical school, osteopathic medicine, and getting into dental school.

(free registration) http://www.studentdoctor.net/

16.2 FELLOWSHIPS AND RESIDENCIES

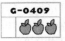

Accreditation Council for Graduate Medical Education The Accreditation Council for Graduate Medical Education (ACGME) reviews and accredits residency programs, establishes standards of performance, and provides a process to consider complaints and possible investigations by the council. The ACGME publishes standards on resident duty hours, citation statistics, and a moonlighting policy. The site also offers information about meetings, workshops, institutional reviews, program requirements, links to residency review committees, and a listing of accredited programs.

http://www.acgme.org

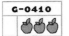

American Medical Association (AMA): Fellowship and Residency Electronic Interactive Database Access (FREIDA) Online System Operated as a service of the AMA, the FREIDA system provides online access to a comprehensive database of information on approximately 7,500 graduate medical educational programs accredited by the Accreditation Council for Graduate Medical Education (ACGME). FREIDA enables the user to search this comprehensive database and offers physician workforce statistics as reported by practicing physicians in a variety of subspecialties.

http://www.ama-assn.org/cgi-bin/freida/freida.cgi

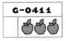

Educational Commission for Foreign Medical Graduates Through its certification program, the commission "assesses the readiness of graduates of foreign medical schools to enter residency or fellowship programs in the United States that are accredited by the Accreditation Council for Graduate Medical Education." The site provides information for foreign students on testing and examination dates, clinical skills required, medical education credentials, visa sponsorship, and certification verification.

http://www.ecfmg.org

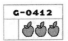

Electronic Residency Application Service The Association of American Medical Colleges (AAMC) provides this application service for students. It transmits residency applications, recommendation letters, deans' letters, transcripts, and other supporting credentials from medical schools to residency program directors via the Internet. At present, the service covers anesthesiology, dermatology, emergency medicine, family practice, internal medicine, nuclear medicine, obstetrics and gynecology, pathology, pediatrics, physical medicine

and rehabilitation, psychiatry, radiology, radiation oncology, and surgery (general, orthopedic, and plastic). The system allows tracking of an application 24 hours a day via a special document tracking system.
(some features fee-based) http://www.aamc.org/eras/news/start.htm

National Residency Matching Program The National Residency Matching Program is a mechanism for the matching of applicants to programs according to the preferences expressed by both parties. Last year this service placed over 20,000 applicants for postgraduate medical training positions into nearly 4,000 residency programs at 700 teaching hospitals in the United States. The applicants and residency programs evaluate and rank each other, producing a computerized pairing of applicants to programs, in ranked order. This process provides applicants and program directors with a uniform date of appointment to positions in March, eliminating decision pressure when options are unknown. The site offers information about the service, publications, and forms for registration. Prospective residents can register with the service for a fee and access the directory of programs.
http://nrmp.aamc.org/nrmp

ResidencySite.com ResidencySite.com provides an online listing of medical residencies organized by specialty, with links to residency program home pages. Program directors can access resumes of residency applicants, and prospective residents can review documents related to residency matching programs and publications offering advice on obtaining a position.
http://www.residencysite.com

16.3 MEDICAL SCHOOL WEB SITES

American Universities All American university home pages are listed at this site. http://www.clas.ufl.edu/CLAS/american-universities.html

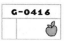

Gradschools.com Sponsored by several universities and other teaching institutions, Gradschools.com offers a listing of graduate programs nationwide. Programs are found by indicating a specific area of study. A directory of distance learning programs is also available.
http://www.gradschools.com/noformsearch.html

Medical Education Accredited medical schools are listed, with links, at this site. http://www.meducation.com/schools.html

MedicalSchoolDirectory.com A directory of medical schools, organized by state, is provided on this site. Contact information and a hyperlink to each school's Web site is offered.
http://www.doctordirectory.com/medicalschools/directory/default.asp

![17]

PATIENT EDUCATION AND PLANNING

17.1 EXERCISE AND PHYSICAL FITNESS

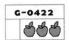

MEDLINEplus Health Information: Exercise/Physical Fitness
Resources on exercise and physical fitness are provided on this Web page, maintained by the National Library of Medicine. The site provides links for overviews on exercise, nutrition for workouts, preventing injuries, specific conditions, organizations, and statistics. Much of the information comes from government agencies or scientific associations, such as the American Heart Association or the American Academy of Family Physicians. Specific aspects of fitness such as tips on buying exercise equipment, stretching, and walking are covered. Information for specific populations is also included with sections for men, women, teenagers, seniors, and children. Some publications are available in Spanish. http://www.nlm.nih.gov/medlineplus/exercisephysicalfitness.html

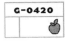

MedNets: Fitness This Web page presents a listing of links on fitness, sponsored by MedNets.com. More than 45 sites are listed in categories including journals and organizations, newsletters, and topics such as weight loss and stretching. http://www.mednets.com/fitness.htm

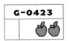

Medscout: Physical Fitness This Web page features a listing of links related to physical fitness for both patients and professionals. More than 100 sites are listed covering associations, nutrition guidelines, exercise guides, and a variety of sports and activities.
http://www.medscout.com/physical_fitness/

President's Council on Physical Fitness and Sports Resources provided at this site include a fitness guide, which details the benefits of physical activity and outlines solutions to common problems interfering with physical fitness. News about physical fitness, an online reading room, scientific research reports on physical activity topics, and resources for coaches and fitness professionals are offered. Details about the national President's Challenge and other programs for physical fitness are presented.
http://www.fitness.gov/

Prevention.com: Weight Loss and Fitness Targeted to consumers, this site from *Prevention* magazine offers information and support for losing weight

and exercising in the form of nutrition news and health articles. A fitness assessment section offers quizzes on topics such as heart health, hiking, and weight. The site also hosts message forums covering a variety of topics, including an online walking club for information and support.

(free registration) http://www.healthyideas.com/weight/

17.2 FOOD AND NUTRITION

American Dietetic Association The American Dietetic Association (ADA) presents this informative site for consumers, students, and dietetic professionals. This site has information on nutrition resources, careers in dietetics, meetings and events, government affairs, current issues, and publications. The "Healthy Lifestyles" section has nutrition tips, fact sheets, and dieting guidelines. The "ADA Press Room" offers an extensive list of resources, including information on ADA campaigns, a link to the *Journal of the ADA*, position papers, and a reading list of consumer publications. There are also links to consumer education and public policy sites; dietetic associations and networking groups; dietetic practice groups; food service and culinary organizations; and medical, health, and other professional organizations.

http://www.eatright.org

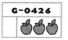

Arbor Nutrition Guide The Arbor Nutrition Guide covers all areas of nutrition including applied and clinical nutrition. The site provides links to information on dietary guidelines, special diets, sports nutrition, individual vitamins and minerals, and cultural nutrition. There are also links relating to food science, such as food labeling in other countries, food regulation, food additives, science journals, phytochemistry, and other related topics. Each link listed is accompanied by a brief description of the site. Arbor also provides links to journals and organizations.

http://www.netspace.net.au/%7Ehelmant/search.htm

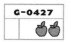

Department of Agriculture: Nutrient Values Visitors can utilize the search engine housed at this site to find the recommended daily allowance (RDA) nutrient values of over 5,000 food items for three different serving sizes for men averaging 174 pounds and for women averaging 138 pounds. The RDAs are calculated for individuals between the ages of 25 and 50.

http://www.rahul.net/cgi-bin/fatfree/usda/usda.cgi

Food and Drug Administration (FDA): Selected Non-FDA Sources of Food and Nutrition Information A list of non-FDA sources of food and nutrition information is featured on this Web page, part of the Food and Drug Administration's Center for Food Safety and Applied Nutrition site. The list contains more than 75 sites categorized as U.S. government sources, non-U.S. government sources, and nutrition journals. There are also links for related LISTSERVs and commercial sites.

(some features fee-based) http://vm.cfsan.fda.gov/~dms/nutrlist.html

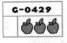

Food and Nutrition Information Center Links to hundreds of Web sites are provided through the A-to-Z food and nutrition listing on this site, maintained by the USDA's Food and Nutrition Information Center. Topics in the listing include food allergies, breastfeeding, child nutrition, eating disorders, and food labeling. Additional sections include resource lists and information on dietary supplements, food composition, dietary guidelines, the food guide pyramid, and FNIC databases. Frequently requested topics are listed in the "Consumer Corner."

http://www.nalusda.gov/fnic/

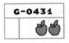

Food Science and Nutrition Journals Visitors to this site will find an alphabetical listing of over 100 food science and nutrition journals. Some provide full-text articles.

(some features fee-based) http://www.sciencekomm.at/journals/food.html

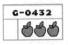

International Food Information Council The International Food Information Council (IFIC) presents resources at this site including current issues, up-to-date information for the media, food safety and nutrition facts, and extensive links to government affairs and agencies. The IFIC library provides an archive of publications geared toward educators, journalists, professionals, students, government officials, and consumers. Also featured is a glossary of food-related terms and *Food Insight*, the council's newsletter.

http://ificinfo.health.org

National Institutes of Health (NIH): Office of Dietary Supplements
The International Bibliographic Information on Dietary Supplements (IBIDS) database is featured on this Web site, courtesy of the NIH. Of interest to consumers and professionals, the IBIDS database contains more than 460,000 citations and abstracts on dietary supplements. The database can be searched via the consumer version, a full version, or peer-reviewed citations only. A journal list is provided to order full-text articles directly from the publisher. In addition, the home page contains links for grant information, a list of publications, and related resources.

http://ods.od.nih.gov/databases/ibids.html

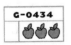

Nutrition and Healthy Eating Advice A broad array of nutrition resources is presented on this Web page. Hundreds of links are offered in categories such as healthy recipes, aging, child nutrition, cultural foods, diet analysis, diseases and conditions, and eating advice. Fad diets, food products including fast food nutrition, food safety, food science, guidelines, and organic foods are also covered. Links to related directories of sites are found as well as a question and answer forum and a free e-mail newsletter.

http://nutrition.about.com/health/nutrition/

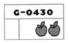

Science Reference Internet Guide to Food Science and Nutrition
Healthcare professionals and consumers may find the listing of food science and nutrition Internet sites on this Web page useful. Maintained by Michigan State University Libraries, the listing covers more than 100 resources. Categories in-

clude associations, comprehensive food and nutrition sites, business and industry resources, composition and nutrient analysis databases, safety and handling, human nutrition and health, and online journal abstracts and publications. (some features fee-based) http://www.lib.msu.edu/science/food.htm

Tufts University: Nutrition Navigator   Presented by the Center on Nutrition Communication in the School of Nutrition Science and Policy at Tufts University, this site offers an up-to-date, rated guide to other nutrition sites. It provides breaking and archived news stories related to nutrition policy and trends as well as information on general nutrition and special dietary needs. There are also sections with sites specifically targeted to parents, children, women, health professionals, educators, and journalists.
http://navigator.tufts.edu

17.3   GRIEF AND BEREAVEMENT

American College of Physicians   Part of a larger *Home Care Guide to Advanced Cancer*, this site features the chapter on grieving. The chapter provides an overview of the grieving process and covers when to get help, self-help issues, common obstacles, and carrying out and adjusting a personal grieving plan. There are also links to related information.
http://www.acponline.org/public/h_care/10-griev.htm

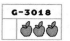

CancerNet: Loss, Grief, and Bereavement   Designed for healthcare professionals, this Physician Data Query (PDQ) from the National Cancer Institute offers guidelines for helping patients cope with loss, grief, and bereavement. A model of life-threatening illness is provided to aid in understanding of the patient's psychological needs. Other topics covered include end-of-life decisions, patterns of dying, and phases of grief. General aspects of grief therapy are described, as well as complicated grief, children and grief, and cross-cultural responses to grief. A bibliography is included, and a link is provided to a patient version of this PDQ.
http://cancernet.nci.nih.gov/cgi-bin/srchcgi.exe?DBID=pdq&
TYPE=search&SFMT=pdq_statement/1/0/0&Z208=208_06750H

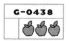

MEDLINEplus Health Information: Bereavement   Bereavement is the focus of this Web page produced by the National Library of Medicine. The site includes overviews on bereavement and grief as well as specific information for dealing with loss due to AIDS, sudden infant death syndrome, stillbirth, and suicide. Tips on helping children, teenagers, and seniors in the grieving process are also included. Some publications are available in Spanish.
http://www.nlm.nih.gov/medlineplus/bereavement.html

17.4 MEDICAL PLANNING

BLOOD BANK INFORMATION

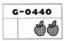

America's Blood Centers America's Blood Centers (ABC) are found in 45 states and collect almost half of the U.S. blood supply. The site provides position papers; *ABC Blood News*, a quarterly awareness publication; and *ABC Blood Bulletin*, a publication written by the ABC Scientific Medical and Technical Committee about current issues in blood banking.
http://www.americasblood.org

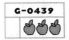

American Association of Blood Banks This site provides a contact list for each state on locating and arranging blood donation, including information on storing blood for an anticipated surgery or emergency (autologous blood transfusion). The association's regulatory affairs, legislative, and legal programs monitor and report on government, congressional, and legal issues affecting the blood banking and transfusion medicine communities. Resources for professionals in these areas include audio conferences, a virtual library, and certification programs. The education department sponsors conferences, workshops, and distance learning programs. Links are also available to AABB's journal *Transfusion*, news magazines, bulletins, and updates.
http://www.aabb.org

CAREGIVER RESOURCES

Family Caregiver Alliance Information on long-term care is featured on the Family Caregiver Alliance (FCA) Web page. Highlights of the site include dealing with hot weather and communicating with your doctor, as well as links to the alliance newsletter, webcasts, and research studies. The "Resource Center" section of the site offers an online support group, FAQs, a discussion forum, and fact sheets regarding issues in long-term care, work, and eldercare. The "Clearinghouse" section contains fact sheets on diseases and disorders, reading lists, and a "News Bureau" to help reporters with background material and interviews. The site also provides information on policy issues, FCA position papers, and a list of related resources.
http://www.caregiver.org/

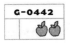

National Family Caregivers Association The National Family Caregivers Association offers education, information, support, public awareness campaigns, and advocacy to caregivers of chronically ill, aged, or disabled loved ones. The address discusses care giving and provides statistics, a survey report, news, an informational pamphlet, a reading list, care giving tips, and contact details. Caregivers will find this site a source of support, encouragement, and information. http://www.nfcacares.org

CHRONIC AND TERMINAL CARE PLANNING

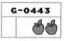
Organ Donation This government site answers frequently asked questions, dispels myths, and presents facts about organ donation. The site also posts information on public affairs and legislative updates, a list of resources on grant applications, and links to related organizations and Web sites. Visitors can also download and print a donor card.
http://www.organdonor.gov

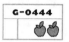
U.S. Living Will Registry This free service electronically stores advance directives and makes them available directly to hospitals by telephone. Registration materials are available to download online or by calling 1-800-LIV-WILL.
http://www.uslivingwillregistry.com

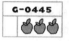
USAhomecare.com USAhomecare.com is a consumer-oriented home care (home health and hospice) site. The site provides answers to common questions, reviews considerations in implementing home care, and discusses the rights and responsibilities of clients and of the elderly population. The site also has an agency locator for the United States, a bookstore, links to related sites, and news. http://www.USAhomecare.com

DIRECTING HEALTHCARE CONCERNS AND COMPLAINTS

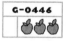
Congress.org This site offers a Capital directory, including members of Congress, the Supreme Court, state governors, and the White House. Users can also find comments on members of Congress by associations and advocacy groups, determine a bill's status through the site's search engine, send messages to Congress members, and find local congressional representatives.
http://congress.org/

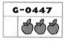
Families USA Families USA is a national, nonprofit, nonpartisan organization dedicated to the achievement of high-quality, affordable healthcare and long-term care for all Americans. The site offers a clearinghouse of information on Medicaid, Medicare, managed care, children's health, and the uninsured. Also included are news and analysis of current issues in healthcare policy. Within the site, at www.familiesusa.org/medicaid/state.htm, a state-specific healthcare information guide is provided, with state-specific issues and contacts for state officials involved with healthcare and/or insurance.
http://www.familiesusa.org

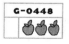
Joint Commission of Accreditation of Healthcare Organizations This independent, nonprofit organization offers an outlet for patients, their families, and caregivers to express concerns about the quality of care at accredited healthcare organizations by mail, fax, or e-mail. Complaints are addressed on issues such as patient rights, patient care, safety, infection control, medication use, and security. The commission may review and investigate warranted

complaints that cannot be resolved by the parties involved using its Quality Incident Review Criteria, also posted online here.
http://www.jcaho.org/compl_frm.html

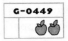

G-0449

Medicare Rights Center The Medicare Rights Center (MRC) is a national, nonprofit organization dedicated to ensuring that seniors and people with disabilities on Medicare have access to quality, affordable healthcare. Specific MRC programs include direct assistance through telephone hotlines, education and training, public policy, and communication to ensure public awareness. Publications available cover topics such as Medicare basics, home health and hospice, and Medicare bills.

(some features fee-based) http://www.medicarerights.org/Index.html

G-0451

State Insurance Commissioners Deloitte and Touche Financial Counseling Services offers the addresses and phone numbers of each state's insurance commissioner at this site.
http://www.dtonline.com/insur/inlistng.htm

Elder and Extended Care

G-0452

Administration on Aging (AOA) Dedicated to providing information on older persons and services for the elderly, the Administration on Aging offers a broad array of resources. Information on the site is divided into sections such as older persons and their families, healthcare professionals, and researchers and students. The older persons section offers a comprehensive listing of Internet resources including an AOA guide for caregivers, an eldercare locator, booklets on health topics, and fact sheets on issues such as age discrimination, longevity, and pensions. Professional resources include information on legal issues, general resources, statistics, and specific program resources such as managed care. A section entitled the "Aging Network" offers a list of general resources, and the research section emphasizes statistics.
http://www.aoa.dhhs.gov

G-0453

American Association for Retired Persons (AARP) This nonprofit group is dedicated to the needs and rights of elderly Americans. Topics discussed at the site include caregiver support, community and volunteer organizations, Medicare, Medicaid, help with home care, finances, health and wellness, independent living, computers and the Internet, and housing options. Benefits and discounts provided to members are described, reference and research materials are available, and users can search the site by keyword.
http://www.aarp.org

G-0454

American Association of Homes and Services for the Aging This association represents nonprofit organizations providing healthcare, housing, and services to the elderly. The site offers tips for consumers and family caregivers on choosing facilities and services, notices of upcoming events, press re-

leases, fact sheets, an online bookstore, and links to sponsors, business partners, an international program, and other relevant sites.
http://www.aahsa.org

Eldercare Locator   The Eldercare Locator is a nationwide directory assistance service designed to help older persons and caregivers locate local support resources for aging Americans. This site helps senior citizens find community assistance and Medicaid information. Interested parties can also contact the Eldercare Locator toll free at 1-800-677-1116.
http://www.aoa.dhhs.gov/aoa/pages/loctrnew.html

Extendedcare.com   This site offers a wide variety of resources related to senior citizens, including information on choosing an extended care provider, a "Senior Health Library" of information resources on health and aging, a glossary of terms related to extended care, and information on over 70,000 care providers searchable by type of care and zip code. Of particular interest, the "Informed Living" section provides in-depth articles on many relevant topics including home adaptation for Alzheimer's sufferers, financial planning, nutrition, exercise, and information on commonly prescribed drugs. Visitors may also participate in online chats with healthcare professionals or with other seniors and caregivers, subscribe to an e-mail newsletter, and read archived newsletters and press releases. A tool for assessing an individual's care needs is also available. A professional section is available to users associated with registered hospitals.
(some features fee-based) http://www.elderconnect.com/asp/default.asp

Insure.com: Answers to Seniors' Health Insurance Questions (on Medicare and Medicaid)   This site provides individual state phone numbers for the State Health Insurance Advisory Program (SHIP). SHIP, a federally funded program found in all states under different names, helps elderly and disabled Medicare and Medicaid recipients understand their rights and options for healthcare. Services include assistance with bills, advice on buying supplement policies, explanation of rights, help with payment denials or appeals, and assistance in choosing a Medicare health plan.
http://www.insure.com/health/ship.html

End-of-Life Decisions

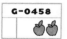

American Medical Association (AMA): Education for Physicians on End of Life Care (EPEC)   Supported by a grant from the Robert Wood Johnson Foundation, EPEC is a program designed to educate physicians nationwide on "the essential clinical competencies in end-of-life care." Visitors will find an overview of the project's purpose, design, and scope; a call for EPEC training conference applications; previous conference details; a mailing list; and an annotated list of educational resource materials. EPEC resources such as the *Participant's Handbook,* a guide to end-of-life care, can be downloaded from the site. http://www.epec.net

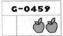

Before I Die The Web companion to a public television program exploring the medical, ethical, and social issues associated with end-of-life care in the United States is featured at this address. Personal stories, a bulletin board, a glossary of terms, contact details for important support sources and organizations, and suggestions on forming a discussion group are available at the site. A program description, viewer's guide, outreach efforts and materials, and credits for the program are also provided.
http://www.pbs.org/wnet/bid

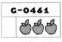

End of Life: Exploring Death in America National Public Radio's "All Things Considered" presents transcripts of a recent series on death and dying and other resources at this informative site. Contact information and links to organizations and other support sources; a bibliography of important publications; texts related to death, dying, and healing; and a forum for presenting personal stories are found at this address.
http://www.npr.org/programs/death

Last Acts Designed to improve end-of-life care, Last Acts seeks to "bring end-of-life issues out in the open and to help individuals and organizations pursue the search for better ways to care for the dying." The site presents information on Last Acts activities, a newsletter, press releases, and discussion forums. Links are available to details of recent news headlines, sites offering additional information resources, grant-making organizations, and a directory of Robert Wood Johnson Foundation end-of-life grantees.
http://www.lastacts.org

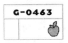

Living Wills A brief description of a living will is offered on this Web site, written by attorney Michelle M. Arostegui. The purpose of the living will is described along with when it is used and what options may be included, such as "Do Not Resuscitate" and removal of nutrition and hydration.
http://estateplanning.about.com/library/weekly/aa080401a.htm?rnk=r3&terms=living+will

Partnership for Caring: America's Voices for the Dying Partnership for Caring is a national nonprofit organization dedicated to improving the way society cares for dying people and their loved ones. The organization promotes communication by hosting live chats and moderated discussions. Resources at the site include a glossary of terms, fact sheets, and articles on topics related to end-of-life issues as well as downloads for state-specific documents on advance directives. Visitors may also access news, press releases, and *Voices*, the organization's newsletter.
http://www.partnershipforcaring.org/HomePage/

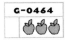

Project on Death in America: Transforming the Culture of Dying The Project on Death in America supports initiatives in research, scholarship, the humanities, and the arts in transforming the American culture in the experience of dying and bereavement. The PDIA also promotes innovations in care, public education, professional education, and public policy. Information is presented on the project's Faculty Scholars Program, as well as on various other

funding initiatives, past and present, in such areas as nursing, social work, arts and humanities, public policy, legal issues, and community-based issues. Other resources described at the site include Grantmakers Concerned with Care at the End of Life, media resources, and other publications offered by the PDIA.
http://www.soros.org/death

HOSPICE AND HOME CARE

 G-0465

American Academy of Hospice and Palliative Medicine This national nonprofit organization is composed of physicians "dedicated to the advancement of hospice/palliative medicines, its practice, research, and education." Academy details, news, press releases, position statements, events and meetings notices, employment listings, and links to related sites are found at this address. Publications, CME opportunities, and conference tapes are also available.
http://www.aahpm.org

 G-0466

Hospice Association of America Serving the needs of the most seriously ill patients suffering from cancer and other diseases, the HAA offers a full menu of information about the field of hospice care including fact sheets and statistics for consumers; legislative, regulatory, research, and legal updates; hospice publications; and education programs offered at conferences.
http://www.hospice-america.org

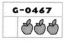 **G-0467**

Hospice Foundation of America The Hospice Foundation of America offers a range of books and training services for hospice professionals and the general public. The Web site provides information on hospices, patients and staff, services and expenses, myths and facts, and volunteering. There is also a reading list, with descriptions, and links related to organizations and resources for both the healthcare provider and the patient are also available.
http://www.hospicefoundation.org

 G-0468

Hospice Net Hospice Net is dedicated to helping patients and families facing life-threatening illnesses. The site contains a listing of useful articles, FAQ sheets, caregiver information, and a listing of select links to other major Web resources. Information is categorized as services, patients, caregivers, and bereavement. Topics and resources covered include finding a local hospice, pain control, the Family and Medical Leave Act, and dealing with grief.
http://www.hospicenet.org

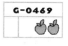 **G-0469**

HospiceWeb This site contains general information, a list of frequently asked questions, a discussion board, a hospice locator, and an extensive list of links to related sites. Links to other hospice organizations are categorized by state. http://www.hospiceweb.com/index.htm

 G-0470

National Association for Home Care The National Association for Home Care (NAHC) is a trade association representing more than 6,000 home care agencies, hospices, and home care aide organizations and medical equipment suppliers. General information offered includes news and association announcements, a newsletter on pediatric home care, and links to affiliates. Departments within NAHC cover legislative and regulatory information, meetings and conferences, statistics and technical papers, and directories of related state associations. Visitors can access a home care and hospice search tool for finding local service providers, as well as a consumer section offering information on choosing a home care provider. This section includes descriptions of agencies providing home care; tips for finding information about agencies; and discussions of services, payment, patients' rights, accrediting agencies, and state resources. One section is restricted to members.

(some features fee-based) http://www.nahc.org

National Hospice and Palliative Care Organization The National Hospice and Palliative Care organization offers a comprehensive site providing information on all aspects of hospice care for the seriously and terminally ill. Areas covered include communicating end-of-life wishes, the Medicare hospice benefit, and details on the organization's public engagement campaign. Other site features include a career center, conference listings, news, and a state-by-state and city-by-city guide to hospice organizations in the United States.

http://www.nhpco.org

MEDICAL INSURANCE AND MANAGED CARE

Agency for Healthcare Research and Quality (AHRQ): Checkup On Health Insurance Choices This discussion of health insurance choices informs consumers on topics such as why individuals need insurance, sources of health insurance, group and individual insurance, making a decision of coverage, and managed care. Types of insurance described at the site include fee-for-service and "customary" fees, health maintenance organizations, preferred provider organizations, Medicaid, Medicare, disability insurance, hospital indemnity insurance, and long-term-care insurance. The site also includes a checklist and worksheet to determine features important to an individual when choosing insurance. A glossary of terms is available for reference.

http://www.ahcpr.gov/consumer/insuranc.htm

American Association of Health Plans Located in Washington, D.C., the American Association of Health Plans represents more than 1,000 HMOs, PPOs, and other network-based plans. Geared toward professionals, the site's "Patient Care" section provides information on clinical practice guidelines, health plan operations, news, conferences, grants and awards, care delivery and disease management, prevention, public health, accreditation, industry standards, and performance measurement. The site also offers resources on government and advocacy activities, public relations materials, reports and statistics, selected bibliographies listed by subject, information on services and products, conference details, and training program information. Consumer resources in-

clude information on choosing a health plan, descriptions of different types of health plans, women's health resources, and fact sheets about health plans.
http://www.aahp.org

drkoop.com: Insurance Center   Part of drkoop.com, this site features an insurance library covering areas such as disability, workers' compensation, and long-term care. A glossary of insurance terms and health insurance news updates are also featured at the site.
http://www.drkoop.com/hcr/insurance

Employer Quality Partnership   The Employer Quality Partnership (EQP) is a volunteer coalition of employer organizations interested in promoting positive change in the healthcare marketplace and in educating employees regarding their employer-based healthcare plans. This site offers a guide for employees on selecting and understanding healthcare plans, assistance for employers in evaluating healthcare plans, and guides for employers on ways to improve the quality of their health plans.
http://www.eqp.org

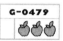

Healthcare Financing Administration   This federal site provides a wealth of information on Medicare, Medicaid, and the State Children's Health Insurance Program (SCHIP) for both patients and healthcare professionals. It covers the basic features of each program and discusses laws, regulations, and statistics about federal healthcare programs. Information is also provided at the state level (state Medicaid), providing a list of sites with important state information.
http://www.hcfa.gov

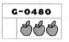

Joint Commission of Accreditation of Healthcare Organizations   The Joint Commission of Accreditation of Healthcare Organizations evaluates and accredits nearly 19,000 healthcare organizations and programs. "Quality Check," a service offered by the commission, allows consumers to check ratings and evaluations of accredited organizations at the site. Information is available for the general public, employers, healthcare purchasers, and unions; the international community; and healthcare professionals and organizations. The site also contains information on filing complaints, career opportunities, news, and links to related sites.
http://www.jcaho.org

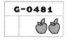

Managed Care Glossary   Designed to be used for professional training purposes or as a general information source, this managed care glossary contains a continuously updated compilation of new terminology related to managed care, with additional items in the field of information technology continuously being added. Physicians and other healthcare professionals may want to bookmark this site to ensure a more complete understanding of modern health maintenance and preferred provider organization structure and service delivery.
http://mentalhelp.net/articles/glossary.htm

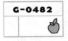

Medical Insurance Resources This site offers a large index of medical insurance resources on the Internet. Links are provided to major insurance companies and other related sites. Each link is accompanied by a brief explanation of the resources that can be found at that particular site.
http://www.nerdworld.com/trees/nw1654.html

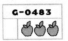

Medicare The Health Care Financing Administration (HCFA) administers Medicare, the nation's largest health insurance program, which covers nearly 40-million Americans. This site answers Medicare questions regarding eligibility, additional insurance, Medicare amounts, and enrollment. Consumer information includes answers to frequently asked questions on Medicare and help regarding health plan options. Those interested in additional information can call 1-800-MEDICARE to receive help in organizing Medicare health options.
http://www.medicare.gov

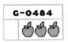

National Committee for Quality Assurance The National Committee for Quality Assurance (NCQA) is a private, nonprofit organization dedicated to assessing and reporting on the quality of managed healthcare plans. These activities are accomplished through accreditation and performance measurement of participating plans. Almost half the HMOs in the nation, covering three-quarters of all HMO enrollees, are involved in the NCQA accreditation process. A set of more than 50 standardized performance measures, called the Health Plan Employer Data and Information Set (HEDIS), is used to evaluate and compare health plans. The NCQA Web site allows the user to search the accreditation status list; results returned include the accreditation status designation and a summary report of the strengths and weaknesses of the plan. NCQA accreditation results allow users to evaluate healthcare plans in such key areas as quality of care, member satisfaction, access, and service.
http://www.ncqa.org

U.S. News Online: America's Top HMOs This site helps consumers to rate their managed care plan by ranking HMOs by state. Other useful tools include an HMO glossary, a medical dictionary, a best-hospitals finder, and a list of the 40 highest-rated HMOs in the United States. Fitness tips, articles related to HMOs, and an ask-the-doctor forum are all found at this site.
http://www.usnews.com/usnews/nycu/health/hetophmo.htm

17.5 ONLINE DRUG STORES

Accurate Pharmacy.com Accurate Pharmacy provides home care services to referred patients, supplying medical equipment, infusion products, oxygen and respiratory therapy products, and pharmaceuticals. The company also offers a 24-hour answering service, discharge assistance, and patient assessment. Patients may complete a Medication Profile to help pharmacists monitor their medications. http://www.accuratepharmacy.com

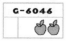

Caremark Therapeutic Services Caremark provides pharmacy benefit services and therapeutic pharmaceutical services, specializing in the management of chronic or genetic disorders. The company covers over a dozen chronic conditions including cystic fibrosis, multiple sclerosis, and rheumatoid arthritis. Each condition is linked to an information sheet on the disorder, services offered by Caremark, and related links. Users may also freely access a drug database for information on drug indications and contraindications, dosages, interactions, and side effects. Caremark's online pharmacy services are available only to patients enrolled in participating healthcare organizations.
http://www.rxrequest.com

ClickPharmacy.com ClickPharmacy seeks to enhance communication between patients, physicians, and independent pharmacies through services at their Web site. ClickPharmacy offers both personal products and prescription products. Prescriptions ordered online may be received by mail or picked up at a local independent pharmacy. Patients may also submit questions to a pharmacist online. http://www.clickpharmacy.com

CVS Pharmacy Consumers can order prescription and nonprescription drugs, along with other pharmacy items, on this Web page. The prescription section offers an extensive description of the purpose of the drug, side effects, precautions, drug interactions, and other prescribing information. Nonprescription drugs, vitamins, first aid, home care, and personal care items are also available. http://www.cvs.com

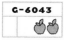

DrugEmporium.com Powered by WebRx, DrugEmporium.com offers personal care products, prescription and over-the-counter medications, vitamins, and contact lenses for home delivery with online ordering. The site also features products in their "Specialty Store" such as home test kits, air purifiers for allergy sufferers, and diabetes test strips. Patients using the DrugEmporium.com pharmacy may view their prescription request history and check on the status of their prescriptions. The site also features an index of drug prices and an interaction checker.
http://www.drugemporium.com

Drugstore.com As one of the first online drugstores, drugstore.com has developed an extensive and informative site that provides prescription and non-prescription medicine, personal care products, vitamins, and other products. There are also articles on solutions to health and beauty problems, an opportunity to ask a drugstore.com pharmacist questions, and opinions on products from customers.
http://www.drugstore.com

Eckerd.com In addition to providing vitamins, beauty products, and health products, this online service allows visitors to place an order online and pick it up at their local store. A drug information and pricing database, home delivery, and "Ask the Pharmacist" departments are available.
http://www.eckerd.com

Don't type in long URLs – add the site number to the eMedguides URL: www.eMedguides.com/**G-1234**.

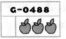

Familymeds.com   Familymeds is a prescription retailer with "brick and mortar" pharmacies as well as a Web address. This online drugstore can be used for both prescription and nonprescription needs. A personal health section features the latest news for topics such as asthma, diabetes, infant health, and women's health. A nutrition section offers fact sheets on vitamins, minerals, and herbal remedies, as well as on therapies such as acupuncture and yoga. For information and clinical recommendations on more than 200 common health concerns, the "Health Clinics" section provides fact sheets that cover causes, symptoms, natural remedies, and prescription remedies. Visitors have the option to view the entire site in Spanish. http://www.familymeds.com/familymeds

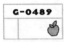

HomePharmacy.com   At Home Pharmacy visitors can perform a site-specific search for products or browse an A-to-Z listing of shopping categories. Popular products are displayed at the home page of this online drugstore, which provides a variety of healthcare products and several price specials.
http://www.homepharmacy.com

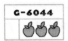

Merck-Medco   This Web site offers an online pharmacy where patients can order, refill, and renew prescriptions and purchase over-the-counter medications and personal care products. Patients can also access drug information and view their 12-month prescription history. In addition, the Merck-Medco site offers a wealth of health-related information directed to consumers. The "Health and Wellness" section contains a listing of health topics such as allergies, mental health, and skin disorders, as well as focused centers for arthritis, cardiovascular health, digestive health, respiratory health, wellness and prevention, and women's health. Each health center contains its own list of topics with articles, audio clips, practical tips, and drug information. "Health and Wellness" also offers health news, product alerts, and a variety of tools such as a health journal, allergy alerts, and a health profile calculator.
(free registration) http://www.merckmedco.com

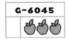

OnlineDrugstore.com   The online pharmacy at this Web site allows patients to fill, refill, and transfer prescriptions; pose questions to a pharmacist; check drug interactions; and view an A-to-Z list of drug prices and information. The site has sections for over-the-counter medications and vitamins, as well as for pet medications. OnlineDrugstore.com also features a health center powered by MedicineNet.com, where consumers may link to articles on a variety of conditions, get first aid tips for injuries, read doctors' views on healthcare and prevention, and access health news and a medical dictionary.
http://www.onlinedrugstore.com/

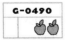

PRESCRIPTIONOnline.com   After registering, visitors can shop for prescriptions on this Web page. When requesting a medication, a close-up photo of the medication appears along with drug information and price. Pharmacists are available through an online chat room or by e-mail, phone, or fax. The site contains a list of state licenses, as well as health plans accepted.
http://prescriptiononline.com/

SafeWeb Medical   SafeWeb Medical is unique in offering patients the ability to consult online with SafeWeb physicians to obtain nonessential medications, sometimes called "embarrassment" drugs. Patients participate in an anonymous, secure, online professional consultation in cases in which a physical exam may not be required. Medications available include Viagra, Xenical, Zyben, Valtrex, Retin-A, Vioxx, and Propecia.
http://www.safewebmedical.com/

Savon.com   Savon is a retail outlet offering consumer products and prescription drugs. The site features the "Health Shopper," which provides premade shopping lists for over 40 health conditions including cataracts, fibromyalgia, hypoglycemia, and ulcerative colitis. The online pharmacy fills prescriptions and hosts an "Ask the Pharmacist" forum, as well as providing drug pricing and interactions links. In addition, a "Health" section offers tools, assessments, and health information covering dozens of health topics in more than 15 categories such as emotional health, men's health, skin health, and women's health.
(free registration) http://www.sav-ondrugs.com/default.asp

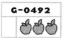

Tel-Drug Rx   Tel-Drug Rx is a mail order pharmacy program focusing on medications prescribed for periods of 30 days or longer in the treatment of chronic conditions. Pharmacy services are available only to patients participating in the CIGNA HealthCare managed pharmacy program.
http://www.cigna.com/consumer/services/pharmacy/tel_drug.html

Verified Internet Pharmacy Practice Sites Program   The Verified Internet Pharmacy Practice Sites (VIPPS) Program of the National Association of Boards of Pharmacy was developed in 1999 out of public concern for the safety of pharmacy practices on the Internet. This site contains a menu with links providing information on the criteria for VIPPS certification; a VIPPS list (which includes the pharmacy name and Web site address); VIPPS definitions; and links to Web sites of state boards of pharmacy, state medical boards, federal agencies, and professional organizations.
http://www.nabp.net/vipps/intro.asp

VitaRx.com   Physicians can use the VitaRx.com site to order prescriptions or injectable drugs for their patients. Patients can refill their prescription online or place orders for over-the-counter medications. A disease support center provides patients with fact sheets on diseases such as Crohn's disease and rheumatoid arthritis, as well as directions on self-injection. There are also "Ask a Pharmacist" and "Ask a Nurse" services where answers are posted online.
http://vitarx.com/

Walgreens   Walgreens allows patients to fill and refill prescriptions online, as well as offering an automatic refill service. Patients can view and print prescription records and histories and keep a health history online. The site also features immunization recommendations, customized e-mail reminders, and an online pharmacist who fields consumer questions. Additionally, the Walgreens

Specialty Pharmacy provides disease-specific care for patients with HIV/AIDS, multiple sclerosis, cystic fibrosis, growth hormone deficiency, and hepatitis. (free registration) http://www.walgreens.com/

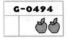

WebRx   This Web site offers customers a wide variety of products, including over-the-counter medicine, personal care items, vitamins, electronics, and prescription medicine. New patients must register by filling out an online form and provide a way to contact their doctors for prescription information. Prescriptions are processed by a registered pharmacist. News and information on more than 90 health topics are included at this resource.
http://www.webrx.com

17.6 Patient Education

General Resources

Patient information regarding various medical conditions and health issues can be obtained at any of the general medical search engines that are included. Below are listings of health Web sites accessible through the well-known search engines, as well as other sites that cover wide-ranging topics of interest to patients.

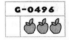

American Family Physician: Health Information for the Whole Family
Directed toward consumers, this site provides a collection of fact sheets on a variety of conditions that can be searched by keyword, population group, or region of the body. The fact sheets can also be browsed alphabetically under the "Health Information Handouts" section. Advice on topics such as lowering cholesterol, preventing flus and colds, and pain relief for lower back pain can be found under the family health facts section. Self-care flowcharts for health concerns covering symptoms, diagnosis, self-care, and when to see a doctor are also provided. In addition, there are databases for conventional drug information, herbal and alternative drugs, and drug interactions that explain proper use, side effects, and reactions. A national directory of family doctors is found, and the site can be translated into Spanish.
http://familydoctor.org

Columbia University College of Physicians and Surgeons: Complete Home Medical Guide   Patients will find this site to be a comprehensive resource for healthcare information. Topics include receiving proper medical care, the correct use of medications, first aid and safety, preventative medicine, and good nutrition. Chapters containing more specific information on health concerns for men, women, and children; disorders; infectious diseases; mental and emotional health; and substance abuse are also available.
http://cpmcnet.columbia.edu/texts/guide

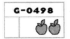

DiscoveryHealth.com   From the producers of the Discovery Channel, this site offers consumer health resources for all groups. News items, feature articles

and reports, links to health reference materials, chat forums, a forum for asking health questions, and descriptions of recent research advances are all found at this site. Visitors can access information specific to men, women, senior citizens, children, mental health, and health in the workplace. Nutrition, fitness, and weight management tools are also available at this site.
http://health.discovery.com/

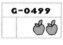

Federal Health Agencies   Consumers will find a list of links to federal health agencies on this Web site, part of a larger Patient Rights.com Web page. Each link is preceded by a short explanation of what the federal agency does. On the same page, there are links to elected officials, state health organizations, state insurance commissions, and state medical boards. Visitors can also research medical conditions through a list of links on conditions.
http://www.patientrights.com/links/links4.htm

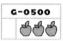

HealthAnswers.com   This site provides consumers with informational resources on a wide range of health topics including senior health, pregnancy, cancer, and STDs in the form of articles, news, and streaming videos. The site also hosts a library with encyclopedia articles that can be searched or browsed on topics such as diseases and conditions, drugs, laboratory tests, nutrition, surgeries and procedures, and symptoms.
http://www.healthanswers.com

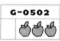

HealthTalk Interactive   Consumers will find articles, interviews, audio clips, and live interactive events with health experts on a variety of health topics on this site. Information on specific diseases can be accessed through the section titled "Disease Education Networks." Diseases covered include asthma, breast cancer, diabetes, lymphoma, menopause, multiple sclerosis, and rheumatoid arthritis. http://www.healthtalk.com/

InteliHealth   This comprehensive site offers consumers tips on healthy living, information and other resources on specific conditions, health news by topic, special reports, an online newsletter, pharmaceutical drug information, and an online store offering health items for the home. Other features include interactive diaries for specific health conditions, free e-mails on nearly 20 health topics, health assessments, and a medical dictionary. Conditions and health topics discussed at the site include allergy, arthritis, asthma, diabetes, mental health, pregnancy, nutrition, and weight management. Links are available to other sites offering consumer health resources. The site obtains its information from various sources, including the Harvard Medical School and the University of Pennsylvania School of Dental Medicine.
(free registration) http://www.intelihealth.com

MayoClinic.com   Visitors to this informative site will find answers to patient questions, news and articles on featured topics, registration details for e-mail alerts of site updates, and site search engines for health information and prescription drug information. Specific information centers are devoted to allergy and asthma, Alzheimer's disease, cancer, children's health, digestive health, and

heart health; the site also features an A-to-Z index of diseases and conditions. A library of answers to health questions, a glossary of medical terms, and a forum for asking specific questions are also available at the site.
http://www.mayohealth.org/home

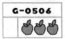

MDAdvice.com   Information on a broad array of health topics is featured on this Web page, targeted for consumers. The "Health Center" section offers a health library with patient fact sheets covering symptoms, conditions, medical tests, and surgeries; a drug information database; an ask-the-expert forum; and in-depth articles under the "Informative Material" link. A section titled "Condition Centers" features a center on cancer and one on heart disease. Each center offers fact sheets, support groups, clinical trial information, and expert advice. There are also community message boards and live chats.
http://www.mdadvice.com

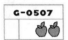

Med Help International   Visitors will find resources on a broad array of health topics on this consumer-oriented site. A comprehensive consumer health information library can be searched by keyword or browsed alphabetically and covers topics such as asthma, Hodgkin's disease, and diabetes. Each topic contains articles, a medical glossary, related questions and answers from an ask-the-expert forum, support groups, treatment options, and clinical trials. The site also features a patient-to-patient network designed to serve as an online support group, along with medical and health news updates.
http://www.medhelp.org

Medical Library   Of interest to consumers and professionals, the Medem site features a medical library, with information drawn from medical societies such as the American Academy of Pediatrics and the American Medical Association. The library is separated into four categories: life stages, diseases and conditions, therapies and health strategies, and health and society. Information in the library is further categorized into subtopics with links to articles, news, journals, and professional resources. In addition to the library, under the "Products and Services" section, physicians can develop their own Web site with secure e-mail messaging to patients. The site also offers a physician finder.
http://www.medem.com/MedLB/medlib_entry.cfm/

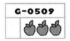

MedicineNet.com   An efficient and thorough source of information on hundreds of diseases and medical conditions, MedicineNet enables the user to click on subjects in an alphabetical list of diseases and conditions. The site's medical content is produced by board-certified physicians and allied health professionals. Other topics include procedures and tests, a pharmacy section, a medical dictionary, first aid information, and a list of poison control centers.
http://www.medicinenet.com

MEDLINEplus   A service of the National Library of Medicine, this consumer health site offers a wide variety of information categorized as health topics, drug information, dictionaries, directories, organizations, and publications. Under "Health Topics," there are hundreds of diseases and disorders, such as

asthma, AIDS, epilepsy, and sickle cell anemia. Each condition contains links for more information such as overviews, symptoms, treatment, diagnostic tests, and research. The "Drug Information" section contains a guide to more than 9,000 prescription and over-the-counter medications. Also notable is a link to MEDLINE, the National Library of Medicine's bibliographic database of more than 11-million articles.
http://www.medlineplus.gov

NetWellness NetWellness is a Web-based health information service with a large group of medical and health experts available to answer consumer questions online. Developed by the University of Cincinnati Medical Center, the Ohio State University, and Case Western Reserve University, the site has nearly 200 health faculty available to answer questions on over 40 topics. Responses are usually provided within two to three days. Visitors can also browse and search archives of articles listed under "Health Topics" or use the site's library which provides encyclopedias, patient education materials, handbooks, and magazines. (some features fee-based) http://www.netwellness.org

New York Online Access to Health (NOAH): Health Topics and Resources This site is offered as a public resource by many providers, including hospitals, institutes, foundations, research centers, and city and state agencies. Users can access information concerning over 40 health topics including diseases, mental health, and nutrition, with links provided to patient resources. A health information database containing abstracts and articles from selected health-related periodicals is only available to users accessing the site from specific institutions, including the New York Public Library branches.
http://www.noah-health.org/english/qksearch.html

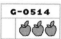

Quackwatch Quackwatch is a nonprofit corporation combating "health-related frauds, myths, fads, and fallacies." The group investigates questionable health claims, answers consumer inquiries, distributes publications, reports illegal marketing, generates consumer-protection lawsuits, works to improve the quality of health information on the Internet, and attacks misleading Internet advertising. Operation costs are generated solely from the sales of publications and individual donations. Sister sites, Chirobase and MLM Watch, offer a consumer's guide to chiropractors and a skeptical guide to multilevel marketing. Information for cancer patients includes alerts of questionable alternative health treatments, a discussion of how questionable practices may harm cancer patients, and other related discussions. Visitors to the site can purchase publications, read general information about questionable medical practices, and view details about specific questionable products and services. Links to government agencies and other sites providing information about health fraud are available at this site, which can be translated into several foreign languages.
http://www.quackwatch.com

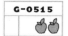

Virtual Hospital: Common Problems in Adults The Virtual Hospital Web page offers consumers and professionals resources for information on

common medical problems in adults. Provided by the University of Iowa, the site contains a table of links, with separate professional and patient sections. It covers more than 45 problems such as abdominal pain, arthritis, cancer, diabetes, pregnancy, and stroke. A link is provided to a similar site for pediatrics.
http://www.vh.org/CommonProblems/CommonProblems.html#Art

ADOLESCENT HEALTH

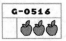

Adolescent Health Resources for Professionals Provided by the Leadership Institute on Adolescent Health, this Web site offers a listing of more than 35 sites that provide adolescent health resources for professionals. The listing includes subject guides about adolescents, general subject guides, lists of resources from associations, adolescent health programs, and special topics such as accidents, drug abuse, and teen pregnancy. There are also professional organizations, philanthropic organizations, databases, and statistics, as well as pages from the federal government.
http://corc.oclc.org/WebZ/XPathfinderQuery?sessionid=0:term=196:xid=UMM

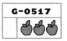

Centers for Disease Control and Prevention (CDC): Adolescent and School Health Hosted by the CDC, this site focuses on adolescent and school health. Healthcare professionals and consumers may find the resources on the site of interest. A report on adolescent health is featured that covers pregnancy, sexually transmitted diseases, and risk behaviors among adolescents. The report offers statistics, state profiles, and trend information. The site also has information on grant funding, along with publications. School health initiatives are described, as well as ongoing research.
http://www.cdc.gov/nccdphp/dash/ahson/ahson.htm

Medscout: Adolescent Health Dedicated to adolescent health, this site offers a comprehensive listing of Internet resources. There are more than 50 sites listed drawn from both domestic and international sources. Links are provided to many organizations dealing with adolescent health-related issues.
http://www.medscout.com/health/adolescent/

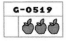

Society for Adolescent Medicine Directed to professionals, the home page of the Society for Adolescent Medicine (SAM) offers information on special interest groups for adolescent healthcare professionals, the SAM newsletter, and a list of fellowships in adolescent medicine. Several position papers can be found in the "Activities" section. Of interest to consumers and professionals, there is a list of more than 50 related links covering eating disorders, gay and lesbian teens, adolescent health, sexuality, social development, substance abuse, and violence.
http://www3.uchc.edu/~sam/samfinal/introduction-low.html

INFANT AND CHILDREN'S HEALTH

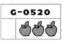

Centers for Disease Control and Prevention (CDC): Infants and Children   Parents will find more than 65 fact sheets on infants' and children's health on this Web page, part of a larger CDC site. The fact sheets cover a variety of topics such as air bags, breastfeeding, child abuse, dog bites, fifth disease, immunizations, and swimming pool safety. Some Spanish-language articles are available.   http://www.cdc.gov/health/nfantsmenu.htm

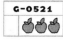

KidsGrowth.com   This site offers a wealth of resources on parenting and child development. A section on parenting offers hundreds of articles and answers from experts on a variety of topics, including discipline, parent skills, and school health. Articles and answers can be found in a child development section, categorized by age group. A section on growth milestones offers parental guidance on development, with related articles arranged chronologically from the prenatal visit to the 10-year-old child. Also available are a free weekly e-mail newsletter, growth tables, an interactive car seat selector, and parent guides for vomiting, fever, coughing, and diarrhea. In addition, the site posts book reviews, poison control resources, and information on product recalls.
http://www.kidsgrowth.com/index2.cfm

KidsHealth.org   This site, created by the Nemours Foundation Center for Children's Health Media, provides expert health information about children from the prenatal period through adolescence. Specific sections target children, teens, and parents, with age-appropriate information and language. Within each section are categories containing a large number of links to articles on specific topics. Categories in the "Parents" section include emotions and behavior, positive parenting, and the healthcare system.
http://kidshealth.org

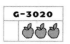

Medem Medical Library: Children's Health   Provided by the American Academy of Pediatrics, information at this page includes coverage of more than 35 child-related health topics. The directory of subjects can be browsed by category and includes topics ranging from asthma to youth violence. Medical news and a site-specific search engine are provided.
http://www.medem.com/MedLB/bufferpage_aap.cfm

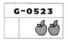

Medscout: Children's Health   A comprehensive listing of more than 100 links related to children's health are provided on this Web page, courtesy of Medscout. The sites are appropriate for both consumers and professionals and cover a broad range of topics relating to infants and children.
http://www.medscout.com/health/childrens/

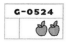

Virtual Children's Hospital: Common Problems in Pediatrics   Parents and professionals will find information on common health problems in children on this Web page, courtesy of the Virtual Children's Hospital. More than 45 health topics are covered such as asthma, behavior problems, diabetes, and sleep

problems. Resources for consumers and health providers are in different sections of the table of resources.
http://www.vh.org/VCH/CommonProblems/CommonProblems.html#An

MEN'S HEALTH

MEDLINEplus Health Information: Men's Health Topics   Information on a variety of men's health topics is provided on this Web page, maintained by the National Library of Medicine. Topics include circumcision, STDs, infertility, and prostate diseases. Each topic has links for additional information categorized as an overview, clinical trials, diagnosis/symptoms, prevention, specific aspects, and related organizations.
http://www.nlm.nih.gov/medlineplus/menshealth.html

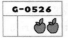

Men's Health Network   Dedicated to education and advocacy on behalf of men's health, the Men's Health Network produces this Web page to provide information on their activities including education, advocacy, and health screening efforts. A library section contains links such as data and statistics on men's high-risk-job injuries, along with resources on prostate disease issues, stroke, diabetes, STDs, and parenting. The "Men's Links" section offers a long list of links covering health resources, workplace safety, domestic violence, and suicide, as well as journals and organizations.
http://www.menshealthnetwork.org/

New York Online Access to Health (NOAH): Men's Health   Directed at consumers, more than 35 links related to men's health are offered on this site, maintained by the New York Online Access to Health project. The links cover basic information, such as anatomy and primary care for men; specific issues, such as fertility, impotence, prostate diseases, and testicular diseases; and information resources, including the Mayo Clinic.
http://www.noah-health.org/english/wellness/healthyliving/menshealth.html

MINORITY HEALTH

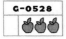

Department of Health and Human Services: Office of Minority Health   Located within the U.S. Department of Health and Human Services, the Office of Minority Health focuses on public health issues affecting minorities. Their Web page offers information on conferences, a list of online publications from federal and nonfederal sources, data and statistics, and related links. There is also a section on federal clearinghouses that can be searched by topic. The "What's New" section covers legislation and funding announcements. Visitors can also learn more about the office's initiatives, programs, and work on health disparities. A resource center offers publications, funding information, and databases of organizations, programs, and documents related to minority health. http://www.omhrc.gov/

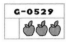

Health Information for Minority Women The National Women's Health Information Center has provided this Web site dedicated to health information for minority women. In addition to an overview of minority health, there are sections of the site dedicated to health information specific to African Americans, Asian/Pacific Islanders, American Indian/Alaskan Natives, and Hispanic/Latinas. Each minority section contains fact sheets on a variety of health topics such as asthma, cancer, and diabetes. Each fact sheet also offers links to publications and related organizations. In addition, there is a link for a list of federal minority offices. A fact sheet on leading causes of death among minority women, as well as a link to the Office on Women's Health site that describes that office's activities to promote minority health, is provided.
http://www.4woman.gov/minority/

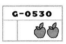

HealthWeb: Minority Health Examining minority health, this Web page offers a directory with hundreds of sites of interest to both professionals and the public. The sites are accessed by clicking on topics in the table of contents, which include general resources, education and training opportunities, African Americans, Asian Americans, Hispanic Americans, Native Americans, and research in minority health.
http://healthweb.org/browse.cfm?subjectid=53

Senior Health

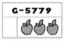

American Association for Retired Persons (AARP) The feature finder at this site connects visitors to a variety of services of the American Association for Retired Persons (AARP), including guides to health and wellness, life transitions, and legislative issues of interest to older Americans. The Web edition of the *AARP Bulletin* offers stories for those entering their middle and later years, and a department on making educated healthcare choices is provided. An online discussion center, links to local AARP chapters, and the current online edition of *Modern Maturity* are also found.
http://www.aarp.org/

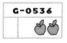

Hardin MD: Geriatrics and Senior Health The Hardin Meta Directory on this site features geriatrics and senior health. Categorized as large and medium lists, there are links to Web pages that contain lists of relevant Internet resources. The lists are drawn from both domestic and international sources and cover hundreds of sites. There are also links to additional directories of lists on Alzheimer's and Parkinson's disease.
http://www.lib.uiowa.edu/hardin/md/ger.html

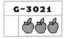

National Institute on Aging (NIA) The NIA, a division of the National Institutes of Health, leads the research effort to extend healthy lives and better understand the processes associated with aging. News and events about the division, a publications and resource list, and details of their research programs can be located from the site's links. The Alzheimer's Disease Education and Referral

(ADEAR), a service of the NIA, offers additional information on Alzheimer's disease and related conditions. The site also provides press releases, funding opportunities, and conference information.

http://www.nih.gov/nia

WOMEN'S HEALTH

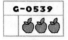

About: Women's Health   A comprehensive consumer-oriented directory of links related to women's health is offered on this Web site. The site offers an A-to-Z listing of health topics, along with commonly referenced topics such as birth control, dieting, menopause, and STDs. Each section lists Internet resources with a description of site content. Also available are a physician locator, a section on surgical procedures, and a calculator/tools section with interactive quizzes on risk factors for disease.

http://womenshealth.about.com/health/womenshealth/library/blaward.htm

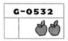

African American Women's Health   Visitors will find a variety of resources dedicated to the health of African American women. There is an A-to-Z listing of health topics such as alcohol addiction, diabetes, and fibroids; each topic has a fact sheet with references and resource links. There are also fact sheets in sections categorized as nutrition and fitness, spiritual and mental health, and finances. In addition, there are a discussion forum and a business directory. Physicians can add their names to a physician locator service.

http://www.blackwomenshealth.com/

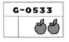

allHealth.com   Primarily directed toward female consumers, a variety of health resources are found at this iVillage Web page. The site offers "Health Tools," where visitors can take quizzes to test their knowledge of breast cancer or learn the difference between allergies and colds. The site also offers educational modules on managing conditions such as asthma, diabetes, and hypertension. Access to MEDLINE and related health databases is provided, as are articles, expert advice, and message boards on specific health concerns. Health topics can be browsed under an A-to-Z directory of conditions or researched in an illustrated medical encyclopedia.

http://www.allhealth.com

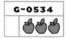

Department of Health and Human Services: National Women's Health Information Center   Focused on women's health, the National Women's Health Information Center offers resources for professionals and the public. The site can be searched by health topic or by keyword. Information on programs such as breastfeeding, violence against women, and healthy pregnancy is provided; each has consumer materials, publications, and a list of related links. A health professionals section offers links to medical journals, clinical trials, publications, and patient fact sheets. Also available are a media section with facts and statistics on women's health, a directory of residential and fellowship

programs, and information on funding opportunities. Some areas of the site can also be viewed in Spanish.
http://www.4woman.org/index.htm

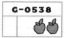

iVillageHealth   Primarily for consumers, the iVillageHealth site offers information on a variety of women's health topics. Visitors can access articles and fact sheets related to topics such as allergies, breast cancer, heart disease, pregnancy, and sexual dysfunction. A "tool kit" on the home page offers interactive tools such as quizzes, a health calculator, and access to MEDLINE. An ask-the-expert section is available on a variety of health topics. Chats, message boards, and support groups are also available.
http://www.ivillagehealth.com/

Medscape: Women's Health   A variety of clinical information related to women's health is featured on this Web page, primarily for professionals. Resources on this site include the latest news, treatment updates, clinical management, and practice guidelines. There is also CME information with some online CME courses. A resource center provides condition-specific information. In addition, there are journals, related links, and an "Exam Room" with interactive case studies. Consumers can find disease information under a patient resources section. (free registration)
http://www.medscape.com/Home/Topics/WomensHealth/WomensHealth.html

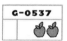

University of Maryland: Women's Health Web Sites   Resources on women's health are featured on this site, maintained by the University of Maryland. The site contains a listing of links to more than 70 women's health Web pages. A short description of each site is provided.
http://research.umbc.edu/~korenman/wmst/links_hlth.html

17.7 SUPPORT GROUPS

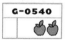

Genetic Alliance: Member Directory   The Genetic Alliance, formerly the Alliance of Genetic Support Groups, offers their membership directory of support groups on this site. The directory can be searched by genetic condition, organization name, or services offered. Alternatively, one can browse the entire directory. A resources section contains links to disease information and genetic issues. http://www.geneticalliance.org/diseaseinfo/search.html

New York Online Access to Health (NOAH): Support Groups   This directory of Web resources includes links to other directories, general health sites, toll-free telephone numbers, face-to-face support groups, support organizations, newsgroups, mailing lists, chat forums, and other online support resources. Visitors can browse listings by type of resource or by specific medical conditions. http://www.noah-health.org/english/support.html

SupportPath.com   SupportPath.com allows people with health, personal, and relationship issues to share their experiences through bulletin boards and online chats and also provides links to support-related information on the Internet. The A-to-Z listing offers hundreds of connections to areas such as disease-related support, bereavement assistance, marriage and family issue groups, and women's/men's issues. The "Message Board Tracker" lists the most recent messages and provides a complete cross-reference of topics.
http://www.supportpath.com

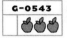

University of Kansas Medical Center: Genetic and Rare Conditions
Organized by the Medical Genetics Department of the University of Kansas Medical Center, this site offers a comprehensive listing of links on genetics and rare conditions. The home page features an A-to-Z listing of rare diseases and conditions. Hyperlinks at the top of the site lead to hundreds of resources categorized as national and international organizations, specific conditions, genetic counselors, children and teens, and advocacy. Information on support groups can be found in the national and international organizations section.
http://www.kumc.edu/gec/support/groups.html

18

WEB SITE AND
TOPICAL INDEX

APPENDICES

Appendix A

Avandia

#1 prescribed TZD...Over 12 million Rxs...Over 2 million patients...Over 2 years on the market*

AVANDIA® (rosiglitazone maleate) tablets
Before prescribing, see complete prescribing information. The following is a brief summary.

INDICATIONS AND USAGE: *Avandia* is indicated as an adjunct to diet and exercise to improve glycemic control in patients with type 2 diabetes mellitus. *Avandia* is indicated as monotherapy. *Avandia* is also indicated for use in combination with a sulfonylurea or metformin when diet, exercise, and a single agent do not result in adequate glycemic control. For patients inadequately controlled with a maximum dose of a sulfonylurea or metformin, *Avandia* should be added to, rather than substituted for, a sulfonylurea or metformin. Prior to initiation of therapy with *Avandia*, investigate and treat secondary causes of poor glycemic control, e.g., infection.

CONTRAINDICATIONS: *Avandia* is contraindicated in patients with known hypersensitivity to this product or any of its components.

WARNINGS: Cardiac Failure and Other Cardiac Effects: *Avandia*, like other thiazolidinediones, alone or in combination with other antidiabetic agents, can cause fluid retention, which may exacerbate or lead to heart failure. Patients should be observed for signs and symptoms of heart failure. *Avandia* should be discontinued if any deterioration in cardiac status occurs. Patients with New York Heart Association (NYHA) Class 3 and 4 cardiac status were not studied during the clinical trials. *Avandia* is not recommended in patients with NYHA Class 3 and 4 cardiac status. In two 26-week U.S. trials involving 611 patients with type 2 diabetes, *Avandia* plus insulin therapy was compared with insulin therapy alone. These trials included patients with long-standing diabetes and a high prevalence of pre-existing medical conditions, including peripheral neuropathy (34%), retinopathy (19%), ischemic heart disease (14%), vascular disease (9%), and congestive heart failure (2.5%). In these clinical studies an increased incidence of cardiac failure and other cardiovascular adverse events were seen in patients on *Avandia* and insulin combination therapy compared to insulin and placebo. Patients who experienced heart failure were on average older, had a longer duration of diabetes, and were mostly on the higher 8 mg daily dose of *Avandia*. In this population, however, it was not possible to determine specific risk factors that could be used to identify all patients at risk of heart failure on combination therapy. Three of 10 patients who developed cardiac failure on combination therapy during the double blind part of the studies had no known prior evidence of congestive heart failure, or pre-existing cardiac condition. **The use of *Avandia* in combination therapy with insulin is not indicated (see ADVERSE REACTIONS).**

PRECAUTIONS: General: Due to its mechanism of action, *Avandia* is active only in the presence of endogenous insulin. Therefore, *Avandia* should not be used in patients with type 1 diabetes or for the treatment of diabetic ketoacidosis. ***Hypoglycemia:*** Patients receiving *Avandia* in combination with other hypoglycemic agents may be at risk for hypoglycemia, and a reduction in the dose of the concomitant agent may be necessary. ***Edema:*** *Avandia* should be used with caution in patients with edema. In a clinical study in healthy volunteers who received *Avandia* 8 mg once daily for 8 weeks, there was a statistically significant increase in median plasma volume compared to placebo. Since thiazolidinediones, including rosiglitazone, can cause fluid retention, which can exacerbate or lead to congestive heart failure, *Avandia* should be used with caution in patients at risk for heart failure. Patients should be monitored for signs and symptoms of heart failure (see WARNINGS, Cardiac Failure and Other Cardiac Effects and PRECAUTIONS, Information for Patients). In controlled clinical trials of patients with type 2 diabetes, mild to moderate edema was reported in patients treated with *Avandia*, and may be dose related. Patients with ongoing edema are more likely to have adverse events associated with edema if started on combination therapy with insulin and *Avandia* (see ADVERSE REACTIONS).

Weight Gain: Dose-related weight gain was seen with *Avandia* alone and in combination with other hypoglycemic agents. The mechanism of weight gain is unclear but probably involves a combination of fluid retention and fat accumulation.

Table 1. Weight Changes (kg) from Baseline During Clinical Trials with *Avandia*

		Control Group		***Avandia* 4 mg**	***Avandia* 8 mg**
Monotherapy	**Duration**		**Median (25th, 75th percentile)**	**Median (25th, 75th percentile)**	**Median (25th, 75th percentile)**
	26 weeks	placebo	-0.9 (-2.8, 0.9)	1.0 (-0.9, 3.6)	3.1 (1.1, 5.8)
	52 weeks	sulfonylurea	2.0 (0, 4.0)	2.0 (-0.6, 4.0)	2.6 (0, 5.3)
Combination therapy					
sulfonylurea	26 weeks	sulfonylurea	0 (-1.3, 1.2)	1.8 (0, 3.1)	—
metformin	26 weeks	metformin	-1.4 (-3.2, 0.2)	0.8 (-1.0, 2.6)	2.1 (0, 4.3)
insulin	26 weeks	insulin	0.9 (-0.5, 2.7)	4.1 (1.4, 6.3)	5.4 (3.4, 7.3)

lematologic: Across all controlled clinical studies, decreases in hemoglobin and hematocrit (mean decreases in ndividual studies ≤1.0 gram/dL and ≤3.3%, respectively) were observed for *Avandia* alone and in combination with ther hypoglycemic agents. The changes occurred primarily during the first 3 months following initiation of *Avandia* ierapy or following an increase in *Avandia* dose. White blood cell counts also decreased slightly in patients treated vith *Avandia*. The observed changes may be related to the increased plasma volume observed with treatment with *vandia* and may be dose related (see ADVERSE REACTIONS, Laboratory Abnormalities).

vulation: Therapy with *Avandia*, like other thiazolidinediones, may result in ovulation in some premenopausal novulatory women. As a result, these patients may be at an increased risk for pregnancy while taking *Avandia* (see RECAUTIONS, Pregnancy, Pregnancy Category C). Thus, adequate contraception in premenopausal women should recommended. This possible effect has not been specifically investigated in clinical studies so the frequency of is occurrence is not known. Although hormonal imbalance has been seen in preclinical studies (see PRECAUTIONS, arcinogenesis, Mutagenesis, Impairment of Fertility), the clinical significance of this finding is not known. If unexcted menstrual dysfunction occurs, the benefits of continued therapy with *Avandia* should be reviewed.

epatic Effects: Another drug of the thiazolidinedione class, troglitazone, was associated with idiosyncratic hepatoxicity, and very rare cases of liver failure, liver transplants, and death were reported during clinical use. In preproval controlled clinical trials in patients with type 2 diabetes, troglitazone was more frequently associated with nically significant elevations in liver enzymes (ALT >3X upper limit of normal) compared to placebo. Very rare cases reversible jaundice were also reported. In pre-approval clinical studies in 4598 patients treated with *Avandia*, compassing approximately 3600 patient years of exposure, there was no signal of drug-induced hepatotoxicity or vation of ALT levels. In pre-approval controlled trials, 0.2% of patients treated with *Avandia* had elevations in ALT X the upper limit of normal compared to 0.2% on placebo and 0.5% on active comparators. The ALT elevations in ients treated with *Avandia* were reversible and were not clearly causally related to therapy with *Avandia*. In postrketing experience with *Avandia*, reports of hepatitis and of hepatic enzyme elevations to three or more times the er limit of normal have been received. Very rarely, these reports have involved hepatic failure with and without l outcome, although causality has not been established. Rosiglitazone is structurally related to troglitazone, a zolidinedione no longer marketed in the United States, which was associated with idiosyncratic hepatotoxicity rare cases of liver failure, liver transplants, and death during clinical use. Pending the availability of the results dditional large, long-term controlled clinical trials and additional postmarketing safety data, it is recommended patients treated with *Avandia* undergo periodic monitoring of liver enzymes. Liver enzymes should be checked to the initiation of therapy with *Avandia* in all patients. Therapy with *Avandia* should not be initiated in patients increased baseline liver enzyme levels (ALT >2.5X upper limit of normal). In patients with normal baseline liver mes, following initiation of therapy with *Avandia*, it is recommended that liver enzymes be monitored every 2 ths for the first 12 months, and periodically thereafter. Patients with mildly elevated liver enzymes (ALT levels X upper limit of normal) at baseline or during therapy with *Avandia* should be evaluated to determine the cause e liver enzyme elevation. Initiation of, or continuation of, therapy with *Avandia* in patients with mild liver me elevations should proceed with caution and include close clinical follow-up, including more frequent liver me monitoring, to determine if the liver enzyme elevations resolve or worsen. If at any time ALT levels increase X upper limit of normal in patients on therapy with *Avandia*, liver enzyme levels should be rechecked as soon ssible. If ALT levels remain >3X the upper limit of normal, therapy with *Avandia* should be discontinued. There o data available from clinical trials to evaluate the safety of *Avandia* in patients who experienced liver abnores, hepatic dysfunction, or jaundice while on troglitazone. *Avandia* should not be used in patients who expeed jaundice while taking troglitazone. If any patient develops symptoms suggesting hepatic dysfunction, which include unexplained nausea, vomiting, abdominal pain, fatigue, anorexia and/or dark urine, liver enzymes d be checked. The decision whether to continue the patient on therapy with *Avandia* should be guided by clindgment pending laboratory evaluations. If jaundice is observed, drug therapy should be discontinued.

ratory Tests: Periodic fasting blood glucose and HbA1c measurements should be performed to monitor therc response. Liver enzyme monitoring is recommended prior to initiation of therapy with *Avandia* in all patients eriodically thereafter (see PRECAUTIONS, *Hepatic Effects* and ADVERSE REACTIONS, Serum Transaminase).

nation for Patients: Patients should be informed of the following. It is important to adhere to dietary instrucnd to regularly have blood glucose and glycosylated hemoglobin tested. Patients should be advised that it can weeks to see a reduction in blood glucose and 2 to 3 months to see full effect. Patients should be informed ood will be drawn to check their liver function prior to the start of therapy and every 2 months for the first 12 s, and periodically thereafter. Patients with unexplained symptoms of nausea, vomiting, abdominal pain, , anorexia, or dark urine should immediately report these symptoms to their physician. Patients who experi unusually rapid increase in weight or edema or who develop shortness of breath or other symptoms of heart while on *Avandia* should immediately report these symptoms to their physician.

nteractions: Drugs Metabolized by Cytochrome P_{450}: *Avandia* was shown to have no clinically relevant eractions with nifedipine and oral contraceptives, which are predominantly metabolized by CYP3A4; glyburide, nin, acarbose, digoxin, warfarin, ethanol and ranitidine. See full prescribing information.

Carcinogenesis, Mutagenesis, Impairment of Fertility: *Carcinogenesis:* Rosiglitazone was not carcinogenic in the mouse. There was an increase in incidence of adipose hyperplasia in the mouse at doses ≥1.5 mg/kg/day (approximately 2 times human AUC at the maximum recommended human daily dose). In rats, there was a significant increase in the incidence of benign adipose tissue tumors (lipomas) at doses ≥0.3 mg/kg/day (approximately 2 times human AUC at the maximum recommended human daily dose). These proliferative changes in both species are considered due to the persistent pharmacological overstimulation of adipose tissue.

Mutagenesis: Rosiglitazone was not mutagenic or clastogenic in the *in vitro* bacterial assays for gene mutation, the *in vitro* chromosome aberration test in human lymphocytes, the *in vivo* mouse micronucleus test, and the *in vivo/in vitro* rat UDS assay. There was a small (about 2-fold) increase in mutation in the *in vitro* mouse lymphoma assay in the presence of metabolic activation.

Impairment of Fertility: Rosiglitazone had no effects on mating or fertility of male rats given up to 40 mg/kg/day (approximately 116 times human AUC at the maximum recommended human daily dose). Rosiglitazone altered estrous cyclicity (2 mg/kg/day) and reduced fertility (40 mg/kg/day) of female rats in association with lower plasma levels of progesterone and estradiol (approximately 20 and 200 times human AUC at the maximum recommended human daily dose, respectively). No such effects were noted at 0.2 mg/kg/day (approximately 3 times human AUC at the maximum recommended human daily dose). In monkeys, rosiglitazone (0.6 and 4.6 mg/kg/day; approximately 3 and 15 times human AUC at the maximum recommended human daily dose, respectively) diminished the follicular phase rise in serum estradiol with consequential reduction in the luteinizing hormone surge, lower luteal phase progesterone levels, and amenorrhea. The mechanism for these effects appears to be direct inhibition of ovarian steroidogenesis.

Animal Toxicology: Heart weights were increased in mice (3 mg/kg/day), rats (5 mg/kg/day), and dogs (2 mg/kg/day) with rosiglitazone treatments (approximately 5, 22, and 2 times human AUC at the maximum recommended human daily dose, respectively). Morphometric measurement indicated that there was hypertrophy in cardiac ventricular tissues, which may be due to increased heart work as a result of plasma volume expansion.

Pregnancy: Pregnancy Category C. There was no effect on implantation or the embryo with rosiglitazone treatment during early pregnancy in rats, but treatment during mid-late gestation was associated with fetal death and growth retardation in both rats and rabbits. Teratogenicity was not observed at doses up to 3 mg/kg in rats and 100 mg/kg in rabbits (approximately 20 and 75 times human AUC at the maximum recommended human daily dose, respectively). Rosiglitazone caused placental pathology in rats (3 mg/kg/day). Treatment of rats during gestation through lactation reduced litter size, neonatal viability, and postnatal growth, with growth retardation reversible after puberty. For effects on the placenta, embryo/fetus, and offspring, the no-effect dose was 0.2 mg/kg/day in rats and 15 mg/kg/day in rabbits. These no-effect levels are approximately 4 times human AUC at the maximum recommended human daily dose. There are no adequate and well-controlled studies in pregnant women. *Avandia* should not be used during pregnancy unless the potential benefit justifies the potential risk to the fetus. Because current information strongly suggests that abnormal blood glucose levels during pregnancy are associated with a higher incidence of congenital anomalies as well as increased neonatal morbidity and mortality, most experts recommend that insulin monotherapy be used during pregnancy to maintain blood glucose levels as close to normal as possible.

Labor and Delivery: The effect of rosiglitazone on labor and delivery in humans is not known. **Nursing Mothers:** Drug-related material was detected in milk from lactating rats. It is not known whether *Avandia* is excreted in human milk. Because many drugs are excreted in human milk, *Avandia* should not be administered to a nursing woman.

ADVERSE REACTIONS: In clinical trials, approximately 4600 patients with type 2 diabetes have been treated with *Avandia*; 3300 patients were treated for 6 months or longer and 2000 patients were treated for 12 months or longer. The following adverse events (occurring at rates ≥5% in any treatment group) were reported by patients in double-blind clinical trials with *Avandia* as monotherapy (N=2526), compared to events seen in patients treated with placebo (N=601), metformin (N=225) or sulfonylureas (N=626), respectively: Upper respiratory tract infection (9.9%, 8.7%, 8.9%, 7.3%); injury (7.6%, 4.3%, 7.6%, 6.1%); headache (5.9%, 5.0%, 8.9%, 5.4%); back pain (4.0%, 3.8%, 4.0%, 5.0%); hyperglycemia (3.9%, 5.7%, 4.4%, 8.1%); fatigue (3.6%, 5.0%, 4.0%, 1.9%); sinusitis (3.2%, 4.5%, 5.3%, 3.0%); diarrhea (2.3%, 3.3%, 15.6%, 3.0%), and hypoglycemia (0.6%, 0.2%, 1.3%, 5.9%). The sulfonylurea group includes patients receiving glyburide (N=514), gliclazide (N=91) or glipizide (N=21).

A small number of patients treated with *Avandia* had adverse events of anemia and edema. Overall, these events were generally mild to moderate in severity and usually did not require discontinuation of treatment with *Avandia*. In double-blind studies, anemia was reported in 1.9% of patients receiving *Avandia* compared to 0.7% on placebo, 0.6% on sulfonylureas and 2.2% on metformin. Edema was reported in 4.8% of patients receiving *Avandia* compared to 1.3% on placebo, 1.0% on sulfonylureas, and 2.2% on metformin. Overall, the types of adverse experiences reported when *Avandia* was used in combination with a sulfonylurea or metformin were similar to those during monotherapy with *Avandia*. Reports of anemia (7.1%) were greater in patients treated with a combination of *Avandia* and metformin compared to monotherapy with *Avandia* or in combination with a sulfonylurea. Lower pre-treatment hemoglobin/hematocrit levels in patients enrolled in the metformin combination clinical trials may have contributed to the higher reporting rate of anemia in these studies (see ADVERSE REACTIONS, Laboratory Abnormalities, Hematologic). In 26-week double-blind studies, edema was reported with higher frequency in the *Avandia* plus insulin combination trials (insulin, 5.4%; and *Avandia* in combination with insulin, 14.7%). Reports of new onset or exacerbation of congestive heart failure occurred at rates of 1% for insulin alone, and 2% (4 mg) and 3% (8 mg) for insulin in combination with *Avandia* (see WARNINGS, Cardiac Failure and Other Cardiac Effects). In postmarketing experience with *Avandia*, adverse events potentially related to volume expansion (e.g., congestive heart failure, pulmonary edema, and pleural effusions) have been reported.

Laboratory Abnormalities: Hematologic: Decreases in mean hemoglobin and hematocrit occurred in a dose-related fashion in patients treated with *Avandia* (mean decreases in individual studies up to 1.0 gram/dL hemoglobin and up to 3.3% hematocrit). The time course and magnitude of decreases were similar in patients treated with a combination of *Avandia* and other hypoglycemic agents or *Avandia* monotherapy. Pre-treatment levels of hemoglobin and hematocrit were lower in patients in metformin combination studies and may have contributed to the higher reporting rate of anemia. White blood cell counts also decreased slightly in patients treated with *Avandia*. Decreases in hematologic parameters may be related to increased plasma volume observed with treatment with *Avandia*.

Lipids: Changes in serum lipids have been observed following treatment with *Avandia* (see CLINICAL STUDIES in the full prescribing information).

Serum Transaminase Levels: In clinical studies in 4598 patients treated with *Avandia* encompassing approximately 3600 patient years of exposure, there was no evidence of drug-induced hepatotoxicity or elevated ALT levels. In controlled trials, 0.2% of patients treated with *Avandia* had reversible elevations in ALT >3X the upper limit of normal compared to 0.2% on placebo and 0.5% on active comparators. Hyperbilirubinemia was found in 0.3% of patients treated with *Avandia* compared with 0.9% treated with placebo and 1% in patients treated with active comparators. In the clinical program including long-term, open-label experience, the rate per 100 patient years exposure of ALT increase to >3X the upper limit of normal was 0.35 for patients treated with *Avandia*, 0.59 for placebo-treated patients, and 0.78 for patients treated with active comparator agents. In pre-approval clinical trials, there were no cases of idiosyncratic drug reactions leading to hepatic failure. In postmarketing experience with *Avandia*, reports of hepatic enzyme elevations three or more times the upper limit of normal and hepatitis have been received (see PRECAUTIONS, *Hepatic Effects*).

DOSAGE AND ADMINISTRATION: The management of antidiabetic therapy should be individualized. *Avandia* may be administered either at a starting dose of 4 mg as a single daily dose or divided and administered in the morning and evening. For patients who respond inadequately following 8 to 12 weeks of treatment, as determined by reduction in FPG, the dose may be increased to 8 mg daily as indicated below. Reductions in glycemic parameters by dose and regimen are described under CLINICAL STUDIES in the full prescribing information. *Avandia* may be taken with or without food. **Monotherapy:** The usual starting dose of *Avandia* is 4 mg administered either as a single dose once daily or in divided doses twice daily. In clinical trials,the 4 mg twice daily regimen resulted in the greatest reduction in FPG and HbA1c. **Combination Therapy with a Sulfonylurea or Metformin:** When *Avandia* is added to existing therapy, the current dose of sulfonylurea or metformin can be continued upon initiation of *Avandia* therapy. ***Sulfonylurea:*** When used in combination with sulfonylurea, the recommended dose of *Avandia* is 4 mg administered as either a single dose once daily or in divided doses twice daily. If patients report hypoglycemia, the dose of the sulfonylurea should be decreased. ***Metformin:*** The usual starting dose of *Avandia* in combination with metformin is 4 mg administered as either a single dose once daily or in divided doses twice daily. It is unlikely that the dose of metformin will require adjustment due to hypoglycemia during combination therapy with *Avandia*.

Maximum Recommended Dose: The dose of *Avandia* should not exceed 8 mg daily, as a single dose or divided twice daily. The 8 mg daily dose has been shown to be safe and effective in clinical studies as monotherapy and in combination with metformin. Doses of *Avandia* greater than 4 mg daily in combination with a sulfonylurea have not been studied in adequate and well-controlled clinical trials. *Avandia* may be taken with or without food. No dosage adjustments are required for the elderly. No dosage adjustment is necessary when *Avandia* is used as monotherapy in patients with renal impairment. Since metformin is contraindicated in such patients, concomitant administration of metformin and *Avandia* is also contraindicated in patients with renal impairment. Therapy with *Avandia* should not be initiated if the patient exhibits clinical evidence of active liver disease or increased serum transaminase levels (ALT >2.5X upper limit of normal at start of therapy) (see PRECAUTIONS, *Hepatic Effects* and CLINICAL PHARMACOLOGY, Hepatic Impairment in full prescribing information). Liver enzyme monitoring is recommended in all patients prior to initiation of therapy with *Avandia* and periodically thereafter (see PRECAUTIONS, *Hepatic Effects*). There are no data on the use of *Avandia* in patients under 18 years of age; therefore, use of *Avandia* in pediatric patients is not recommended.

BRS-AV:L6   Rx only

* Based on overall physician population, Scott-Levin SPA, May 2001;

Appendix B

Augmentin

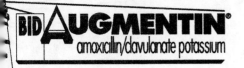

BID AUGMENTIN®
amoxicillin/clavulanate potassium

NTIN ® amoxicillin/clavulanate potassium
MMARY. FOR FULL PRESCRIBING INFORMATION, SEE PACKAGE INSERT.
NS AND USAGE: *Augmentin* is indicated in the treatment of infections caused by susceptible strains of
ited organisms in the conditions listed below:
iratory Tract Infections caused by β-lactamase-producing strains of *Haemophilus influenzae* and *Moraxella*
la) catarrhalis. Otitis Media caused by β-lactamase-producing strains of *Haemophilus influenzae* and *Morax-*
amella) catarrhalis. Sinusitis caused by β-lactamase-producing strains of *Haemophilus influenzae* and *Mo-*
nhamella) catarrhalis. Skin and Skin Structure Infections caused by β-lactamase-producing strains of *Staphy-*
reus, Escherichia coli, and *Klebsiella* spp. *Urinary Tract Infections* caused by β-lactamase-producing strains
ebsiella spp. and *Enterobacter* spp. While *Augmentin* is indicated only for the conditions listed above, infec-
d by ampicillin-susceptible organisms are also amenable to *Augmentin* treatment due to its amoxicillin con-
ore, mixed infections caused by ampicillin-susceptible organisms and β-lactamase-producing organisms
to *Augmentin* should not require the addition of another antibiotic. Because amoxicillin has greater *in vitro*
nst *Streptococcus pneumoniae* than does ampicillin or penicillin, the majority of *S. pneumoniae* strains with
susceptibility to ampicillin or penicillin are fully susceptible to amoxicillin and *Augmentin.* (See Microbiol-
on.)
al studies to determine the causative organisms and their susceptibility to *Augmentin* should be performed
h any indicated surgical procedures. Therapy may be instituted prior to obtaining the results from bacterio-
usceptibility studies to determine the causative organisms and their susceptibility to *Augmentin* when there
believe the infection may involve any of the β-lactamase-producing organisms listed above. Once results
djust therapy, if appropriate.
ICATIONS: Patients with a history of allergic reactions to any penicillin; or patients with a history of
ssociated cholestatic jaundice/hepatic dysfunction.
SERIOUS AND OCCASIONALLY FATAL HYPERSENSITIVITY (ANAPHYLACTIC) REACTIONS HAVE BEEN
PATIENTS ON PENICILLIN THERAPY. THESE REACTIONS ARE MORE LIKELY TO OCCUR IN INDIVIDUALS
ORY OF PENICILLIN HYPERSENSITIVITY AND/OR A HISTORY OF SENSITIVITY TO MULTIPLE ALLERGENS.
BEEN REPORTS OF INDIVIDUALS WITH A HISTORY OF PENICILLIN HYPERSENSITIVITY WHO HAVE EXPE-
VERE REACTIONS WHEN TREATED WITH CEPHALOSPORINS. BEFORE INITIATING THERAPY WITH
CAREFUL INQUIRY SHOULD BE MADE CONCERNING PREVIOUS HYPERSENSITIVITY REACTIONS TO
CEPHALOSPORINS OR OTHER ALLERGENS. IF AN ALLERGIC REACTION OCCURS, *AUGMENTIN* SHOULD
NUED AND THE APPROPRIATE THERAPY INSTITUTED. **SERIOUS ANAPHYLACTIC REACTIONS**
MEDIATE EMERGENCY TREATMENT WITH EPINEPHRINE. OXYGEN, INTRAVENOUS STEROIDS
MANAGEMENT, INCLUDING INTUBATION, SHOULD ALSO BE ADMINISTERED AS INDICAT-
nembranous colitis has been reported with nearly all antibacterial agents, including
nd has ranged in severity from mild to life-threatening. Therefore, it is important to consider
s in patients who present with diarrhea subsequent to the administration of antibacterial
nent with antibacterial agents alters the normal flora of the colon and may permit overgrowth of
ies indicate that a toxin produced by *Clostridium difficile* is one primary cause of "antibiotic associated
the diagnosis of pseudomembranous colitis has been established, appropriate therapeutic measures
ted. Mild cases of pseudomembranous colitis usually respond to drug discontinuation alone. In moderate
, consideration should be given to management with fluids and electrolytes, protein supplementation
with an antibacterial drug clinically effective against *Clostridium difficile* colitis. Use *Augmentin* cau-
nts with evidence of hepatic dysfunction. Hepatic toxicity associated with *Augmentin* use is usually
are occasions, deaths have been reported (less than 1 death reported per estimated 4 million prescrip-
e). These have generally been cases associated with serious underlying diseases or concomitant
ee CONTRAINDICATIONS and ADVERSE REACTIONS.)
: General: While *Augmentin* possesses the characteristic low toxicity of the penicillin group of antibi-
ssessment of organ system functions, including renal, hepatic and hematopoietic function, is advisable
d therapy.
ge of patients with mononucleosis who receive ampicillin develop an erythematous skin rash. Thus,
antibiotics should not be administered to patients with mononucleosis. The possibility of superinfec-
ic or bacterial pathogens should be kept in mind during therapy. If superinfections occur (usually involv-
s or *Candida*), the drug should be discontinued and/or appropriate therapy instituted.
ns: Probenecid decreases the renal tubular secretion of amoxicillin. Concurrent use with *Augmentin*
reased and prolonged blood levels of amoxicillin. Co-administration of probenecid cannot be recom-
current administration of allopurinol and ampicillin increases substantially the incidence of rashes in
both drugs as compared to patients receiving ampicillin alone. It is not known whether this potentia-
rashes is due to allopurinol or the hyperuricemia present in these patients. There are no data with
llopurinol administered concurrently.
ther broad-spectrum antibiotics, *Augmentin* may reduce the efficacy of oral contraceptives.
Test Interactions: Oral administration of *Augmentin* will result in high urine concentrations of
urine concentrations of ampicillin may result in false-positive reactions when testing for the presence
e using Clinitest®, Benedict's Solution or Fehling's Solution. Since this effect may also occur with
erefore *Augmentin,* it is recommended that glucose tests based on enzymatic glucose oxidase reac-
istix® or Tes-Tape®) be used.
tration of ampicillin to pregnant women a transient decrease in plasma concentration of total conju-
iol-glucuronide, conjugated estrone and estradiol has been noted. This effect may also occur with
erefore *Augmentin.*
Mutagenesis, Impairment of Fertility: Long-term studies in animals have not been performed to
enic potential. **Mutagenesis:** The mutagenic potential of *Augmentin* was investigated *in vitro* with
man lymphocyte cytogenetic assay, a yeast test and a mouse lymphoma forward mutation assay, and
e micronucleus tests and a dominant lethal test. All were negative apart from the *in vitro* mouse
here weak activity was found at very high, cytotoxic concentrations.
rtility: *Augmentin* at oral doses of up to 1200 mg/kg/day (5.7 times the maximum human dose, 1480
on body surface area) was found to have no effect on fertility and reproductive performance in rats
tio formulation of amoxicillin:clavulanate.
cts: Pregnancy (Category B): Reproduction studies performed in pregnant rats and mice given
dosages up to 1200 mg/kg/day, equivalent to 7200 and 4080 mg/m^2/day, respectively (4.9 and 2.8
human oral dose based on body surface area), revealed no evidence of harm to the fetus due to
are, however, no adequate and well-controlled studies in pregnant women. Because animal repro-
not always predictive of human response, use this drug during pregnancy only if clearly needed.
y: Oral ampicillin class antibiotics are generally poorly absorbed during labor. Studies in guinea pigs
ravenous administration of ampicillin decreased the uterine tone, frequency of contractions, height
duration of contractions. However, it is not known whether the use of *Augmentin* in humans during
immediate or delayed adverse effects on the fetus, prolongs the duration of labor, or increases the
ps delivery or other obstetrical intervention or resuscitation of the newborn will be necessary.
Ampicillin class antibiotics are excreted in the milk; therefore, caution should be exercised when
stered to a nursing woman.
ONS: *Augmentin* is generally well tolerated. The majority of side effects observed in clinical trials
ent; <3% of patients discontinued therapy because of drug-related side effects. The most frequently
ects were diarrhea/loose stools (9%), nausea (3%), skin rashes and urticaria (3%), vomiting (1%)
he overall incidence of side effects, and in particular diarrhea, increased with the higher recom-
less frequently reported reactions include: abdominal discomfort, flatulence and headache.
e reactions have been reported for ampicillin class antibiotics:
miting, indigestion, gastritis, stomatitis, glossitis, black "hairy" tongue, mucocutaneous candidia-
d hemorrhagic/pseudomembranous colitis. Onset of pseudomembranous colitis symptoms may
antibiotic treatment. (See WARNINGS.) Skin rashes, pruritus, urticaria, angioedema, serum sick-
rticaria or skin rash accompanied by arthritis, arthralgia, myalgia and frequently fever), erythema
evens-Johnson Syndrome) and an occasional case of exfoliative dermatitis (including toxic epider-
e reactions may be controlled with antihistamines and, if necessary, systemic corticosteroids.
ons occur, the drug should be discontinued, unless the opinion of the physician dictates otherwise.
al fatal hypersensitivity (anaphylactic) reactions can occur with oral penicillin. (See WARNINGS.)
ST (SGOT) and/or ALT (SGPT) has been noted in patients treated with ampicillin class antibiotics
these findings is unknown. Hepatic dysfunction, including increases in serum transaminases (AST
irubin and/or alkaline phosphatase, has been infrequently reported with *Augmentin.* It has been
nly in the elderly, in males, or in patients on prolonged treatment. The histologic findings on liver
of predominantly cholestatic, hepatocellular, or mixed cholestatic-hepatocellular changes. The
ms of hepatic dysfunction may occur during or several weeks after therapy has been discontin-
nction, which may be severe, is usually reversible. On rare occasions, deaths have been reported
orted per estimated 4 million prescriptions worldwide). These have generally been cases associ-
rlying diseases or concomitant medications. Interstitial nephritis and hematuria have been reported
ng hemolytic anemia, thrombocytopenia, thrombocytopenic purpura, eosinophilia, leukopenia and
been reported during therapy with penicillins. These reactions are usually reversible on discon-
d are believed to be hypersensitivity phenomena. A slight thrombocytosis was noted in less than
ted with *Augmentin.* There have been reports of increased prothrombin time in patients receiving
agulant therapy concomitantly. Agitation, anxiety, behavioral changes, confusion, convulsions,
d reversible hyperactivity have been reported rarely.

DOSAGE AND ADMINISTRATION

Since both the *Augmentin* 250 mg and 500 mg tablets contain the same amount of clavulanic acid (125 mg, as the potassium salt), 2 *Augmentin* 250 mg tablets are not equivalent to 1 *Augmentin* 500 mg tablet. Therefore, 2 *Augmentin* 250 mg tablets should not be substituted for 1 *Augmentin* 500 mg tablet.

Dosage:

Adults: The usual adult dose is 1 *Augmentin* 500 mg tablet every 12 hours or 1 *Augmentin* 250 mg tablet every 8 hours. For more severe infections and infections of the respiratory tract, the dose should be 1 *Augmentin* 875 mg tablet every 12 hours or 1 *Augmentin* 500 mg tablet every 8 hours.

Patients with impaired renal function do not generally require a reduction in dose unless the impairment is severe. Severely impaired patients with a glomerular filtration rate of <30 mL/minute should not receive the 875 mg tablet. Patients with a glomerular filtration rate of 10 to 30 mL/minute should receive 500 mg or 250 mg every 12 hours, depending on the severity of the infection. Patients with a less than 10 mL/minute glomerular filtration rate should receive 500 mg or 250 mg every 24 hours, depending on severity of the infection.

Hemodialysis patients should receive 500 mg or 250 mg every 24 hours, depending on severity of the infection. They should receive an additional dose both during and at the end of dialysis.

Hepatically impaired patients should be dosed with caution and hepatic function monitored at regular intervals. (See WARNINGS.)

Pediatric Patients: Pediatric patients weighing 40 kg or more should be dosed according to the adult recommendations.

Due to the different amoxicillin to clavulanic acid ratios in the *Augmentin* 250 mg tablet (250/125) versus the *Augmentin* 250 mg chewable tablet (250/62.5), the *Augmentin* 250 mg tablet should not be used until the pediatric patient weighs at least 40 kg or more.

Administration: *Augmentin* may be taken without regard to meals; however, absorption of clavulanate potassium is enhanced when *Augmentin* is administered at the start of a meal. To minimize the potential for gastrointestinal intolerance, *Augmentin* should be taken at the start of a meal.

BRS-AG:AL6

Rx only

Appendix C

Coreg

;OREG® (carvedilol) Tablets

;ee complete prescribing information in SmithKline Beecham Pharmaceuticals literature. 'he following is a brief summary.

NDICATIONS AND USAGE: Congestive Heart Failure (CHF): Treatment of mild or moderate NYHA class II or III) heart failure of ischemic or cardiomyopathic origin, in conjunction with igitalis, diuretics, and ACE inhibitor, to reduce the progression of disease as evidenced by ardiovascular death, cardiovascular hospitalization, or the need to adjust other heart failure med- ations. *Coreg* may be used in patients unable to tolerate an ACE inhibitor, and in patients who 'e or are not receiving digitalis, hydralazine or nitrate therapy.

ONTRAINDICATIONS: Patients with NYHA class IV decompensated cardiac failure requiring travenous inotropic therapy, bronchial asthma (two cases of death from status asthmaticus have een reported in patients receiving single doses of *Coreg*) or related bronchospastic conditions, econd- or third-degree AV block, sick sinus syndrome (unless a permanent pacemaker is in place), rdiogenic shock or severe bradycardia. Do not use *Coreg* in patients with clinically manifest patic impairment. Contraindicated in patients with hypersensitivity to the drug.

ARNINGS: Hepatic Injury: Mild hepatocellular injury, confirmed by rechallenge, has occurred ely. In controlled studies of CHF, the incidence of liver function abnormalities reported as verse experiences was 5.0% (38 of 765 *Coreg* patients) and 4.6% (20 of 437 placebo patients). ree *Coreg* patients (0.4%) and two placebo patients (0.5%) in controlled trials withdrew for normal hepatic function. Hepatic injury has been reversible, and has occurred after short- and/or g-term therapy with minimal clinical symptomatology. No deaths due to liver function abnor- ities have been reported. Perform laboratory testing at the first symptom/sign of liver dysfunc- (e.g., pruritus, dark urine, persistent anorexia, jaundice, right upper quadrant tenderness or xplained "flu-like" symptoms). Stop *Coreg* and do not restart if the patient has laboratory evi- ce of liver injury or jaundice. **Peripheral Vascular Disease:** β-blockers can precipitate or aggra- e symptoms of arterial insufficiency in patients with peripheral vascular disease. Use caution in h individuals. **Anesthesia and Major Surgery:** If *Coreg* is to be continued perioperatively, take icular care when anesthetic agents that depress myocardial function, such as ether, cyclopro- e and trichloroethylene, are used. **Diabetes and Hypoglycemia:** β-blockers may mask some ifestations of hypoglycemia, particularly tachycardia. Nonselective β-blockers may potentiate lin-induced hypoglycemia and delay recovery of serum glucose levels. Caution patients sub- to spontaneous hypoglycemia, or diabetic patients receiving insulin or oral hypoglycemic nts, about these possibilities and use *Coreg* with caution. In CHF patients, there is a risk of sening hyperglycemia (see PRECAUTIONS). **Thyrotoxicosis:** β-adrenergic blockade may mask cal signs of hyperthyroidism, such as tachycardia. Abrupt withdrawal of β-blockade may be wed by an exacerbation of the symptoms of hyperthyroidism or may precipitate thyroid storm.

CAUTIONS: General: Since *Coreg* has β-blocking activity, do not discontinue abruptly, partic- y in patients with ischemic heart disease. Instead, discontinue *Coreg* over 1 to 2 weeks. In al trials, *Coreg* caused bradycardia in about 2% of hypertensive patients and 9% of CHF nts. If pulse drops below 55 beats/min., reduce the dosage. Hypotension and postural hypo- on occurred in 9.7% and syncope in 3.4% of CHF patients receiving *Coreg* compared to 3.6% .5% of placebo patients, respectively. The risk for these events was highest during the first ys of dosing, corresponding to the up-titration period and caused discontinuation of therapy % of *Coreg* patients, compared to 0.4% of placebo patients. To decrease the likelihood of pe or excessive hypotension, start treatment with 3.125 mg b.i.d. for CHF patients. Increase e slowly; see DOSAGE AND ADMINISTRATION section. *Coreg* should be taken with food. initiation of therapy, warn the patient to avoid situations such as driving or hazardous tasks, injury could result should syncope occur. Rarely, *Coreg* use in CHF patients has resulted in oration of renal function. Patients at risk appear to be those with low blood pressure (sys- P<100 mm Hg), ischemic heart disease and diffuse vascular disease, and/or underlying renal ciency. Renal function has returned to baseline when *Coreg* was stopped. In patients with risk factors, monitor renal function during *Coreg* up-titration. Discontinue *Coreg* or reduce e if renal function worsens. Worsening cardiac failure or fluid retention may occur during up-titration. If such symptoms occur, increase diuretics; do not advance *Coreg* dose until stability resumes (see DOSAGE AND ADMINISTRATION). Occasionally it is necessary to the *Coreg* dose or temporarily discontinue it. Such episodes do not preclude subsequent sful *Coreg* titration. In pheochromocytoma patients, initiate an α-blocking agent prior to ny β-blocking agent. Although *Coreg* has both α- and β-blocking activities, there has been erience with its use in this condition. Therefore, use caution in administering *Coreg* to s suspected of having pheochromocytoma. Agents with non-selective β-blockade may pro- est pain in patients with Prinzmetal's variant angina. There has been no clinical experience oreg in these patients although the α-blocking activity may prevent such symptoms. er, use caution in administering *Coreg* to patients suspected of having Prinzmetal's variant **Risk of Anaphylactic Reaction:** While taking β-blockers, patients with a history of severe actic reaction to a variety of allergens may be more reactive to repeated challenge, either tal, diagnostic or therapeutic. Such patients may be unresponsive to the usual doses of rine used to treat allergic reaction. **Nonallergic Bronchospasm (e.g., chronic bronchitis physema):** Patients with bronchospastic disease should, in general, not receive β-blockers. ay be used with caution, however, in patients who do not respond to, or cannot tolerate, tihypertensive agents. Use the smallest effective dose, to minimize inhibition of endoge- exogenous β-agonists. Use *Coreg* with caution in CHF patients who have bronchospastic Follow the dosing recommendations closely and lower the dose if bronchospasm is d during up-titration.

nsive Patients with Left Ventricular Failure: In hypertensive patients who have CHF con- ith digitalis, diuretics and/or an angiotensin-converting enzyme inhibitor, *Coreg* may be nce such patients depend, in part, on sympathetic stimulation for circulatory support, fol- ng instructions for CHF patients. In CHF patients with diabetes, *Coreg* therapy may lead ning hyperglycemia, which responds to intensification of hypoglycemic therapy. Monitor cose when *Coreg* dosing is initiated, adjusted, or discontinued.

ion for Patients: Do not interrupt or discontinue *Coreg* without a physician's advice. CHF should consult their physician if they experience signs or symptoms of worsening heart ch as weight gain or increasing shortness of breath. They may experience a drop in blood when standing, resulting in dizziness and, rarely, fainting. Patients should sit or lie down se symptoms of lowered blood pressure occur. If patients experience dizziness or fatigue, ld avoid driving or hazardous tasks and consult a physician, in case the dosage should be They should take *Coreg* with food. Diabetics should report any changes in blood sugar heir physician. Contact lens wearers may experience decreased lacrimation.

ractions: *Inhibitors of CYP2D6; poor metabolizers of debrisoquin:* Interactions of *Coreg* ng inhibitors of CYP2D6 (such as quinidine, fluoxetine, paroxetine, and propafenone) been studied, but these drugs would be expected to increase blood levels of the R(+) er of *Coreg*. Retrospective analysis in clinical trials showed that poor 2D6 metabolizers er rate of dizziness during up-titration, presumably resulting from vasodilating effects of concentrations of the α-blocking R(+) enantiomer. *Catecholamine-depleting agents:* serve patients taking both agents with β-blockade and a drug that can deplete catechol- g., reserpine and MAO inhibitors) for signs of hypotension and/or severe bradycardia. Concomitant administration of clonidine with agents with β-blockade may potentiate sure- and heart-rate-lowering effects. When concomitant treatment with agents with and clonidine is to be terminated, discontinue the β-blocking agent first. Discontinue erapy several days later by gradually decreasing the dosage. *Cyclosporin:* Modest in- mean trough cyclosporin concentrations were observed following initiation of carvedilol in 21 renal transplant patients suffering from chronic vascular rejection. In about 30% the dose of cyclosporin had to be reduced in order to maintain cyclosporin concentra- n the therapeutic range, while in the remainder no adjustment was needed. On the the group, the dose of cyclosporin was reduced about 20% in these patients. Due to dividual variability in the dose adjustment required, it is recommended that cyclosporin ons be monitored closely after initiation of carvedilol therapy and that the dose of cyclo- djusted as appropriate. *Digoxin:* Digoxin concentrations are increased by about 15% in and *Coreg* are administered concomitantly. Both digoxin and *Coreg* slow AV conduc- ore, increase monitoring of digoxin when initiating, adjusting or discontinuing *Coreg*. *d inhibitors of hepatic metabolism:* Rifampin reduced plasma concentrations of *Coreg* %. Cimetidine increased AUC by about 30% but caused no change in C_{max}. *Calcium ckers:* Isolated cases of conduction disturbance (rarely with hemodynamic compro- been observed when *Coreg* is co-administered with diltiazem. As with other agents ade, if *Coreg* is to be administered orally with calcium channel blockers, monitor ECG essure. *Insulin or oral hypoglycemics:* Agents with β-blockade may enhance the blood- ng effect of insulin and oral hypoglycemics. Therefore, monitor blood glucose regularly aking insulin or oral hypoglycemics.

esis, Mutagenesis, Impairment of Fertility: In 2-year rat studies of *Coreg* at doses kg/day (12 times the maximum recommended human dose [MRHD] when compared basis) or in mice given up to 200 mg/kg/day (16 times the MRHD on a mg/m² basis), carcinogenic effect. *Coreg* was negative when tested in a battery of genotoxicity ding the Ames and CHO/HGPRT assays for mutagenicity and *in vitro* hamster micro- nucleus and *in vivo* human lymphocyte cell tests for clastogenicity. At doses ≥200 mg/kg/day (≥32 times the MRHD as mg/m²) *Coreg* was toxic to adult rats (sedation, reduced weight gain) and associated with a reduced number of successful matings, prolonged mating time, significantly fewer corpora lutea and implants per dam and complete resorption of 18% of the litters. The no-observed-effect dose level for overt toxicity and impairment of fertility was 60 mg/kg/day (10 times the MRHD as mg/m²). **Pregnancy: Teratogenic Effects. Pregnancy Category C.:** Studies in pregnant rats and rabbits given *Coreg* revealed increased post-implantation loss in rats at doses of 300 mg/kg/day (50 times the MRHD as mg/m²) and in rabbits at doses of 75 mg/kg/day (25 times the MRHD as mg/m²). In rats, there was also a decrease in fetal body weight at the maternally toxic dose of 300 mg/kg/day (50 times the MRHD as mg/m²), accompanied by an elevation in the frequency of fetuses with delayed skeletal development (missing or stunted 13th rib). In rats, the no-observed-effect level for developmental toxicity was 60 mg/kg/day (10 times the MRHD as mg/m²); in rabbits it was 15 mg/kg/day (5 times the MRHD as mg/m²). There are no adequate and well-controlled studies in pregnant women. Use *Coreg* during pregnancy only if the potential benefit justifies the potential risk to the fetus. **Nursing Mothers:** It is not known whether *Coreg* is excreted in human milk. Rat studies have shown that *Coreg* and/or its metabolites (as well as other β-blockers) cross the placental barrier and are excreted in breast milk. There was increased mortality at one week post-partum in neonates from rats treated with 60 mg/kg/day (10 times the MRHD as mg/m²) and above during the last trimester through day 22 of lactation. Because many drugs are excreted in human milk and because of the potential for serious adverse reactions in nursing infants from β-blockers, especially bradycardia, decide whether to discontinue nursing or to discontinue the drug, taking into account the importance of the drug to the mother. The effects of other α- and β-blocking agents have included perinatal and neonatal distress. **Pediatric Use:** Safety and efficacy in patients younger than 18 have not been established. **Geriatric Use:** 31% and 39% of CHF patients in U.S. and worldwide trials, respectively, were 65 years of age or older. There were no notable differences in efficacy or the incidence of adverse events between older and younger patients. With the exception of dizziness (8.8% in the elderly vs. 6% in younger patients), there were no events where the incidence in the elderly exceeded that in younger patients by over 2.0%. Similar results were observed in a postmarketing surveillance study of 3,328 *Coreg* patients, of whom approximately 20% were over 65.

ADVERSE REACTIONS: Congestive Heart Failure: *Coreg* has been evaluated for safety in CHF in over 1,900 patients worldwide (1,300 participated in U.S. trials). Approximately 54% of the 1,900 received *Coreg* for ≥6 months and 20% received *Coreg* for ≥12 months. The *Coreg* adverse events profile in CHF was consistent with *Coreg* pharmacology and health status of the patients. In U.S. trials comparing *Coreg* in daily doses up to 100 mg (n=765) to placebo (n=437), 5.4% of *Coreg* patients discontinued for adverse experiences vs. 8.0% of placebo patients. Median study medication exposure was 6.33 months for both *Coreg* and placebo.

The following adverse events with an incidence greater than 2% (regardless of causality) were more frequent in *Coreg* patients (n=765) than patients who received placebo (n=437) during U.S. placebo-controlled CHF trials: **Autonomic Nervous System:** sweating increased (2.9% vs. 2.1%); **Body as a Whole:** fatigue (23.9% vs. 22.4%); chest pain (14.4% vs. 14.2%); pain (8.6% vs. 7.6%); injury (5.9% vs. 5.5%); drug level increased (5.1% vs. 3.7%); edema generalized (5.1% vs. 2.5%); edema dependent (3.7% vs. 1.8%); fever (3.1% vs. 2.3%); edema legs (2.2% vs. 0.2%); **Cardiovascular:** bradycardia (8.8% vs. 0.9%); hypotension (8.5% vs. 3.4%); syncope (3.4% vs. 2.5%); hypertension (2.9% vs 2.5%); AV block (2.9% vs. 0.5%); angina pectoris aggravated (2.0% vs. 1.1%); **Central Nervous System:** dizziness (32.4% vs. 19.2%); headache (8.1% vs. 7.1%); paresthesia (2.0% vs. 1.8%); **Gastrointestinal:** diarrhea (11.8% vs. 5.9%); nausea (8.5% vs. 4.8%); abdominal pain (7.2% vs. 7.1%); vomiting (6.3% vs. 4.3%); **Hematologic:** thrombocytopenia (2.0% vs. 0.5%); **Metabolic:** hyperglycemia (12.2% vs. 7.8%); weight increase (9.7% vs. 6.9%); gout (6.3% vs. 6.2%); BUN increased (6.0% vs. 4.6%); NPN increased (5.8% vs. 4.6%); hypercholesterolemia (4.1% vs. 2.5%); dehydration (2.1% vs. 1.6%); hypervolemia (2.0% vs. 0.9%); **Musculoskeletal:** back pain (6.9% vs. 6.6%); arthralgia (6.4% vs. 4.8%); myalgia (3.4% vs. 2.7%); **Resistance Mechanism:** upper respiratoy tract infection (18.3% vs. 17.6%); infection (2.2% vs. 0.9%); **Respiratory:** sinusitis (5.4% vs. 4.3%); bronchitis (5.4% vs. 3.4%); pharyngitis (3.1% vs. 2.7%); **Urinary/Renal:** urinary tract infection (3.1% vs. 2.7%); hematuria (2.9% vs. 2.1%); **Vision:** vision abnormal (5.0% vs. 1.8%).

Withdrawal rates due to adverse events with an incidence greater than 2% (regardless of causality) seen more commonly in *Coreg*-treated patients vs. those receiving placebo during *Coreg* clinical trials were as follows: **Body as a Whole:** fatigue (0.7% vs. 0.7%); chest pain (0.1% vs. 0%); pain (0% vs. 0.2%); drug level increased (0% vs. 0.2%); edema legs (0.1% vs. 0.2%); **Cardiovascular:** bradycardia (0.8% vs. 0%); hypotension (0.4% vs. 0.2%); syncope (0.3% vs. 0.2%); hypertension (0.1% vs. 0%); **Central Nervous System:** dizziness (0.4% vs. 0%); headache (0.3% vs. 0%); paresthesia (0.1% vs. 0%); **Gastrointestinal:** diarrhea (0.3% vs. 0%); abdominal pain (0.3% vs. 0%); vomiting (0.1% vs. 0%); **Hematologic:** thrombocytopenia (0.1% vs. 0%); **Metabolic:** hyperglycemia (0.1% vs. 0%); weight increase (0.1% vs. 0.5%); BUN increased (0.3% vs. 0.2%); NPN increased (0.3% vs. 0.2%); **Musculoskeletal:** arthralgia (0.1% vs. 0.2%); **Respiratory:** bronchitis (0% vs. 0.2%); **Vision:** vision abnormal (0.1% vs. 0%).

Incidence >2%, Regardless of Causality; Withdrawal Rates due to Adverse Events
In addition to the events listed above, asthenia, cardiac failure, flatulence, anorexia, dyspepsia, palpitation, extrasystoles, hyperkalemia, arthritis, angina pectoris, insomnia, depression, anemia, viral infection, dyspnea, coughing, respiratory disorder, rhinitis, rash, and leg cramps were also reported, but rates were equal to, or more common in, placebo-treated patients. The following adverse events with incidence of >1% to <2% were reported more frequently with *Coreg* in U.S. placebo-controlled trials in CHF: **Body as a Whole:** Peripheral edema, allergy, sudden death, malaise, hypovolemia. **Cardiovascular:** Fluid overload, postural hypotension. **Central and Peripheral Nervous System:** Hypesthesia, vertigo. **Gastrointestinal:** Melena, periodontitis. **Liver and Biliary System:** SGPT increased, SGOT increased. **Metabolic and Nutritional:** Hyperuricemia, hypoglycemia, hyponatremia, increased alkaline phosphatase, glycosuria. **Platelet, Bleeding and Clotting:** Prothrombin decreased, purpura. **Psychiatric:** Somnolence. **Reproductive, male:** Impotence. **Urinary System:** Abnormal renal function, albuminuria.

POSTMARKETING EXPERIENCE: The following adverse reaction has been reported in postmarketing experience: reports of aplastic anemia have been rare and received only when carvedilol was administered concomitantly with other medications associated with the event.

DOSAGE AND ADMINISTRATION: Congestive Heart Failure: DOSAGE MUST BE INDIVIDUALIZED AND CLOSELY MONITORED BY A PHYSICIAN DURING UP-TITRATION. Before starting *Coreg*, stabilize dosing of digitalis, diuretics and ACE inhibitors (if used). The recommended *Coreg* starting dose is 3.125 mg twice daily (b.i.d.) for two weeks. If this dose is tolerated, it can then be increased to 6.25 mg b.i.d. Dosing should then be doubled every 2 weeks to the highest level tolerated by the patient. At initiation of each new dose, observe patients for dizziness or light-headedness for one hour. The maximum recommended dose is 25 mg b.i.d. in patients under 85 kg (187 lbs) and 50 mg b.i.d. in patients over 85 kg. Take *Coreg* with food to slow the rate of absorption and reduce the incidence of orthostatic effects.

Before each dose increase, the patient should be seen in the office and evaluated for symptoms of worsening heart failure, vasodilation (dizziness, light-headedness, symptomatic hypotension) or bradycardia, in order to determine *Coreg* tolerability. Treat transient worsening of heart failure with increased doses of diuretics; occasionally it is necessary to lower the *Coreg* dose or temporarily discontinue it. Vasodilation symptoms often respond to reducing the dose of diuretics or ACE inhibitor. If these changes do not relieve symptoms, decrease *Coreg* dose. Do not increase *Coreg* dose until symptoms of worsening heart failure or vasodilation have been stabilized. Initial difficulty with titration should not preclude later attempts to introduce *Coreg*. If CHF patients experience bradycardia (pulse below 55 beats/min.), reduce *Coreg* dose.

BRS-CO:L5

APPENDIX D

PAXIL

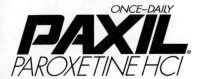

ONCE-DAILY

PAXIL®

PAROXETINE HCl

PAXIL® (brand of paroxetine hydrochloride)

See complete prescribing information in SmithKline Beecham Pharmaceuticals literature. The following is a brief summary.

INDICATIONS AND USAGE: *Paxil* is indicated for the treatment of depression, obsessions and compulsions in patients with obsessive compulsive disorder (OCD) as defined in DSM-IV, panic disorder, with or without agoraphobia, as defined in DSM-IV, social anxiety disorder, as defined in DSM-IV, and generalized anxiety disorder, as defined in DSM-IV.

CONTRAINDICATIONS: Concomitant use in patients taking either monoamine oxidase inhibitors (MAOIs) or thioridazine is contraindicated. (See WARNINGS and PRECAUTIONS.) Contraindicated in patients with a hypersensitivity to paroxetine or any of the inactive ingredients in *Paxil*.

WARNINGS: Interactions with MAOIs may occur. Given the fatal interactions reported with concomitant or immediately consecutive administration of MAOIs and other SSRIs, do not use *Paxil* in combination with a MAOI or within 2 weeks of discontinuing MAOI treatment. Allow at least 2 weeks after stopping *Paxil* before starting a MAOI.

Potential Interaction with Thioridazine

Thioridazine administration alone produces prolongation of the QTc interval, which is associated with serious ventricular arrhythmias, such as torsade de pointes-type arrhythmias, and sudden death. This effect appears to be dose related.

An *in vivo* study suggests that drugs which inhibit $P_{450}IID_6$, such as paroxetine, will elevate plasma levels of thioridazine. Therefore, it is recommended that paroxetine not be used in combination with thioridazine.

PRECAUTIONS: As with all antidepressants, use *Paxil* cautiously in patients with a history of mania.

Use *Paxil* cautiously in patients with a history of seizures. Discontinue it in any patient who develops seizures.

The possibility of suicide attempt is inherent in depression and may persist until significant remission occurs. Close supervision of high-risk patients should accompany initial drug therapy. Write *Paxil* prescriptions for the smallest quantity of tablets consistent with good patient management in order to reduce the risk of overdose.

Reversible hyponatremia has been reported, mainly in elderly patients, patients taking diuretics or those who were otherwise volume depleted. Abnormal bleeding (mostly ecchymosis and purpura), including a case of impaired platelet aggregation, has been reported; the relationship to paroxetine is unclear.

Clinical experience with *Paxil* in patients with concomitant systemic illness is limited. Use cautiously in patients with diseases or conditions that could affect metabolism or hemodynamic responses. Observe the usual cautions in cardiac patients. In patients with severe renal impairment (creatinine clearance <30 mL/min.) or severe hepatic impairment, a lower starting dose (10 mg) should be used.

Caution patients about operating hazardous machinery, including automobiles, until they are reasonably sure that *Paxil* therapy does not affect their ability to engage in such activities. Tell patients 1) to continue therapy as directed; 2) to inform physicians about other medications they are taking or plan to take; 3) to avoid alcohol while taking *Paxil*; 4) to notify their physicians if they become pregnant or intend to become pregnant during therapy, or if they're nursing.

Weakness, hyperreflexia, and incoordination following use of an SSRI and sumatriptan have been rarely reported. Concomitant use of *Paxil* with tryptophan is not recommended. Use cautiously with warfarin. When administering *Paxil* with cimetidine, dosage adjustment of *Paxil* after the 20 mg starting dose should be guided by clinical effect. When co-administering *Paxil* with phenobarbital or phenytoin, no initial *Paxil* dosage adjustment is needed; base subsequent changes on clinical effect. Concomitant use of *Paxil* with drugs metabolized by cytochrome $P_{450}IID_6$ (antidepressants such as nortriptyline, amitriptyline, imipramine, desipramine and fluoxetine; phenothiazines; Type 1C antiarrhythmics such as propafenone, flecainide and encainide) or with drugs that inhibit this enzyme (e.g., quinidine) may require lower doses than usually prescribed for either *Paxil* or the other drug; approach concomitant use cautiously. However, due to the risk of serious ventricular arrhythmias and sudden death potentially associated with elevated plasma levels of thioridazine, paroxetine and thioridazine should not be co-administered. An *in vivo* interaction study revealed that paroxetine had no effect on terfenadine pharmacokinetics. Additional *in vitro* studies showed that the inhibitory effects of paroxetine on other $IIIA_4$ substrates (astemizole, cisapride, triazolam and cyclosporin) was at least 100 times less potent than ketoconazole, a potent $IIIA_4$ inhibitor. Assuming the relationship between paroxetine's *in vitro* Ki and its lack of effect on terfenadine's *in vivo* clearance predicts its effect on other $IIIA_4$ substrates, paroxetine's inhibition of $IIIA_4$ activity should have little clinical significance. Use caution when co-administering *Paxil* with tricyclic antidepressants (TCAs). TCA plasma concentrations need monitoring and the TCA dose may need to be reduced. Administration of *Paxil* with another tightly protein-bound drug may shift plasma concentrations, resulting in adverse effects from either drug. Concomitant use of *Paxil* and alcohol in depressed patients is not advised. Undertake concomitant use of *Paxil* and lithium or digoxin cautiously. If adverse effects are seen when co-administering *Paxil* with procyclidine, reduce the procyclidine dose. Elevated theophylline levels have been reported with *Paxil* co-administration; monitoring theophylline levels is recommended.

In 2-year studies, a significantly greater number of male rats in the 20 mg/kg/day group developed reticulum cell sarcomas vs. animals given doses of 1 or 5 mg/kg/day. There was also a significantly increased linear trend across dose groups for the occurrence of lymphoreticular tumors in male rats. Although there was a dose-related increase in the number of tumors in mice, there was no drug-related increase in the number of mice with tumors. The clinical significance of these findings is unknown. There is no evidence of mutagenicity with *Paxil*.

Rats receiving paroxetine at 15 mg/kg/day (2.4 times the MRHD on a mg/m² basis) showed a reduced pregnancy rate.

Pregnancy Category C. Reproduction studies performed in rats and rabbits at doses up to 6 mg/kg/day, 8.1 (rat) and 1.9 (rabbit) times the MRHD on a mg/m² basis, have revealed no evidence of teratogenic effects or of selective toxicity to the fetus. However, rat pup deaths increased during the first 4 days of lactation when dosing occurred during the last trimester of gestation and continued throughout lactation. The cause of these deaths is not known. There are no adequate and well-controlled studies in pregnant women. *Paxil* should be used in pregnancy only if the potential benefit justifies the potential risk to the fetus. The effect of *Paxil* on labor and delivery in humans is unknown. Paroxetine is secreted in human milk; exercise caution when administering *Paxil* to a nursing woman.

Safety and effectiveness in the pediatric population have not been established.

In worldwide premarketing *Paxil* clinical trials, 17% of *Paxil*-treated patients were ≥65 years of age. Pharmacokinetic studies revealed a decreased clearance in the elderly and a lower starting dose is recommended. However, there were no overall differences in the adverse event profile between older and younger patients.

ADVERSE REACTIONS: Incidence in Controlled Trials—*Commonly Observed Adverse Events in Controlled Clinical Trials:* The most commonly observed adverse events associated with the use of *Paxil* in the treatment of depression (incidence of 5% or greater and incidence for *Paxil* at least twice that for placebo): asthenia (15% vs. 6%), sweating (11% vs. 2%), nausea (26% vs. 9%), decreased appetite (6% vs. 2%), somnolence (23% vs. 9%), dizziness (13% vs. 6%), insomnia (13% vs. 6%), tremor (8% vs. 2%), nervousness (5% vs. 3%), ejaculatory disturbance (13% vs. 0%) and other male genital disorders (10% vs. 0%).

The most commonly observed adverse events associated with the use of paroxetine in the treatment of obsessive compulsive disorder (incidence of 5% or greater and incidence for *Paxil* at least twice that of placebo) were: nausea (23% vs. 10%), dry mouth (18% vs. 9%), decreased appetite (9% vs. 3%), constipation (16% vs. 6%), dizziness (12% vs. 6%), somnolence (24% vs. 7%), tremor (11% vs. 1%), sweating (9% vs. 3%), impotence (8% vs. 1%) and abnormal ejaculation (23% vs. 1%).

The most commonly observed adverse events associated with the use of paroxetine in the treatment of panic disorder (incidence of 5% or greater and incidence for *Paxil* at least twice that for placebo) were: asthenia (14% vs. 5%), sweating (14% vs. 6%), decreased appetite (7% vs. 3%), libido decreased (9% vs. 1%), tremor (9% vs. 1%), abnormal ejaculation (21% vs. 1%), female genital disorders (9% vs. 1%) and impotence (5% vs. 0%).

The most commonly observed adverse events associated with the use of paroxetine in the treatment of social anxiety disorder (incidence of 5% or greater and incidence for *Paxil* at least twice that for placebo) were: sweating (9% vs. 2%), nausea (25% vs. 7%), dry mouth (9% vs. 3%), constipation (5% vs. 2%), decreased appetite (8% vs. 2%), somnolence (22% vs. 5%), tremor (9% vs. 1%), libido decreased (12% vs. 1%), yawn (5% vs. 1%), abnormal ejaculation (28% vs. 1%), female genital disorders (9% vs. 1%) and impotence (5% vs. 1%).

The most commonly observed adverse events associated with the use of paroxetine in the treatment of generalized anxiety disorder (incidence of 5% or greater and incidence for *Paxil* at least twice that for placebo) were: asthenia, infection, constipation, decreased appetite, dry mouth, nausea, libido decreased, somnolence, tremor, sweating, and abnormal ejaculation.

Twenty percent (1,199/6,145) of *Paxil* patients in worldwide clinical trials in depression and 16.1% (84/522), 11.8% (64/542), 9.4% (44/469) and 10.7% (79/735) of *Paxil* patients in worldwide trials in social anxiety disorder, OCD, panic disorder and generalized anxiety disorder, respectively, discontinued treatment due to an adverse event. The most common events (≥1%) associated with discontinuation and considered to be drug related include the following: **depression**–somnolence, agitation, tremor, nausea, diarrhea, dry mouth, vomiting, asthenia, abnormal ejaculation, sweating; **OCD**–insomnia, dizziness, constipation, nausea, asthenia, abnormal ejaculation, impotence; **panic disorder**–somnolence, insomnia, nausea; **social anxiety disorder**–somnolence, insomnia, tremor, anxiety, dizziness, nausea, vomiting, flatulence, asthenia, abnormal ejaculation, sweating, libido decreased; **generalized anxiety disorder**–somnolence, dizziness, nausea, asthenia, abnormal ejaculation, sweating.

The following adverse events occurred in 6-week placebo-controlled trials of similar design at a frequency of 1% or more, in patients dosed (20 to 50 mg/day) for the treatment of depression: headache, asthenia, palpitation; vasodilation; sweating, rash; nausea, dry mouth, constipation, diarrhea, decreased appetite, flatulence, oropharynx disorder, dyspepsia; myopathy, myalgia, myasthenia; somnolence, dizziness, insomnia, tremor, nervousness, anxiety, paresthesia, libido decreased, drugged feeling, confusion; yawn; blurred vision, taste perversion; ejaculatory disturbance, other male genital disorders, urinary frequency, urination disorder, female genital disorders.

The following adverse events occurred at a frequency of 2% or more among OCD patients on *Paxil* who participated in placebo-controlled trials of 12 weeks duration in which patients were dosed in a range of 20 to 60 mg/day or among patients with panic disorder on *Paxil* who participated in placebo-controlled trials of 10 to 12 weeks duration in which patients were dosed in a range of 10 to 60 mg/day or among patients with social anxiety disorder on *Paxil* who participated in placebo-controlled trials of 12 weeks duration in which patients were dosed in a range of 20 to 50 mg/day: asthenia, abdominal pain, chest pain, back pain, chills, trauma; vasodilation, palpitation; sweating, rash; nausea, dry mouth, constipation, diarrhea, decreased appetite, dyspepsia, flatulence, increased appetite, vomiting; myalgia; insomnia, somnolence, dizziness, tremor, nervousness, libido decreased, agitation, anxiety, abnormal dreams, concentration impaired, depersonalization, myoclonus, amnesia, rhinitis, pharyngitis, yawn; abnormal vision, taste perversion; abnormal ejaculation, dysmenorrhea, female genital disorder, impotence, urinary frequency, urination impaired, urinary tract infection.

The following adverse events occurred at a frequency of 2% or more among GAD patients on *Paxil* who participated in placebo-controlled trials of 8 weeks duration in which patients were dosed in a range of 10 mg/day to 50 mg/day; asthenia, headache, infection, vasodilation, sweating, nausea, dry mouth, constipation, diarrhea, decreased appetite, vomiting, insomnia, somnolence, dizziness, tremor, nervousness, libido decreased, respiratory disorder, sinusitis, yawn, abnormal vision, abnormal ejaculation, female genital disorder, impotence.

Studies in depression show a clear dose dependency for some of the more common adverse events associated with *Paxil* use. There was evidence of adaptation to some adverse events with continued *Paxil* therapy (e.g., nausea and dizziness). Significant weight loss may be an undesirable result of *Paxil* treatment for some patients but, on average, patients in controlled trials had minimal (about 1 lb) loss. In placebo-controlled clinical trials, *Paxil*-treated patients exhibited abnormal values on liver function tests no more frequently than placebo-treated patients.

In placebo-controlled clinical trials involving more than 2,500 patients with depression, OCD, panic disorder, social anxiety disorder or generalized anxiety disorder, the following incidences of untoward sexual experiences for patients receiving *Paxil* were reported, varying with the disease state: In males: decreased libido (6% to 15%), ejaculatory disturbance, mostly delayed ejaculation (13% to 28%), impotence (2% to 8%). In females: decreased libido (0% to 9%), orgasmic disturbance (2% to 9%). The reported incidence of each of these adverse events was <5% among male and female patients receiving placebo.

Other Events Observed During the Premarketing Evaluation of *Paxil*: During premarketing assessment in depression multiple doses of *Paxil* were administered to 6,145 patients in phase 2 and 3 studies. During premarketing clinical trials in OCD, panic disorder, social anxiety disorder and generalized anxiety disorder, 542, 469, 522 and 735 patients, respectively, received multiple doses of *Paxil*. The following adverse events were reported. Note: "frequent" = events occurring in at least 1/100 patients; "infrequent"= 1/100 to 1/1000 patients; "rare" = less than 1/1000 patients. Events are classified within body system categories and enumerated in order of decreasing frequency using the above definitions. It is important to emphasize that although the events occurred during *Paxil* treatment, they were not necessarily caused by it.

Body as a Whole: *frequent:* chills, malaise; *infrequent:* allergic reaction, face edema, moniliasis, neck pain; *rare:* adrenergic syndrome, cellulitis, neck rigidity, pelvic pain, peritonitis, ulcer. **Cardiovascular System:** *frequent:* hypertension, tachycardia; *infrequent:* bradycardia, hematoma, hypotension, migraine, syncope; *rare:* angina pectoris, arrhythmia nodal, atrial fibrillation, bundle branch block, cerebral ischemia, cerebrovascular accident, congestive heart failure, heart block, low cardiac output, myocardial infarct, myocardial ischemia, pallor, phlebitis, pulmonary embolus, supraventricular extrasystoles, thrombophlebitis, thrombosis, varicose vein, vascular headache, ventricular extrasystoles. **Digestive System:** *infrequent:* bruxism, colitis, dysphagia, eructation, gastritis, gastroenteritis, gingivitis, glossitis, increased salivation, liver function tests abnormal, rectal hemorrhage, ulcerative stomatitis; *rare:* aphthous stomatitis, bloody diarrhea, bulimia, cholelithiasis, duodenitis, enteritis, esophagitis, fecal impactions, fecal incontinence, gum hemorrhage, hematemesis, hepatitis, ileus, intestinal obstruction, jaundice, melena, mouth ulceration, peptic ulcer, salivary gland enlargement, stomach ulcer, stomatitis, tongue discoloration, tongue edema, tooth caries. **Endocrine System:** *rare:* diabetes mellitus, goiter, hyperthyroidism, hypothyroidism, thyroiditis. **Hemic and Lymphatic Systems:** *infrequent:* anemia, eosinophilia, leukocytosis, leukopenia, lymphadenopathy, purpura; *rare:* abnormal erythrocytes, basophilia, bleeding time increased, hypochromic anemia, iron deficiency anemia, lymphedema, abnormal lymphocytes, lymphocytosis, microcytic anemia, monocytosis, normocytic anemia, thrombocythemia, thrombocytopenia. **Metabolic and Nutritional:** *frequent:* weight gain, weight loss; *infrequent:* alkaline phosphatase increased, edema, peripheral edema, SGOT increased, SGPT increased, thirst; *rare:* bilirubinemia, BUN increased, creatinine phosphokinase increased, dehydration, gamma globulins increased, gout, hypercalcemia, hypercholesteremia, hyperglycemia, hyperkalemia, hyperphosphatemia, hypocalcemia, hypoglycemia, hypokalemia, hyponatremia, ketosis, lactic dehydrogenase increased, non-protein nitrogen (NPN) increased; **Musculoskeletal System:** *frequent:* arthralgia; *infrequent:* arthritis, arthrosis; *rare:* bursitis, myositis, osteoporosis, generalized spasm, tenosynovitis, tetany. **Nervous System:** *frequent:* emotional lability, vertigo; *infrequent:* abnormal thinking, alcohol abuse, ataxia, delirium, dystonia, dyskinesia, euphoria, hallucinations, hostility, hypertonia, hypesthesia, hypokinesia, incoordination, lack of emotion, libido increased, manic reaction, neurosis, paralysis, paranoid reaction, psychosis; *rare:* abnormal gait, akinesia, antisocial reaction, aphasia, choreoathetosis, circumoral paresthesias, convulsion, delusions, diplopia, drug dependence, dysarthria, extrapyramidal syndrome, fasciculations, grand mal convulsion, hyperalgesia, hysteria, manic-depressive reaction, meningitis, myelitis, neuralgia, neuropathy, nystagmus, peripheral neuritis, psychotic depression, reflexes decreased, reflexes increased, stupor, torticollis, trismus, withdrawal syndrome. **Respiratory System:** *infrequent:* asthma, bronchitis, dyspnea, epistaxis, hyperventilation, pneumonia, respiratory flu; *rare:* emphysema, hemoptysis, hiccups, lung fibrosis, pulmonary edema, sputum increased, voice alteration. **Skin and Appendages:** *frequent:* pruritus; *infrequent:* acne, alopecia, contact dermatitis, dry skin, ecchymosis, eczema, furunculosis, herpes simplex, maculopapular rash, photosensitivity, urticaria; *rare:* angioedema, erythema nodosum, erythema multiforme, exfoliative dermatitis, fungal dermatitis, herpes zoster, hirsutism, seborrhea, skin discoloration, skin hypertrophy, skin ulcer, sweating decreased, vesiculobullous rash. **Special Senses:** *frequent:* tinnitus; *infrequent:* abnormality of accommodation, conjunctivitis, ear pain, eye pain, mydriasis, otitis media, photophobia; *rare:* amblyopia, anisocoria, blepharitis, cataract, conjunctival edema, corneal ulcer, deafness, exophthalmos, eye hemorrhage, glaucoma, hyperacusis, keratoconjunctivitis, night blindness, otitis externa, parosmia, ptosis, retinal hemorrhage, taste loss, visual field defect. **Urogenital System:** *infrequent:* abortion, amenorrhea, breast pain, cystitis, dysuria, hematuria, menorrhagia, nocturia, polyuria, urinary incontinence, urinary retention, urinary urgency, vaginal moniliasis, vaginitis; *rare:* breast atrophy, breast enlargement, endometrial disorder, epididymitis, female lactation, fibrocystic breast, kidney calculus, kidney pain, leukorrhea, mastitis, metrorrhagia, nephritis, oliguria, pyuria, urethritis, uterine spasm, urolith, vaginal hemorrhage.

Postmarketing Reports

Voluntary reports of adverse events that have been received since market introduction and not listed above that may have no causal relationship with *Paxil* include–acute pancreatitis, elevated liver function tests (the most severe cases were deaths due to liver necrosis, and grossly elevated transaminases associated with severe liver dysfunction), Guillain-Barré syndrome, toxic epidermal necrolysis, priapism, syndrome of inappropriate ADH secretion, symptoms suggestive of prolactinemia and galactorrhea, neuroleptic malignant syndrome-like events; extrapyramidal symptoms which have included akathisia, bradykinesia, cogwheel rigidity, dystonia, hypertonia, oculogyric crisis (which has been associated with concomitant use of pimozide), tremor and trismus; serotonin syndrome, associated in some cases with concomitant use of serotonergic drugs and with drugs which may have impaired *Paxil* metabolism (symptoms have included agitation, confusion, diaphoresis, hallucinations, hyperreflexia, myoclonus, shivering, tachycardia and tremor), status epilepticus, acute renal failure, pulmonary hypertension, allergic alveolitis, anaphylaxis, eclampsia, laryngismus, optic neuritis, porphyria, ventricular fibrillation, ventricular tachycardia (including torsade de pointes), thrombocytopenia, hemolytic anemia, and events related to impaired hematopoiesis (including aplastic anemia, pancytopenia, bone marrow aplasia and agranulocytosis). There have been spontaneous reports that discontinuation (particularly when abrupt) may lead to symptoms such as dizziness, sensory disturbances, agitation or anxiety, nausea and sweating; these events are generally self-limiting. There has been a report of an elevated phenytoin level after 4 weeks of *Paxil* and phenytoin co-administration, and a report of severe hypotension when *Paxil* was added to chronic metoprolol treatment.

DRUG ABUSE AND DEPENDENCE: Controlled Substance Class: *Paxil* is not a controlled substance. Evaluate patients carefully for history of drug abuse and observe such patients closely for signs of *Paxil* misuse or abuse (e.g., development of tolerance, incrementations of dose, drug-seeking behavior).

BRS–PX:L20

©2001 The GlaxoSmithKline Group of Companies
All rights reserved. PX7463S